Neurology Update

Reviews for continuing professional development

Edited by

Huw Morris
Senior Lecturer in Neurology
School of Medicine, Cardiff University
Consultant Neurologist, Royal Gwent Hospital, Newport

Foreword by

Gordon C Cook
President
The Fellowship of Postgraduate Medicine

Series Editor

John Mayberry

Series Sponsor
THE FELLOWSHIP OF POSTGRADUATE MEDICINE

Radcliffe Publishing
Oxford • Seattle

Radcliffe Publishing Ltd
18 Marcham Road
Abingdon
Oxon OX14 1AA
United Kingdom

www.radcliffe-oxford.com
Electronic catalogue and worldwide online ordering facility.

© 2006 The Fellowship of Postgraduate Medicine

All rights reserved. No part of this publication may be reproduced, stored in a retrieval system or transmitted, in any form or by any means, electronic, mechanical, photocopying, recording or otherwise without the prior permission of the copyright owner.

British Library Cataloguing in Publication Data

A catalogue record for this book is available from the British Library.

ISBN 1 85775 722 X

Typeset by Anne Joshua & Associates, Oxford
Printed and bound by TJ International Ltd, Padstow, Cornwall

Contents

Foreword

Postgraduate Medical Education in London, and indeed Britain generally, in the early years of the twentieth century was dominated by two major government reports: the *Athlone Report* (1921) and *Report of the Postgraduate Medical Education Committee* (1930). But it is important not to underestimate the crucial pioneering role of the Fellowship of Postgraduate Medicine (FPM). This organisation came into existence in 1918 in order to provide postgraduate courses in all of the major specialities in medicine and surgery. Until then, postgraduate medical training in Britain had been seriously neglected, although already viable, prior to the Great War (1914–18), in several cities in mainland Europe.

In the aftermath of the War, men (and a few women) who had served in the armed forces from the British Dominions and Northern America were congregating at the 'heart of the British Empire' in search of postgraduate courses.

Until the FPM took up the challenge, the scenario regarding postgraduate courses in Britain was dire. Only in the latter years of the nineteenth century and very early twentieth was any attempt made to fill this gap. A few luminaries, such as CRB Keetley (1848–1909) and LA Bidwell (1865–1912) at the West London Hospital, Jonathan Hutchinson (1828–1913) at the Medical Graduates' College and Polyclinic, and RHP Crawfurd (1865–1938) at the London Postgraduate Association had attempted to organise courses, but a *clinical* component was invariably missing.

The present venture, i.e. republishing in book format a series of outstanding review articles from the *Postgraduate Medical Journal* (*PMJ*) in the major specialities within medicine, is to be warmly welcomed. It is entirely in line with the FPM's original objectives. The first collection of essays was devoted to recent advances in *Gastroenterology*, and the present one to *Neurology*; both publications owe their genesis to the inspiration and enthusiasm of John Mayberry (the present Editor of the *PMJ*) and Gillian Nineham (Editorial Director at Radcliffe Publishing) – to both of them we are greatly indebted.

Gordon C Cook
President
The Fellowship of Postgraduate Medicine
September 2005

Preface

Like many medical specialties Neurology has undergone dramatic changes in the last 20 years and these changes are likely to continue apace. The emphasis on the clinical neuroanatomy of rare conditions such as syringomyelia and sub-acute combined degeneration is no longer the mainstay of undergraduate teaching in Neurology. Neuroanatomy remains central to neurology and the detailed history and examination remain the most important diagnostic tools for the physician and neurologist evaluating neurological disorders. However, the advent of CT and MR imaging, the introduction of new medications for common chronic conditions such as epilepsy and Parkinson's disease, the increase in the number of neurologists and the progress with developing a therapeutic evidence base has changed the part that neurology plays in general hospital practice.

The contributions in this book come from geriatricians, rheumatologists, psychiatrists and neurologists reflecting the range of doctors with special expertise involved in the care of patients with neurological disease. Unusual presentations in neurological disease continue to fascinate doctors, and Neurology has been well represented in contributions to short answer questions and case reports in the *Postgraduate Medical Journal*. However, the review articles chosen from the Journal for this volume have been selected to be particularly relevant to the management of common neurological problems in general hospital practice. The majority of the articles concern the management of epilepsy/blackouts and stroke, which make up about 15% of admissions on general medical intake in the UK. These articles include areas such as special issues in the management of women with epilepsy, and the evaluation of patients with non-epileptic attack disorders, often poorly covered in textbooks. There are new developments in therapeutics described in the articles on stroke and stroke thrombolysis. The readership of the *Postgraduate Medical Journal* has always been international and this volume covers conditions such as encephalitis and tuberculosis, seen more commonly in the developing world, but becoming increasingly prevalent in Europe and North America.

Lastly, a section is devoted to neurodegeneration, likely to become an increasing public health problem with the projected future increase in the aged population. This is an area in which improvements have been made in both palliative and supportive care and in the molecular and genetic understanding of the basis for these diseases. These advances are exemplified in the articles on motor neurone disease and neurological dysphagia. It is hoped that the developments in the molecular understanding of neurological disease will lead to new disease modifying therapies, which will one day become part of standard medical treatments for patients with devastating conditions such as Parkinson's disease, Alzheimer's disease and motor neurone disease.

Huw Morris
September 2005

List of contributors

Dr V Adhiyaman
Department of Geriatric Medicine
Glan Clwyd District General Hospital
Rhyl

Dr W Arthur
Norfolk and Norwich University Hospital
NHS Trust
Norwich

Dr M Asghar
Department of Elderly Care
Gloucestershire Royal Hospital
Gloucester

Prof AMO Bakheit
Peninsular Medical School
University of Exeter
Plymouth

Dr KP Bhatia
University Department of Clinical Neurology
Sobell Department of Motor Neuroscience
and Movement Disorders
Institute of Neurology
London

Prof BK Bhowmick
Directorate of Medicine
Glan Clwyd District General Hospital
Rhyl

Dr A Chaudhuri
Department of Neurology
University of Glasgow
Glasgow

Dr N Delanty
Department of Neurology
Beaumont Hospital
Dublin

Dr KN Ganeshram
Care of the Elderly
Countess of Chester Hospital
Chester

Dr RK Garg
Department of Neurology
King George's Medical University
Lucknow

Dr SK Gilmour-White
Department of Neurology
Guy's Hospital
London

Dr S Hadjikoutis
Epilepsy Unit
University Hospital of Wales
Cardiff

Dr RS Howard
Guy's and St Thomas' NHS Trust
Department of Neurology
Guy's and St Thomas' Hospital
London

Dr GRV Hughes
Lupus Research Unit
St Thomas' Hospital
London

Dr GC Kaye
Department of Cardiology
Castle Hill Hospital
Cottingham

Prof PGE Kennedy
Department of Neurology
Southern General Hospital
Glasgow

Dr Y Langan
Epilepsy Research Group
Institute of Neurology
London

Dr SM Leary
Rehabilitation Group
Institute of Neurology
London

Prof AJ Lees
Reta Lila Weston Institute of
Neurological Studies
Institute of Neurology
London

Dr SD Lhatoo
Department of Neurology
Institute of Clinical Neurosciences
Frenchay Hospital
Bristol

Dr PJ Martin
Neurology Department
Addenbrooke's Hospital
Cambridge

Dr R McGovern
St Luke's General Hospital
Kilkenny

Dr JDC Mellers
Department of Neuropsychiatry
Maudsley Hospital
London

Dr HR Morris
Neurology (C4)
University of Wales College of Medicine
Cardiff

Dr A Münchau
Neurology Department
Hamburg University
Hamburg

Dr MD O'Brien
Department of Neurology
Guy's Hospital
London

Dr RW Orrell
University Department of Clinical
Neurosciences
Royal Free and University College
Medicine School
London

Dr AC Pereira
Department of Clinical Neurology
St George's Hospital Medical School
London

Dr B Porter
Rehabilitation Group
Institute of Neurology
London

Dr R Renganathan
Department of Neurology
Cork University Hospital
Cork

Prof MN Rossor
Dementia Research Centre
National Hospital for Neurology and
Neurosurgery
London

Dr AG Rudd
Stroke Unit
St Thomas' Hospital
London

Dr EL Sampson
Dementia Research Centre
National Hospital for Neurology
and Neurosurgery
London

Prof JWAS Sander
Department of Clinical and
Experimental Epilepsy
Institute of Neurology
London

Dr SA Schneider
Sobell Department of Motor Neuroscience
and Movement Disorders
Institute of Neurology
London

Dr PEM Smith
Epilepsy Unit
University Hospital of Wales
Cardiff

Dr K Talbot
Clinical Neurology
Radcliffe Infirmary
Oxford

Prof AJ Thompson
Rehabilitation Group
Institute of Neurology
London

Dr EA Warburton
Neurology Department
Addenbrooke's Hospital
Cambridge

Dr JD Warren
Dementia Research Centre
Institute of Neurology
London

Dr AJ Williams
Lane Fox Respiratory Unit
St Thomas' Hospital
London

Prof CD Wolfe
Department of Public Health Sciences
King's College
London

Prof NW Wood
Molecular Neuroscience
Institute of Neurology
London

Part 1

Epilepsy and syncope

Chapter One

Juvenile myoclonic epilepsy: under-appreciated and under-diagnosed

R Renganathan and N Delanty

Juvenile myoclonic epilepsy (JME) is a hereditary, idiopathic, generalised epilepsy and is found in 5%–11% of patients with epilepsy. It is characterised by myoclonic jerks, occasional generalised tonic-clonic seizures, and sometimes absence seizures. JME continues to be under-appreciated and under-diagnosed. Accurate diagnosis is important as it usually responds well to treatment with appropriate anticonvulsants and misdiagnosis often results in unnecessary morbidity. In addition lifelong therapy is usually indicated as the natural history is one of relapse off treatment, even after a prolonged seizure-free period.

In 1822, 'myoclonus' was described by Pritchard as 'a symptom associated with epilepsy'.[1] Delasiave in 1854 termed it 'petit mal moteur'. In 1867, Herpin gave the first detailed description of a patient with juvenile myoclonic epilepsy (JME) calling the myoclonic jerks 'secousses'. In 1881, Gowers classified the jerks among the generalised 'auras' and considered them to be epileptic. Unvericht described progressive myoclonic epilepsy in 1901 but failed to recognise the existence of more benign variants. In 1957, Janz and Christian published their article on 47 patients with 'impulsive petit mal'. Lund in 1975 introduced the term JME and this term was soon admitted into the international classification system thereafter.

Definition

The original description by Janz and Christian distills the essential clinical features of this syndrome: '[epilepsy with] impulsive petit mal appears around puberty and is characterised by seizures with bilateral, single or repetitive arrhythmic, irregular myoclonic jerks, predominantly in the arms. Jerks may cause some patients to fall suddenly. No disturbance of consciousness is noticeable. Often there are GTCS [generalised tonic-clonic seizures] and infrequent absences. The seizures usually occur after awakening and are often precipitated by sleep deprivation. Interictal and ictal EEG [electroencephalogram(s)] have rapid generalised, often irregular spike waves and polyspike waves; there is no close phase correlation between EEG spikes and jerks. Frequently the patients are photosensitive. Response to appropriate drugs is good.'[2]

Aetiopathogenesis

JME is an inherited disorder, but the exact mode of inheritance is not clear. There is a positive family history in 50% of cases or less. One study has confirmed a causative role of EJM1 in the pathogenesis of idiopathic generalised seizures in the majority of German families of JME patients. This study has refined a candidate region of 10.1 cM in the chromosomal region 6p21 between the flanking loci HLA-DQ and D6s1019.[3] However, some studies have revealed controversial results and genetic heterogeneity is suspected. Linkage to chromosome 15 has at most a minor role in JME.[4] Few studies have focused on pathological findings in the brain of JME patients. Some studies suggest that microdysgenesis occurs more frequently in epileptic patients with idiopathic generalised epilepsy; if so, its pathological significance is unknown.[5]

Clinical features

JME may be responsible for about 10% of all epilepsies; exact figures may be higher as it is still an under-diagnosed syndrome. Studies show similar prevalence in males and females.[6] We commonly see patients with a non-specific diagnosis of a 'seizure disorder' for many years before a definitive diagnosis is reached.

Eighty percent of patients with JME begin having seizures between ages 12 and 18 with a mean age of onset of 14.6 years. The mean age of onset for GTCS is 15.5 years, absence seizures 11.5 years, and myoclonic seizures 15.4 years.[7] Earlier onset is seen in photosensitive patients. Absence seizures typically begin between ages 5 and 16 years. Myoclonic jerks follow between one and nine years later followed by GTCS a few months later. Approximately 3–8% of childhood absence epilepsies evolve into JME.

The most important element in the diagnosis of JME is the history. JME is still under-diagnosed because of lack of awareness of the syndrome by doctors who fail to ask patients about the occurrence of myoclonic jerks and about precipitating factors.[8] Atypical EEG findings in some patients also contribute to the misdiagnosis of patients with JME.[9] Myoclonic jerks are seen in 100% of cases of JME and are the *sine qua non* of diagnosis. They occur as the only seizure type in about 3–5% of JME patients. Myoclonic jerks are characterised by short, bilateral, and usually symmetric synchronous muscle contractions predominantly involving the shoulders and arms. They can be single or repetitive and they are usually arrhythmic. The amplitude and the force of the jerks vary. Some jerks occur unilaterally. Sometimes myoclonic seizures of JME are perceived only as a subjective electric shock sensation inside the body. It is important to note that consciousness is preserved. Common symptoms used to describe myoclonic jerks are shakes, clumsiness, twitches, and nervousness. Patients may not volunteer information about their myoclonus unless specifically asked. Sometimes, the myoclonus is noticed only by the patient's family. GTCS occur in 90–95% of patients with JME. GTCS are often preceded by a few minutes of generalised mild to moderate myoclonus of increasing frequency and intensity. GTCS occurring in JME are often characterised by lack of sensory aura, symmetry, remarkable violence, and a long duration of the tonic phase. They occur predominantly after awakening. Some patients may describe a brief dizziness or a funny sensation in the head beforehand.

Absence seizures are a feature in 40% of patients. These seizures are relatively infrequent, brief, and not associated with automatisms. They may occur several times a day without circadian variation. Severity is age dependent with absence seizures of later onset (>10 years) being less severe. Seizures of JME are often precipitated by sleep deprivation, fatigue, emotional stress, menses, and moderate to heavy intake of alcohol. They tend to occur just after morning awakening. Thirty to forty percent of patients with JME are photosensitive. Seizures are precipitated by flashing strobe lights or flickering sunlight (for example, through a line of trees) in patients with photosensitivity. Drugs such as cocaine and amitryptiline, which reduce the seizure threshold, can precipitate seizures of JME. Physical examination is usually normal. Intelligence is preserved.

Investigations

An interictal EEG from a sleep-deprived patient characteristically shows discharges of diffuse bilaterally symmetrical and synchronous 4–6 Hz polyspike and wave complexes lasting between 0.5–10 seconds; these may be predominantly seen over the frontocentral region. The resting awake EEG background activity shows normal alpha rhythm. Continuous video-EEG monitoring reveals 10–16 Hz polyspike discharges often associated with myoclonic jerks. These may be preceded by asymptomatic spike and wave activity and often are followed by 1–3 Hz slow waves. The number of spikes ranges from 5–20 and is evidently more closely related to the intensity than to the duration of the jerks. Absence seizures are associated with 3 Hz spike and wave activity. Intermittent photic stimulation frequently precipitates spike and wave pattern more so in females than males. Subtle focal abnormalities may be seen in 30–50% of JME patients.[10] These may present as focal slow waves, spikes, or sharp waves or a focal onset of a generalised discharge. If clinical and EEG data are consistent with JME, there is no need for imaging. High resolution magnetic resonance imaging (MRI) is normal in patients with JME. It may be reasonable to obtain MRI in those with refractory JME.

Electrophysiological studies have shown higher P25 and N33 amplitudes in somatosensory evoked potentials.[11] Voxel-based analysis MRI data are only a research tool at present. Some studies using this technique have shown abnormal cerebral structure in JME with involvement of mesiofrontal cortical structures.[12] Magnetic resonance spectroscopy studies show reduced frontal lobe concentration of *N*-acetyl aspartate in JME, which may suggest prefrontal neuronal dysfunction in JME.[13] Positron emission tomography studies indicate that patients with JME may have cortical disorganisation that affects both the epileptogenic potential and frontal lobe cognitive functioning.[14] Such patients may exhibit abnormal patterns of cortical activation that are associated with subtle cognitive dysfunction. However, magnetic resonance spectroscopy and positron emission tomography studies are currently only research tools.

Box 1.1   **Learning points**

- JME is an idiopathic generalised epilepsy characterised by myoclonic jerks, generalised tonic-clonic seizures, and sometimes absence seizures.

- JME is frequently under-diagnosed and under-appreciated.
- Myoclonic jerks are seen in 100% of cases of JME and are the *sine qua non* of diagnosis.
- JME responds to treatment with sodium valproate. Newer broad spectrum drugs such as topiramate, and possibly levetiracetam, may also be of benefit.
- Lifelong treatment is needed.

Differential diagnosis

JME should be distinguished from hypnagogic myoclonus, which is a normal phenomenon. The progressive myoclonic epilepsies are symptomatic generalised epilepsies which are characterised by progressive neurological deterioration, dementia, and ataxia. Epilepsy with grand mal seizures upon awakening is an important condition that should be considered in the differential diagnosis. This syndrome is closely related to JME, but myoclonic seizures are not present. Non-epileptic seizures may sometimes resemble seizures of JME.

Management

The goal of pharmacological management is to render the individual seizure-free without side effects of the medication. Sodium valproate has traditionally been the drug of choice. Eighty-five to ninety percent of patients with JME become seizure-free with valproate monotherapy. All patients with JME require lifelong treatment because seizures invariably return after withdrawal of therapy. Absence seizures alone may be treated with ethosuximide. Myoclonic jerks respond well to clonazepam. Primidone, vigabatrin, gabapentin, and tiagabine have been unsuccessful in treatment of JME. Phenytoin and carbamazepine have shown to aggravate the myoclonic and absence seizures of JME and therefore should be avoided.[15] The response to lamotrigine has shown unpredictable results.[16,17] Topiramate appears to be of benefit in JME, and levetericetam is currently being investigated.[18,19] Vagal nerve stimulation has been used as in refractory JME.[20] JME is difficult to treat in about 15% of patients. The predictors of pharmacoresistance include:

1 the coexistence of all three seizure types (myoclonic jerks, absence seizures, and GTCS) and
2 the existence of associated psychiatric problems.[21]

Precipitating factors for seizures should be avoided. These include avoiding moderate to heavy consumption of alcohol, fatigue, and photosensitising lights. Patients should be encouraged to develop regular sleeping habits. Advice regarding driving restrictions, working at height, and supervised swimming is appropriate. During pregnancy, the risks of discontinuing treatment outweigh the benefits. The importance of pre-pregnancy counselling and the addition of folic acid is an essential part of management in women of childbearing potential.

Prognosis

Although JME has been described as a benign condition, it should be borne in mind that any condition that places the patient at risk for GTCS increases morbidity and mortality. Failure to diagnose the condition increases the patient's morbidity. All patients require lifelong treatment. As mentioned, patients with JME are at increased risk of relapse if treatment is discontinued.

References

1 Genton P, Gelisse P. Juvenile myoclonic epilepsy. *Arch Neurol* 2001; **58**: 1487–90.
2 Janz D, Durner M. Juvenile myoclonic epilepsy. In: Engel J Jr, Pedley TA, eds. *Epilepsy: a comprehensive textbook*. Philadelphia: Lippincott-Raven, 1997: 2389–400.
3 Sander T, Bockenkamp B, Hildmann T, *et al*. Refined mapping of the epilepsy susceptibility locus EJM1 on chromosome 6. *Neurology* 1997; **49**: 842–7.
4 Durner M, Shinnar S, Resor SR, *et al*. No evidence for a major susceptibility locus for juvenile myoclonic epilepsy on chromosome 15q. *Am J Med Genet (Neuropsychiatric Genetics)* 2000; **96**: 49–52.
5 Meencke HJ, Janz D. The significance of microdysgenesia in primary generalised epilepsy: an answer to the considerations of Lyon and Gastaut. *Epilepsia* 1985; **26**: 368–71.
6 Panyiotopoulos CP, Obeid T, Tahan R. Juvenile myoclonic epilepsy: a 5 year prospective study. *Epilepsia* 1994; **35**: 285–96.
7 Delgado-Escueta AV, Serratosa JM, Medina MT. Juvenile myoclonic epilepsy. In: Wylie E, ed. *The treatment of epilepsy: principles and practice*. 2nd edn. Baltimore: Williams & Wilkins, 1996: 484–51.
8 Gruenwald Ra, Chroni E, Panayiotopoulos CP. Delayed diagnosis of juvenile myoclonic epilepsy. *J Neurol Neurosurg Psychiatry* 1992; **55**: 497–9.
9 Lancman ME, Asconape JJ, Penry JK. Clinical and EEG asymmetries in juvenile myoclonic epilepsy. *Epilepsia* 1994; **35**: 302–6.
10 Alibert V, Grunewald A, Panayiotopoulos CP, *et al*. Focal electroencephalographic abnormalities in juvenile myoclonic epilepsy. *Epilepsia* 1994; **35**: 297–301.
11 Salas-Pung J, Tunon A, Diaz M, *et al*. Somatosensory evoked potentials in juvenile myoclonic epilepsy. *Epilepsia* 1992; **33**: 527–30.
12 Woermann FG, Free SL, Koepp MJ, *et al*. Abnormal cerebral structure in juvenile myoclonic epilepsy demonstrated with voxel-based analysis of MRI. *Brain* 1999; **122**: 2101–7.
13 Savic I, Lekvall A, Greitz D, *et al*. MR Spectroscopy shows reduced frontal lobe concentrations of N-acetyl aspartate in patients with juvenile myoclonic epilepsy. *Epilepsia* 2000; **41**: 290–6.
14 Swartz BE, Simpkins F, Halgren E, *et al*. Visual working memory in primary generalised epilepsy: an [18]FDG-PET study. *Neurology* 1996; **47**: 1203–12.
15 Genton P, Gelisse P, Thomas P, *et al*. Do carbamazepine and phenytoin aggravate juvenile myoclonic epilepsy? *Neurology* 2000; **55**: 1106–9.
16 Buchanan N. The use of lamotrigine in juvenile myoclonic epilepsy. *Seizure* 1996; **5**: 149–51.
17 Biraben A, Allain H, Scarabin JM, *et al*. Exacerbation of juvenile myoclonic epilepsy with lamotrigine. *Neurology* 2000; **55**: 1758.
18 Biton V, Montouris GD, Ritter F, *et al*. A randomized, placebo-controlled study of topiramate in primary generalized tonic-clonic seizures. *Neurology* 1999; **52**: 1330.

19 Smith K, Bettz T. The effect of add on therapy with leveteracetam (UCBL059) on patients with resistant juvenile myoclonic epilepsy (abstract). *Fourth Eilat Conference on New Antiepileptic Drugs* 1998: 57.

20 Disabato JA, Barnhurst RF, Levisohn PM. Efficacy of vagus nerve stimulation in young children with generalized epilepsies (abstract). *Epilepsia* 2001; **42**: 171.

21 Gelisse P, Genton P, Thora P, *et al*. Clinical factors of drug resistance in juvenile myoclonic epilepsy. *J Neurol Neurosurg Psychiatry* 2001; **70**: 240–3.

Chapter Two

Sudden unexpected death in epilepsy

SD Lhatoo, Y Langan and JWAS Sander

The majority of persons with epilepsy develop lasting remission from seizures, although mortality is significantly greater than that of the age-matched general population. Of the deaths that are thought to be directly related to seizures, sudden unexpected death in epilepsy is probably the commonest category; more so than status epilepticus or seizure-related accidents. Annual incidence rates vary from 1 in 200 patients with chronic epilepsy to about 1 in 1000 in more population-based studies. Young adults with severe, intractable epilepsy appear to be the most frequently affected group and may have even higher incidence rates. Other risk factors may also be important. An area of great research interest, several pathogenetic mechanisms have been postulated, centring mainly around cardiac rhythm and central hypoventilation. Given the frequent devastation caused by sudden unexpected death in epilepsy, the importance of seizure control is emphasised.

It has become increasingly clear that epilepsy can kill, not only through status epilepticus and accidents caused by seizures but through other mechanisms that cause sudden unexpected deaths. Sudden death is a real problem in the management of epilepsy and is now perhaps the commonest category of seizure-related death in patients with chronic epilepsy, often affecting young adults in this group.[1] Sudden unexpected death in epilepsy (SUDEP) is defined as a sudden, unexpected, non-accidental death in an individual with epilepsy with or without evidence of a seizure having occurred (excluding documented status epilepticus) and where autopsy does not reveal an anatomical or toxicological cause of death.[2] In 1910, Munson reported on mortality from the Craig Colony in New York which housed patients with intractable epilepsy and found that 99 out of 582 deaths were 'sudden'.[3] Though some of these were seizure-related *accidental* deaths, he concluded that most had occurred in the midst of a seizure, noting that 'these deaths occur very rapidly at times, seizures not infrequently take place silently'. Since then, there has been a somewhat reluctant acceptance of a small but significant risk of death directly attributable to seizures, and sudden death has appeared sporadically through the decades in several epilepsy mortality series as a category of death.[4] With present day knowledge of an increased mortality in epilepsy,[5–7] there has been renewed interest in the phenomenology of SUDEP and several studies have attempted to describe this enigma.

Box 2.1   SUDEP: definition

A sudden, unexpected, non-accidental death in an individual with epilepsy, with or without evidence of a seizure having occurred (excluding status epilepticus), where autopsy does not reveal an anatomical or toxicological cause of death.

Epidemiological studies

It is clear from outcome studies of epilepsy that more than 70% of all patients with epilepsy enter lasting remission from the condition and up to 30% suffer chronic seizures that are difficult to control. Approximately 1 out of every 200 such patients with chronic epilepsy die suddenly and unexpectedly every year. But how common is this phenomenon in the community where the majority of patients do not have difficult, intractable epilepsy? The National GP Study of Epilepsy in the UK (NGPSE), which is an observational study of epilepsy in the community,[8] has had only one confirmed SUDEP death in a prospective cohort of 564 patients with definite epilepsy followed up for approximately 8000 person years.[9] The MRC Antiepileptic Drug Withdrawal Study had just two deaths attributable to SUDEP after 5000 person years of follow-up.[10] These figures are reflective of the relative rarity of this phenomenon in patients who do not have chronic epilepsy, as in the NGPSE almost 70% of the cohort had achieved 5-year remission from seizures.[11] Similarly, the MRC study population was in remission and there is strong evidence that SUDEP is mainly a problem in the patient with intractable epilepsy.

Case ascertainment methods to determine the exact incidence of SUDEP have varied in different studies, but can be broadly categorised into studies that have used death certificates and coroner's registers,[12–15] studies that have used treatment data, either medical,[16–19] surgical,[20–22] or palliative,[23] and those that have been based on data from epilepsy clinics or institutions.[24–27] Coroner-based studies have shown incidences varying between 1:370 and 1:2100. Many of these studies, however, are flawed due to the fact that death certificates are notoriously unreliable; a large number do not accurately record the cause of death or the underlying conditions that could have contributed.[28] In addition, the prevalent epilepsy population is used as denominator – a presumed figure prone to variation and inaccuracy.[28] A recent case-control study found that annual incidence figures for SUDEP were 1.4 per 1000 patient years in both males and females.[29]

SUDEP incidence rates of up to 1:200 per year have been reported by studies based on tertiary epilepsy clinic data,[30] and slightly higher figures have been reported from institutionalised patients who share features of seizure intractability with clinic subjects.[24,26] These figures are probably close to the true incidence of SUDEP in patients with chronic epilepsy.

Several studies have used anti-epileptic drug therapy lists for case ascertainment.[17,16,19] More recent studies have been based on newer anti-epileptic drug registers such as those on lamotrigine,[18] gabapentin[31] and tiagabine.[32] Some studies based on surgical data have shown particularly high incidences of sudden death (up to 1:50 per year), especially in post-surgical patients where

Table 2.1   The incidence of SUDEP in different populations

Population studied	Annual incidence in population studied	Incidence in person years	Type of epilepsy	Comments
Epilepsy surgery patients[20]	1 in 150	–	Chronic	Severe epilepsy
Epilepsy clinic patients[30]	1 in 200	–	Chronic	Moderate to severe epilepsy
Patients from coroners' lists[13]	1 in 1100	–	All	Mild, moderate and severe epilepsy
Patients from community-based studies of epilepsy[9]	–	1 in 8000	All	Mild, moderate and severe epilepsy
Patients from a case control study[29]	1.4 in 1000	–	All	Mild, moderate and severe epilepsy

the operative procedure has not been successful in containing seizures, reflective of a group with particularly bad epilepsy.[20] In a more recent study, 791 patients who had received vagal nerve stimulation system implants (a seizure-reducing device that acts by stimulating the left vagal nerve) were followed up for 1335 person years and showed an incidence of definite or probable SUDEP of 4.5/1000 person years of follow-up.[23] The high mortality and incidence figures in most of these studies may reflect the severe epilepsy suffered by patients in these study populations and is likely to indicate the increasingly high risk of SUDEP in patients with chronic epilepsy.

Risk factors

Seizure status

It is obvious from most studies that seizure control or the lack thereof is vitally important in the mortality statistics of SUDEP and incidence figures are considerably higher in cohorts of patients with refractory and chronic seizures (hospital- or clinic-based) as compared to studies that are more community-based. One surgical study found a particularly high incidence of SUDEP in patients unsuccessfully treated surgically for their epilepsy, with mortality approaching 1:50, in contrast to 1:150 when both pre- and post-surgical candidates were analysed together.[21] In contrast, the NGPSE and MRC Drug Withdrawal studies, which both have large numbers of patients with mild epilepsy, have shown very low incidence figures for sudden death. It is important to note, however, that there have been reports of patients dying suddenly during their first-ever or second-ever seizure, though these are obviously uncommon occurrences. A recent case-control study showed that the relative risk of SUDEP increased with number of seizures per year (10.16; 95% CI=2.94–35.18), appearing substantially higher in patients with more than 50 seizures per year than in patients with two or less seizures per year.[29]

Age, sex and race

Patients with epilepsy within the 20 to 40 year age group appear to suffer higher mortality from this entity, and this has been a consistent finding in many studies.[12,13,27] However, this does not mean that other age groups are immune and studies in children as well as older patients with epilepsy have shown significant mortality due to SUDEP. Apart from one study of children with epilepsy in a residential school, most studies have shown a male preponderance.[13,25,27,30] One study found a higher incidence of sudden death in the African American population but this could reflect the higher incidence of epilepsy in this group.[13]

Medication

Non-compliance with prescribed anti-epileptic medication has been implicated in the occurrence of sudden death and several patients have been found to have sub-therapeutic serum levels of anti-epileptic drugs.[12,13,22,33] The significance of drug levels, however, is arguable as patients with well-controlled epilepsy can have low drug levels and vice versa. Conversely, there are reported instances of patients experiencing sudden arrhythmic deaths due possibly to the cardiac side effects of carbamezepine,[34] though this is obviously not the case in the majority of SUDEP cases. The above-mentioned case-control study showed that patients on three anti-epileptic drugs were more likely to suffer SUDEP than patients on monotherapy, although it could be argued that patients with bad epilepsy are more likely to be prescribed polytherapy and the increased mortality reflects on refractory epilepsy rather than drug therapy.[29]

Box 2.2   Possible pathogenetic mechanisms of SUDEP

- cardiovascular
- central hypoventilation
- combined mechanisms

Neurological status

A higher incidence of SUDEP has been found in patients with neurological deficits and learning difficulties.[24] This may be attributed to the severity of epilepsy that is usually present in these patient groups and the higher all-cause mortality generally found in such patients.

Other

Alcohol abuse has also been implicated in some patients,[13] as have psychotropic drugs.[19] Recent head injuries have also been mentioned as a possible risk factor.

Circumstances of death

There is considerable evidence that the majority of sudden deaths in epilepsy are seizure-related and circumstantial evidence of a generalised tonic-clonic seizure having occurred is often found in the form of superficial injuries, a bitten tongue or characteristic postures.[13,30,35] This is strongly borne out by witnessed accounts of sudden death, one of which occurred during direct observation at a telemetry unit.[36] However, less than half of sudden deaths in epilepsy are witnessed and it is yet unclear whether all such deaths are due to seizures.

Autopsy findings

Autopsy findings, by definition, should not indicate an anatomical or toxico-logical cause of death, though this does not necessarily imply that no abnorm-alities are found on post-mortem examination. Pulmonary oedema is often found, although this is usually of insufficient severity to be an attributable cause of death.[12,13,37,38] Similarly, increased liver, cardiac and brain weights are also found. Some studies have found brain lesions on autopsy[12,13,38] that could have caused seizures in those cases. A recent study noted the presence of interstitial cardiac fibrosis in patients who had epilepsy-related sudden deaths.[39]

Pathogenetic mechanisms

Seizure activity remains central in the various hypotheses that have been put forward to explain the pathogenetic mechanisms that underlie sudden death. These studies can be broadly categorised into those that have looked at cardiovascular causes and those that have emphasised the role of central hypoventilation during seizures.

Various rhythm abnormalities have been implicated in SUDEP, but although autonomic disturbances are common enough observations in the fitting, hospi-talised patient, there is no convincing evidence that malignant tachyarrhythmias cause significant mortality in epilepsy. There are case reports, however, of significant bradyarrhythmias and sinus arrest occurring in patients with temporal lobe epilepsy, suggesting that these could be a cause of death.[40–42] Significant ST segment changes[43] and QTc interval prolongations have been observed with epileptiform electroencephalogram (EEG) discharges in patients with chronic epilepsy, although the investigators also found that this prolongation remained within normal limits in almost all cases.[44] Intrinsic cardiac disease has been implicated and in one recent study a significant number of patients were found to have interstitial cardiac fibrosis, though whether this is directly related to a mechanism of death is debatable.[39] The influence of cardio-active anti-epileptic drugs, too, remains speculative.[45]

In an interesting study where seizures were chemically induced in sheep, central hypoventilation was found to be a mechanism of death.[46] Endogenous opioids that may be released during seizures have been implicated in the causation of this central hypoventilation and could well account for the suppres-sion of respiratory drive.[47] In another study on anaesthetised and ventilated animals, elevated left atrial and pulmonary vascular pressures were found – a possible mechanism for the pulmonary oedema found in patients who have died from SUDEP, though why this should happen in the first place is unclear.[48]

In another study, transient bradyarrhythmias were found to occur in associ-ation with apnoea and/or a change in respiratory pattern in patients experiencing seizures, suggesting that both cardiovascular as well as central mechanisms are important and that cardiorespiratory brainstem reflexes may play a role in SUDEP.[49] In summary, however, although there are several postulates, the true mechanism of sudden death remains unclear.

Box 2.3   Epilepsy Bereaved

PO Box 112, Wantage OX2 8XT, UK
Tel 01235 772852/772850

Epilepsy Bereaved is a registered charity that provides valuable support and information to friends and relatives of patients with epilepsy who have suffered sudden unexpected death. Information packs on epilepsy are available from the National Society for Epilepsy helpline at 01494 601400.

Box 2.4   Learning points

- 30% of all patients with epilepsy develop chronic seizures
- approximately 1 out of every 200 patients with chronic, severe epilepsy suffer SUDEP every year
- central hypoventilation and cardiac arrhythmias are possible mechanisms
- control of epilepsy is likely to be an important preventive measure
- all chronic epilepsy patients should be referred to specialist epilepsy units

---

Conclusion

Seizure control is likely to be an important issue in SUDEP and evidence from many studies strongly suggests an important role played by uncontrolled epilepsy. There is no doubt that the traditional emphases on drug compliance, minimisation of potential seizure precipitants, and referral of appropriate patients to epilepsy specialist units are as important as ever.[50] Although the incidence of SUDEP in community-based populations may be low, its occurrence is often devastating to relatives, carers and physicians. In patients with chronic epilepsy, where the incidence is considerably higher, the role of adequate supervision is equally important, especially amongst children and the institutionalised. As newer anti-epileptics appear on the market and the provision of both curative and palliative surgery for intractable epilepsy becomes more established, the incidence of this often tragic complication will hopefully lessen. The role of further studies examining the risk factors involved in SUDEP in this cannot be under-emphasised and detailed studies, such as a case-control study presently under way at this centre, should be encouraged.

References

1 Nashef L, Sander JWAS. Sudden unexpected deaths in epilepsy – where are we now? *Seizure* 1996; **5**: 235–8.
2 Nashef L. Sudden unexpected death in epilepsy: Terminology and definitions. *Epilepsia* 1997; **38**: S6–S8.
3 Munson JF. Death in epilepsy. *Med Rec* 1910; **77**.

4 Rodin EA. *The prognosis of patients with epilepsy.* Springfield: Charles Thomas, 1968.

5 Cockerell OC, Johnson AL, Sander JW, Hart YM, Goodridge DM, Shorvon SD. Mortality from epilepsy: results from a prospective population-based study [see comments]. *Lancet* 1994; **344**: 918–21.

6 Hauser WA, Annegers JF, Elveback LR. Mortality in patients with epilepsy. *Epilepsia* 1980; **21**: 399–412.

7 O'Donoghue MF, Sander JW. A historical perspective on the mortality associated with chronic epilepsy. *Acta Neurol Scand* 1997; **96**: 138–41.

8 Sander JW, Hart YM, Johnson AL, Shorvon SD. National General Practice Study of Epilepsy: newly diagnosed epileptic seizures in a general population. *Lancet* 1990; **336**: 1267–71.

9 Lhatoo SD, Langan Y, MacDonald BK, Zeidan S, Sander JWAS. Sudden unexpected death: a rare event in a large community based prospective cohort with newly diagnosed epilepsy and high remission rates. *J Neurol Neurosurg Psychiatry* 1999; **66**: 692.

10 Medical Research Council Antiepileptic Drug Withdrawal Study Group. Randomised study of antiepileptic drug withdrawal in patients in remission. *Lancet* 1991; **337**: 1175–80.

11 Cockerell OC, Johnson AL, Sander JW, Shorvon SD. Prognosis of epilepsy: a review and further analysis of the first nine years of the British National General Practice Study of Epilepsy, a prospective population-based study. *Epilepsia* 1997; **38**: 31–46.

12 Leestma JE, Kalelkar MB, Teas SS. Sudden unexpected death associated with seizures: analysis of 66 cases. *Epilepsia* 1984; **25**: 84–8.

13 Leestma JE, Walczak T, Hughes JR, Kalelkar MB, Teas SS. A prospective study on sudden unexpected death in epilepsy. *Ann Neurol* 1989; **26**: 195–203.

14 Terrence CF, Wisotzkey HM, Perper JA. Unexpected, unexplained death in epileptic patients. *Neurology* 1975; **25**: 594–8.

15 Langan Y, Nolan N, Hutchinson M. The incidence of sudden unexpected death in epilepsy in South Dublin and Wicklow. *Seizure* 1998; **7**: 355–8.

16 Derby LE, Tennis PS, Jick H. Sudden unexplained death among subjects with refractory epilepsy. *Epilepsia* 1996; **37**: 931–5.

17 Jick SS, Cole TB, Mesher MD, Tennis PS, Jick H. Sudden unexplained death in young persons with primary epilepsy. *Pharmacoepidemiol Drug Safety* 1992; **1**: 59–64.

18 Leestma JE, Annegers JF, Brodie MJ, *et al.* Sudden unexplained death in epilepsy: observations from a large clinical development program. *Epilepsia* 1997; **38**: 47–55.

19 Tennis PS, Cole TB, Annegers JF, Leestma JE, McNutt M, Rajput A. Cohort study of incidence of sudden unexplained death in persons with seizure disorder treated with antiepileptic drugs in Saskatchewan, Canada. *Epilepsia* 1995; **36**: 29–36.

20 Dasheiff RM. Sudden unexpected death in epilepsy: a series from an epilepsy surgery program and speculation on the relationship to sudden cardiac death. *J Clin Neurophysiol* 1991; **8**: 216–22.

21 Sperling MR, O'Connor MJ, Saykin AJ, Plummer C. Temporal lobectomy for refractory epilepsy. *JAMA* 1996; **276**: 470–5.

22 Vickery BG. Mortality in a consecutive cohort of 248 adolescents who underwent diagnostic evaluation for epilepsy surgery. *Epilepsia* 1997; **38**: S67–S69.

23 Annegers JF, Coan SP, Hauser WA, Leestma JE, Duffel W, Tarver B. Epilepsy, vagal nerve stimulation by the NCP system, mortality, and sudden, unexpected, unexplained death. *Epilepsia* 1998; **39**: 206–12.

24 Klenerman P, Sander JW, Shorvon SD. Mortality in patients with epilepsy: a study of patients in long term residential care. *J Neurol Neurosurg Psychiatry* 1993; **56**: 149–52.

25 Lip GY, Brodie MJ. Sudden death in epilepsy: an avoidable outcome? *J R Soc Med* 1992; **85**: 609–11.

26 Nashef L, Fish DR, Garner S, Sander JW, Shorvon SD. Sudden death in epilepsy: a study of incidence in a young cohort with epilepsy and learning difficulty. *Epilepsia* 1995; **36**: 1187–94.

27 Timmings PL. Sudden unexpected death in epilepsy: a local audit. *Seizure* 1993; **2**: 287–90.

28 Zielinski JJ. Epilepsy and mortality rate and causes of death. *Epilepsia* 1974; **15**: 191–201.

29 Nilsson L, Farahmand BY, Persson PG, Tomson T. Risk factors for sudden unexpected death in epilepsy: a case control study. *Lancet* 1999; **353**: 888–93.

30 Nashef L, Sander JWAS, Fish DR, Shorvon SD. Incidence of sudden unexpected death in an adult outpatient cohort with epilepsy at a tertiary referral centre. *J Neurol Neurosurg Psychiatry* 1995; **58**: 462–4.

31 Anon. Neurontin. In: *Physician's Desk Reference*. Montvale NJ: Medical Economics, 1996.

32 Leppick IE. Tiagabine: the safety landscape. *Epilepsia* 1995; **36**(suppl 6): S10–S13.

33 George GR, Davis GG. Comparison of antiepileptic drug levels in different cases of sudden death. *J Forensic Sci* 1998; **43**: 598–603.

34 Roesen F, Andersen EB, Kehn E, *et al.* Cardiac conduction disturbances during carbamezepine therapy. *Acta Neurol Scand* 1983; **68**: 49–52.

35 Nashef L, Garner S, Sander JW, Fish DR, Shorvon SD. Circumstances of death in sudden death in epilepsy: interviews of bereaved relatives. *J Neurol Neurosurg Psychiatry* 1998; **64**: 349–52.

36 Bird JM, Dembny KAT, Sandeman D, Butler S. Sudden unexplained death in epilepsy. *Epilepsia* 1997; **38**: S52–S56.

37 Earnest MP, Thomas GE, Eden RA, Hossack KF. The sudden unexplained death syndrome in epilepsy: demographic, clinical, and postmortem features. *Epilepsia* 1992; **33**: 310–16.

38 Hirsch CS, Martin DL. Unexpected death in young epileptics. *Neurology* 1971; **21**: 682–90.

39 Natelson BH, Suarez RV, Terrence CF, Turizo R. Patients with epilepsy who die suddenly have cardiac disease. *Arch Neurol* 1998; **55**: 857–60.

40 Dasheiff RM, Dickinson LJ. Sudden unexpected death of epileptic patient due to cardiac arrhythmia after seizure. *Arch Neurol* 1986; **43**: 194–6.

41 Fincham RW, Shivapour ET, Leis AA, Martins JB. Ictal bradycardia with syncope: a case report. *Neurology* 1992; **42**: 2222–3.

42 Howell SJ, Blumhardt LD. Cardiac asystole associated with epileptic seizures: a case report with simultaneous EEG and ECG. *J Neurol Neurosurg Psychiatry* 1989; **52**: 795–8.

43 Tiagaran S, Rasmussen V, Dam M, Pedersen S, Hogenhaven H. ECG changes in epilepsy patients. *Acta Neurol Scand* 1997; **96**: 72–5.

44 Tavernor SJ, Brown SW, Tavernor RME, Gifford C. Electrocardiograph QT lengthening associated with epileptiform EEG discharges – a role in sudden unexplained death in epilepsy? *Seizure* 1996; **5**: 79–83.

45 Tomson T, Kenneback G. Arrhythmia, heart rate variability and antiepileptic drugs. *Epilepsia* 1997; **38**: S48–S51.

46 Johnston SC, Horn JK, Valente J, Simon RP. The role of hypoventilation in a sheep model of epileptic sudden death. *Ann Neurol* 1995; **37**: 531–7.

47 Ramabadran K, Bansinath M. Endogenous opioid peptides and epilepsy. *J Clin Pharm Ther Toxicol* 1990; **28**: 47–62.

48 Johnston SC, Darragh TM, Simon RP. Postictal pulmonary edema requires pulmonary vascular pressure increases. *Epilepsia* 1996; **37**: 428–32.

49 Nashef L, Walker F, Allen P, Sander JW, Shorvon SD, Fish DR. Apnoea and bradycardia during epileptic seizures: relation to sudden death in epilepsy. *J Neurol Neurosurg Psychiatry* 1996; **60**: 297–300.

50 Langan Y, Nashef L. Sudden unexpected death. *Neurol Rev Int* 1999.

Chapter Three

Important points in the clinical evaluation of patients with syncope

W Arthur and GC Kaye

A careful history, physical examination, and an electrocardiogram (ECG) are the most important components of the evaluation of a syncopal episode. These three components will provide a diagnosis or determine whether diagnostic testing is necessary in most patients.[1] The potential cost savings made by avoiding unnecessary and expensive investigations are obvious when one considers that good clinical skills lead to the identification of the cause of syncope in 75–85% of cases in which a successful diagnosis is made.[2]

History

A comprehensive account of the events preceding the syncopal spell is invaluable for diagnosis (*see* Box 3.1). The premonitory (prodromal) symptoms, precipitating factors, rate of onset, witnessed accounts, features during the recovery phase, past medical history, and the frequency and previous history of syncope will assist in the diagnosis and direct the physician in the evaluation of patients. The differential diagnosis for syncope varies with age; this fact coupled with other historical findings can help to pinpoint the diagnosis (*see* Table 3.1).

Box 3.1   History preceding syncope

- Neurally mediated syncope

    Premonitory symptoms: pallor, diaphoresis, nausea, visual blurring, light-headedness, hearing loss

    Situation: neck turning, stress, pain, fear, crowding, prolonged upright posture, cough, micturition, swallowing, defecation

- Cardiac syncope

    Abrupt onset, effort, or exertion, preceding chest pain, palpitations

    Drug-related arrhythmia: antiarrhythmics, neuroleptics, digoxin, β-blockers, alcohol, illicit drugs

- Orthostatic syncope

    Abrupt changes in posture

    Drug-related: angiotensin converting enzyme (ACE) inhibitors, nitrates, diuretics, alcohol

    Postprandial

    Haemorrhage

Prodromal symptoms

Most persons with neurocardiogenic syncope have premonitory symptoms before losing consciousness; usually nausea, diaphoresis and pallor.[3] Yawning, visual blurring, weakness, and a feeling of impending doom are consistent with neurally mediated syncope. The presence of palpitations preceding syncope is highly suggestive of an arrhythmia. Syncope caused by ventricular tachycardia typically occurs without a prodrome, although some patients may report brief palpitations, with light-headedness preceding loss of consciousness. Supraventricular tachycardia may occasionally lead to loss of consciousness; in these rare cases palpitations are frequently noticed by the patient.[4] A characteristic aura immediately preceding syncope might implicate epileptiform activity.

Precipitating factors

Syncope on exertion implies left ventricular outflow tract obstruction, left ventricular dysfunction, or ventricular dysrrhythmia. Loss of consciousness after the completion of exercise maybe due to a strong vagal response producing a significant bradycardia. Sudden symptom onset unrelated to posture or effort is suggestive of a cardiac arrhythmia. Coexistent sudden onset pleuritic chest pain and/or dyspnoea may indicate a pulmonary embolism. Diagnosis of carotid sinus syncope requires that spontaneous symptoms of presyncope or syncope be reproduced by carotid sinus massage.[5] Correlation between symptoms and precipitating factors such as neck twisting, wearing a tight collar, shaving, or previous neck surgery reinforces the diagnosis. Syncope occurring after abrupt changes in posture would implicate orthostatic syncope. This diagnosis may frequently be missed due to concurrent hypertension in the supine position.[6] Postprandial hypotension and even syncope may occur as a consequence of splanchnic shunting of blood and the intake of alcoholic beverages.[7] Episodes related to stressful or emotional situations point

Table 3.1   Age distribution of syncope

Young (<35 years)	Middle aged (35–65 years)	Elderly (>65 years)
Neurally mediated: Neurocardiogenic	Neurally mediated	Cardiac: Arrhythmic Mechanical
Psychiatric	Cardiac: Arrhythmic Mechanical	Orthostatic: Drug induced
[Hypertrophic cardiomyopathy]		Neurally mediated: Carotid sinus hypersensitivity
[WPW syndrome]		
[Long QT syndrome]		

[ ] indicates less common but important causes of syncope. WPW = Wolff-Parkinson-White. Reproduced with permission from Olshansky.[17]

towards neurally mediated syncope; in these circumstances the patient is often aware of losing consciousness.

Witnessed accounts

In addition to the history given by the patient, information available from an observer of the event is crucial. The duration of syncope is, by definition, transient. After a seizure loss of consciousness may be prolonged. Full assessment of the patient is not complete until eyewitness accounts of the events preceding and following the patient's loss of consciousness are taken from those accompanying the patient to the emergency department or the clinic. If the patient is unaccompanied at initial presentation potential witnesses should be encouraged to attend as they may hold the clues to the diagnosis. It must be remembered of course that witnessed accounts, while often heavily relied upon, may be inaccurate.

Recovery phase

The account of the observer is particularly invaluable when trying to differentiate between types of syncope and seizure. The presence of confusion after the event is the single most powerful discriminator between seizure and syncope.[8] Mental function is usually quickly recovered after a syncopal episode, whereas seizures are followed by a postictal period of residual confusion which can last from minutes to hours. Differentiating the recovery time between causes of syncope is more difficult but recovery after neurocardiogenic syncope can take minutes in comparison with postural hypotension or a long sinus pause after which the patient is alert within seconds. Dizziness or headache in the recovery phase (in the absence of head trauma) points towards a neurological cause.

Past medical history

The patient with depressed left ventricular function and/or ischaemic heart disease in association with syncope is at high risk of sudden death.[9] Obtaining a cardiac history and elucidating associated risk factors for ischaemic heart disease is mandatory during clinical evaluation. The presence of diabetes mellitus frequently causes silent myocardial ischaemia and may mask a myocardial infarction giving rise to a ventricular arrhythmia. Diabetic peripheral neuropathy may also lead to orthostatic syncope. Features suggestive of *multiple system atrophy* may be elicited from the history in patients with orthostatic syncope.

Risk can be assessed at the initial presentation by examining the frequency of syncope. If recurrent episodes are spread out over a number of years malignant arrhythmias are unlikely to be the cause. Multiple syncopal recurrences are most likely due to neurally mediated syncope or psychiatric causes. In contrast, patients with isolated (<3) episodes of syncope or with a short history of recurrence are at risk of cardiac death.[10] New onset syncope may herald a new serious cardiovascular cause.

Drug history

Medications, particularly in the elderly, may be causal for syncope in a substantial number of patients. A detailed drug history should be taken; in particular changes in medication or the initiation of a new drug maybe implicated in the aetiology of the event. Antihypertensives, nitrates, and diuretics are frequently contributory to orthostatic hypotension. Vasodilatation and/or volume depletion may trigger enhanced central mechanoreceptor responses leading to neurocardiogenic syncope. Ophthalmic preparations, mostly β-blockers, can aggravate bradyarrhythmias or heart block. Antiarrhythmics, antidepressants, psychotropic drugs, many non-sedating antihistamine drugs, and other preparations may independently, or in interaction, prolong the QT interval predisposing to polymorphic ventricular tachycardia.

Miscellaneous points

Patients with a family history of syncope or sudden death raise the possibility of the congenital long QT syndromes, hypertrophic cardiomyopathy or Wolff-Parkinson-White syndrome. There may be a familial history of neurocardiogenic syncope. A detailed family history should therefore be taken including data relating to distant relatives who died unexpectedly and any relevant familial disease. A psychiatric history may reveal anxiety disorders, major depression, and hysterical personality disorder. Patients with syncope and psychiatric disorders are younger (more often female), have a high number of syncopal episodes and have a variety of other complaints. In young patients with no structural heart disease those with multiple episodes of syncope (>5 in preceding year) are less likely to have an arrhythmia and are more likely to have psychiatric illnesses.[11] A full social history is also important to exclude illicit drug use as a cause of syncope and to pinpoint risk factors for ischaemic heart disease. The occupation of the patient is essential information as urgent diagnosis and therapy is required in those whose careers and safety are compromised by syncope.

Physical examination

During a thorough physical examination attention should be directed to the vital signs, the cardiovascular and neurological examination. After a supine period of at least five minutes blood pressure and pulse measurements should be taken; these should be repeated after the patient has been standing for three minutes. An abrupt drop in systolic blood pressure of between 20–30 mm Hg with standing associated with reproduction of symptoms suggests orthostatic syncope as a cause.[12] In a volume depleted patient the heart rate should rise on standing. In those with dysautonomic syncope the blood pressure can drop over several minutes while upright with no concomitant change in heart rate.

Because the prognosis after syncope is worse if there is underlying cardiac disease, the principal objective of the examination is to determine whether there is evidence for underlying cardiovascular abnormality. The cardiovascular examination may reveal a pulse character or murmurs consistent with left ventricular outflow tract obstruction. Mitral valve prolapse, left atrial myxoma, pulmonary hypertension, or prosthetic valve dysfunction may also be suspected after auscultation of the precordium. A third or fourth heart sound consistent with cardiac disease and/or congestive cardiac failure may be heard.

In the absence of contraindications (carotid bruit, stroke, or myocardial infarction within the previous 6 months, or a history of ventricular tachycardia or ventricular fibrillation) carotid sinus massage (CSM) should be performed in all individuals with unexplained syncope, particularly those who are elderly with features suggestive of carotid sinus syncope.[13,14] Massage to the carotid sinus is performed by applying longitudinal digital pressure at the bifurcation of the internal and external carotid artery for five seconds. CSM is applied to the right then the left side after a two minute interval. Pressure should never be applied to both sides simultaneously. A standard technique of carotid sinus stimulation with applied exclusion criteria, as outlined above, causes infrequent complications most of which are transient and result in full recovery.[14] Potential complications of CSM include ventricular arrhythmias and prolonged asystole, therefore continuous ECG monitoring and venous access is required.

Pulmonary examination and assessment of the jugular venous pressure may reveal congestive heart failure. The response to voluntary hyperventilation may be useful in certain patients and has been advocated as part of standard evaluation of syncope.[15] In the context of an acute syncopal episode a rectal examination should be performed to look for evidence of an occult gastrointestinal bleed. The neurological examination should look to identify focal neurological signs that may offer an immediate diagnosis and redirect investigations accordingly.

Electrocardiogram

An ECG should be performed in all patients with syncope. An abnormal ECG is found in up to 50% of patients with syncope, but in most patients it is not diagnostic.[16] In a person with a normal ECG there is a low likelihood that an arrhythmia is the cause of syncope, and these persons are at low risk of sudden death.[11] Despite being a brief investigation the ECG together with a rhythm strip can identify potential causes of syncope in 2–11% of patients.[16] Acquired or congenital disease of the atrioventricular node or the distal conduction (His-Purkinje) system may be evident from second or third degree heart block. There may be evidence of conduction system disease in the His-Purkinje system with a prolonged P-R interval and associated bundle branch block and fascicular block. This pattern might implicate intermittent complete heart block as a cause of syncope and give a clue to underlying structural heart disease. The presence of bundle branch block increases the likelihood that significant sustained mono-morphic ventricular tachycardia will be inducible at electrophysiological testing.[17] The ECG may indicate sinus node dysfunction, myocardial infarction, ventricular pre-excitation, or a long QT interval. The electrical criteria for left ventricular hypertrophy may be fulfilled raising the suspicion of left ventricular outflow tract obstruction.

Summary points

* The history and examination are the most important stages involved in stratifying the patient into high and low risk groups and identifying the cause of syncope.

- Those with a history of structural or ischaemic heart disease or with recent onset, isolated episodes of syncope have a high risk of sudden death.
- Obtaining an eyewitness account is a vital component of the initial assessment of the cause of syncope.
- Postural hypotension and carotid sinus syncope can be reliably and safely diagnosed at the time of examination if a standard technique is adhered to.
- An abnormal ECG is found in up to 50% of patients with syncope and should therefore be part of the initial clinical assessment.

Conclusion

When a cause of syncope is determined, it is most frequently established on the basis of clinical data available at the time of initial contact with the physician. A diagnostic strategy should utilise these data as a guide to further investigation thereby minimising costly procedures that may ultimately be misleading. Such a strategy requires a thorough account of the episode(s) of syncope from the individual affected and witnesses present. The age of the patient is useful to broadly stratify causes of syncope. The routine ECG is part of the initial clinical assessment and can identify potential causes of syncope or patients with structural heart disease in significant numbers. The crux of stratifying those at high risk depends on whether or not structural heart disease is present. Gaining this information at the earliest possible opportunity should expedite the successful management of the patient.

References

1 Linzer M, Yang EH, Estes NA 3rd, *et al*. Diagnosing syncope. Part 1: value of history, physical examination, and electrocardiography. Clinical efficacy assessment project of the American College of Physicians. *Ann Intern Med* 1997; **126**: 989–96.
2 Day SC, Cook EF, Funkenstein H, *et al*. Evaluation and outcome of emergency room patients with transient loss of consciousness. *Am J Med* 1982; **73**: 15–23.
3 Calkins H, Shyr Y, Frumin H, *et al*. The value of the clinical history in the differentiation of syncope due to ventricular tachycardia, atrioventricular block, and neurocardiogenic syncope. *Am J Med* 1995; **98**: 365–73.
4 Leitch JW, Klein GJ, Yee R, *et al*. Syncope associated with supraventricular tachycardia: an expression of tachycardia rate or vasomotor response? *Circulation* 1992; **85**: 1064–71.
5 Hammill SC. Value and limitations of noninvasive assessment of syncope. *Cardiol Clin* 1997; **15**: 195–218.
6 Robertson D, Robertson RM. Causes of chronic orthostatic hypotension. *Arch Intern Med* 1994; **154**: 1620–4.
7 Lipsitz LA, Ryan SM, Parker A, *et al*. Hemodynamic and autonomic nervous system responses to mixed meal ingestion in healthy young and old subjects and dysautonomic patients with postprandial hypotension. *Circulation* 1993; **87**: 391–400.
8 Gastaut H, Fischer-Williams M. Electroencephalographic study of syncope: its differentiation from epilepsy. *Lancet* 1957; **ii**: 1018–25.
9 Middlekauff HR, Stevenson WG, Saxon LA. Prognosis after syncope: impact of left ventricular function. *Am Heart J* 1993; **125**: 121–7.
10 Krol RB, Morady F, Flaker GC, *et al*. Electrophysiological testing in patients with unexplained syncope: clinical non-invasive predictors of outcome. *J Am Coll Cardiol* 1987; **10**: 358–63.

11 Kapoor WN. Diagnostic evaluation of syncope. *Am J Med* 1991; **90**: 91–106.

12 Atkins D, Hanusa B, Sefcik C, *et al.* Syncope and orthostatic hypotension. *Am J Med* 1991; **91**: 179–85.

13 Wagshal AB, Huang SKS. Carotid sinus hypersensitivity. In: Grubb BP, Olshansky B, eds. *Syncope: mechanisms and management.* Armonk, NY: Futura, 1998: 281–95.

14 Davies AJ, Kenny RA. Frequency of neurologic complications following carotid sinus massage. *Am J Cardiol* 1998; **81**: 1256–7.

15 Linzer M, Varia I, Pontinen M, *et al.* Medically unexplained syncope: relationship to psychiatric illness. *Am J Med* 1992; **92**: 18–25.

16 Kapoor WN. Evaluation and outcome of patients with syncope. *Medicine* 1990; **69**: 160–75.

17 Olshansky B. Syncope: overview and approach to management. In: Grubb BP, Olshansky B, eds. *Syncope: mechanisms and management.* Armonk, NY: Futura, 1998: 15–71.

Chapter Four

The approach to patients with 'non-epileptic seizures'

JDC Mellers

Up to one fifth of patients who present to specialist clinics with seizures do not have epilepsy. The majority of such patients suffer from psychologically mediated attacks; dissociative seizures, often referred to as 'non-epileptic seizures'. This paper describes the diagnostic evaluation of seizure disorders, including clinical assessment and the role of special investigations. The organic and psychiatric imitators of epilepsy are outlined and findings on psychiatric assessment are reviewed. This group of patients often proves difficult to engage in appropriate treatment and an approach to explaining the diagnosis is described. As yet there are no controlled trials of treatment in this disorder but preliminary evidence suggests cognitive behavioural treatment is both a rational and promising way forward.

Up to one in five patients with apparently intractable epilepsy referred to specialist centres are found to have no organic cause for their seizures.[1–4] It has been widely supposed that this high prevalence reflects referral bias but a recent community-based study found a similar proportion among patients with recent-onset seizures.[5] This group of patients suffer from psychologically mediated paroxysmal behavioural disturbances which are often dramatic, alarming for bystanders and all too easily mistaken for epilepsy. Diagnostic errors are the rule rather than an exception. Most patients are treated for epilepsy for several years[6,7] and by the time the correct diagnosis is made they will commonly have taken more anti-epileptic drugs (AEDs) at higher doses and experience more side effects than an equivalent cohort of patients with epilepsy.[8,9] One in 10 patients will present in apparent status epilepticus.[1,7,8] Astonishingly, approximately one quarter of referrals to a specialist neurological intensive care unit with refractory status were found to have 'pseudostatus'.[10]

What this disorder should be called has been the subject of considerable debate. Some terms (hysterical seizures, pseudoseizures) are pejorative, unacceptable to patients[11] and have largely been abandoned. Others (non-epileptic seizures (NES), non-epileptic attack disorder) merely describe what the condition is not, rather than conveying what it is. Furthermore, these terms have been used with different meanings: the term NES, for example, is sometimes used to refer to the group of neurological, cardiological and other medical conditions, in addition to psychiatric disorders, which constitute the differential diagnosis for epilepsy,[4] while on other occasions the term is used as a form of loose shorthand to refer to the psychological attacks alone.[12] The terms psychogenic non-epileptic seizures and functional seizures overcome some of these objections but formal psychiatric classification systems provide clearly defined labels. Unfortunately, though, there are still inconsistencies: thus, within DSM IV[13] such attacks are classified under somatoform disorder and in ICD 10[14] the diagnostic label 'Dissociative Convulsions' is classified within the group of conversion disorders. It is the latter terminology that will be adopted here.

As we have seen, dissociative convulsions or seizures (DS) are common, the diagnosis is often missed, and when it is, patients not only fail to receive appropriate treatment but are subject to unnecessary, costly[15] and potentially harmful medical interventions. In considering the management of this disorder we will therefore focus on assessment and diagnosis before considering contemporary approaches to treatment.

Clinical assessment

It should be emphasised from the start that epilepsy is primarily a clinical diagnosis. Great care must be taken in establishing the precise sequence of

Table 4.1   The differential diagnosis of epilepsy

A. Medical causes of transient neurological dysfunction (with or without loss of consciousness)

1. Syncope
     – vasovagal
     – cardiogenic

2. Neurological
     – cerebrovascular
     – migraine
     – vertigo
     – cataplexy
     – parasomnias
     – movement disorders
     – startle-induced phenomena

3. Endocrine and metabolic
     – hypoglycaemia
     – hypocalcaemia
     – hereditary fructose intolerance
     – pheochromocytoma
     – drugs and alcohol

B. Psychiatric disorders

1. Psychiatric disorders that may be mistaken for epilepsy
     – panic disorder
     – psychosis
     – Attention Deficit Hyperactivity Disorder
     – depersonalisation disorder

2. Dissociative seizures

3. Factitious disorder

---

events during an attack and history taking is not complete until an eyewitness account has been obtained. The duration of each phase of symptoms, including recovery from the attack, should be determined. Any habitual pattern in the circumstances which trigger attacks should be sought. Patients and eyewitnesses should be prompted for specific symptoms because significant features may not be mentioned spontaneously (e.g. psychic and cognitive symptoms, automatisms, occurrence during sleep).

Medical differential diagnosis

The medical and psychiatric differential diagnosis for epilepsy is listed in Table 4.1 (*see* reviews[16,17]). Of medical disorders mistaken for epilepsy, syncope is the most common[3] and in non-specialist settings is the condition most likely to be misdiagnosed as epilepsy. It is important to note that tonic or clonic movements may be seen during syncope.[18] However, characteristic prodromal symptoms (lightheadedness, clammy sweatiness, a sense of receding sound and vision, nausea), associated cardiac symptoms and a relationship in some cases to postural changes or valsalva usually make identifying cases of syncope straightforward.[19,20] In patients with cerebrovascular disease the differentiation of transient ischaemic attacks from partial seizures may sometimes be difficult. Ischaemic episodes may last for seconds to minutes but usually occur with preserved consciousness, are associated only with a loss of function and are not followed by more typical epileptic features. A relatively long duration of symptoms is useful in recognizing migraine, migraine equivalents (the latter featuring prodromal symptoms but no headache)[21] and vertigo. Abnormal startle phenomena, including hyperekplexia, are rare but often mistaken for epilepsy and need to be distinguished from startle-induced seizures.[17,22] Paroxysmal movement disorders may be mistaken for epilepsy.[23] Sudden loss of muscle tone which may produce falls in response to an emotional trigger suggest cataplexy which is usually found in association with other features of the narcolepsy syndrome (narcolepsy, hypnopompic or hypnogogic hallucinations and sleep paralysis). Other parasomnias giving rise to complex behavioural episodes arising from sleep may be confused with epileptic automatisms although the former lack any preceding ictus and are usually of relatively long duration.[24] Space occupying lesions in the 3rd ventricle may produce intermittent cerebrospinal fluid (CSF) obstruction associated with visual symptoms and are a rare cause of sudden episodes of collapse with loss of consciousness. Metabolic disorders associated with loss of consciousness usually have a protracted time course and are suggested by other features in the history.

Psychiatric differential diagnosis

Once epilepsy and other organic causes of seizures have been excluded there are three categories of psychiatric diagnoses that must be considered:

1 dissociative seizures
2 factitious disorder
3 other psychiatric disorders that have been mistaken for epilepsy.

Dealing with the last category first, paroxysmal symptoms of psychiatric disorders may sometimes raise the question of epilepsy. The most common example of this is panic disorder.[25] Patients may report depersonalization, derealisation and tremulousness during panic attacks while partial epileptic seizures may include both emotional and somatic symptoms of anxiety.[26] Features that are useful in distinguishing the two conditions include a longer duration, cognitive symptoms and the presence of specific environmental triggers in panic disorder and, in partial seizures, the unique quality of the emotional symptoms ('ictal fear') together with associated more characteristic epileptic features in partial seizures. Paroxysmal symptoms in psychosis may sometimes raise the question of epilepsy but such symptoms (e.g. hallucinations) lack the highly stereotyped quality of epileptic phenomena and episodes are usually of long and variable duration. Other psychiatric disorders sometimes confused with epilepsy include depersonalisation disorder and Attention Deficit Hyperactivity Disorder in which failing school performance and poor concentration may sometimes raise the possibility of juvenile absence epilepsy.

In the majority of cases, however, the seizures will be the principle symptom and cannot be accounted for by another psychiatric condition. The two diagnostic possibilities are dissociative seizures and factitious disorder distinguished from one another by whether the seizures are thought to arise through unconscious processes (DS) or are deliberately enacted. In factitious disorder the patient is held to be deliberately simulating epilepsy for reasons understandable in terms of their psychological background. It is distinguished from malingering (not a medical diagnosis) in which individuals are simulating illness for some obvious practical gain (e.g. compensation, avoidance of criminal responsibility).

The semiology of dissociative seizures

A careful history will usually provide sufficient grounds for suspecting DS, which is by far the commonest psychiatric imitator of epilepsy. Since the introduction of video electroencephalographic monitoring (v-EEG telemetry) 30 years ago countless studies have compared DS with epilepsy aiming to find clinical features which distinguish one condition from the other.[27] Unfortunately, no one symptom or sign allows the diagnosis to be made with absolute certainty. Some of the more useful clinical features, together with important 'red herrings', are listed in Table 4.2.

Some two thirds of DS involve prominent motor features. The remainder may mimic partial seizures or involve a period of unresponsiveness with little in the way of motor activity.[7,8,28,36,37,41,44] The hallmark of epileptic seizures (ES) is that they are brief, temporary alterations of neurological function that follow a highly stereotyped pattern in a single individual from one occasion to the next. Furthermore, epileptic seizures conform to a number of familiar syndromes which have now been clearly defined.[45] It is any variation from these well described syndromes that will alert the experienced clinician to suspect DS. In addition to recognizing an 'atypical sequence of events'[7] the most helpful objective features distinguishing DS from epileptic seizures are long duration (over 2 minutes), a gradual onset with motor features that wax and wane throughout the seizure and, on recovery, evidence that the patient is able to recall events for a period of unresponsiveness. An episode of motionless unresponsiveness (that is reversible) lasting over 5 minutes is unlikely to have an organic explanation.[7] Additional features on history which favour (and only that) a diagnosis of DS

Table 4.2 Some clinical semiological features of epileptic and dissociative seizures

	Dissociative seizures	Epileptic seizures
Duration over 2 minutes	common[1,7,28–30]	rare
[a]Stereotyped attacks	common[7,31,32]	common
Motor features		
Gradual onset	common[7,28,31,33,34]	rare
Fluctuating course	common[7]	very rare
Thrashing, violent movements	common[28,35–37]	rare
Side to side head movement	common[29,35]	rare
Asynchronous movements	common[29,38]	very rare
Eyes closed	common[28,39]	rare
Pelvic thrusting	occasional[1,29,40]	rare
Opisthotonus, 'arc de cercle'	occasional[28,31,41]	very rare
Automatisms	rare[41]	common
Weeping	occasional[42,43]	very rare
[a]Incontinence	occasional[7,35,44]	common
[a]Injury		
Biting inside of mouth	occasional[7,35,39,41,44]	common
Severe tongue biting[b]	very rare[7,35,39,41,44]	common
Recall for period of unresponsiveness	common[1,7,41]	very rare

Note:

[a] Three features ('red herrings') that are commonly misinterpreted as evidence for epilepsy have been included in this table for emphasis. Otherwise the table lists clinical features that are often useful in distinguishing DS from ES. Figures for frequency of these features are approximate: common > 30%; occasional = 10–30%; rare < 10%; very rare < 5%.

[b] Injuries to the tongue in epilepsy usually involve the side of the tongue. Bite injuries to the tip of the tongue or lip are rare in epilepsy and suggest DS.[39]

rather than epilepsy include onset of seizures after the age of 10, a failed response to AEDs and the presence of risk-factors for DS (including a history of previous unexplained medical symptoms, a psychiatric history and a history of childhood traumatic experiences – see below). An absence of risk factors for epilepsy is reassuring in making a diagnosis of DS but their presence may be misleading[32] as, for example, DS are common in patients with learning difficulties (also associated with epilepsy) and a family history of seizures is common in patients with DS.[46]

Between 10 and 30% of patients with DS also have epilepsy[1,7,28,36,38,41,43,44,47] which may create problems in diagnosis and management. A history of multiple seizure types is not a reliable indicator of comorbid epilepsy as some 20 percent of patients with DS alone report more than one type of seizure.[35,36,41] Special mention should also be made of frontal lobe epilepsy which is frequently mistaken for DS. Frontal lobe seizures may involve bizarre emotional and behavioural features highly suggestive of DS.[47,48] These include intense emotional reactions, asymmetrical motor posturing, kicking and thrashing, body rocking, side-to-side head movements and complex behavioural paroxysms such as pelvic thrusting, undressing, masturbatory activity and uttering obscenities. Furthermore, despite the complexity of behaviours involved patients will often claim some preservation of awareness during attacks and there is frequently an extensive past psychiatric history (not least because these patients are often initially misdiagnosed as having DS). Characteristics of frontal lobe seizures which help distinguish them from DS are short ictal duration, stereotyped patterns of movements and occurrence during sleep (sometimes associated with secondary generalisation).

An opportunity to observe a seizure first-hand and to examine the patient during a seizure may provide invaluable information.[1,7,28,29,35] Careful note should be taken of the type of movements seen, their distribution and whether apparent clonic movements are rhythmic and synchronous (as they usually are in epilepsy) or not (DS). After a generalised tonic-clonic seizure the corneal reflex will usually be impaired and plantar responses extensor. If the patient's eyes are shut the examiner should attempt to open them and note any resistance to this (DS). A simple test to look for avoidance of a noxious stimulus is to hold the patient's hand over their face and drop it: in DS the patient may be seen to control their arm movement so their hand falls to one side. If the eyes are open, evidence of visual fixation may be sought in two ways. The first involves rolling the patient onto their side. In a patient with DS the eyes will often be deviated to the ground. The patient should then be rolled onto the other side and note taken if the eyes are still directed towards the ground (The 'Henry and Woodruff Sign').[49] A second useful manoeuvre is to place a small mirror in front of the patient and look for evidence of convergent gaze and fixation on the reflection. This procedure may also prove useful in stopping the seizure. All of these examination findings must however be interpreted with caution: the 'correct' response to any of these tests may be learned by patients who are simulating illness.

Following careful clinical assessment the experienced clinician may often be in a position to reach a confident diagnosis. Sometimes, however, doubt remains, even if a seizure is witnessed: in one study an experienced epileptologist viewing

Table 4.3 A checklist of examination procedures that may help differentiate DS from ES. The findings in the first three tests indicate some preservation of intact awareness and volition. By general consensus, however, these examination findings should not be interpreted as proving the patient is fabricating their illness. As a cautionary note, some patients may learn to produce the 'correct' neurological response with any of these examinations.

Examination procedure	Finding in DS
Drop patient's hand over their face	hand falls to the side
If eyes closed, attempt to open them	resistance to eye-opening
If eyes open	evidence of visual fixation
Place mirror in front of patient	
Roll patient from one side to the other (*see* text)	
Corneal reflex	intact neurological reflexes
Plantar reflex	

videotapes of seizures correctly identified only 73% of DS and 71% of ES.[38] Special investigations therefore have an important role in diagnosis but there are pitfalls and limitations which will be considered next.

Special investigation

EEG

According to Chadwick,[50] the EEG is 'one of the most abused investigations in clinical medicine and is unquestionably responsible for great human suffering'. While a single routine EEG may be normal in some 30% of patients with epilepsy (the false negative rate falls to around 15%, or even less in patients with repeated studies or sleep recordings[51]), Chadwick was highlighting the problem of false positives. Anything up to 15% of the normal population may have a 'non-specific' abnormality noted on EEG. There is clearly a danger both that an EEG may be 'over-reported', especially if the request form sent to the electrophysiologist expresses no doubt about the diagnosis, and also that such non-specific abnormalities might be misunderstood by inexperienced clinicians as backing a diagnosis of epilepsy when they do no such thing. This problem is compounded by the fact that such non-specific abnormalities (principally a slow background rhythm) are more common in patients with DS than in healthy volunteers[52] and in patients with borderline personality disorder,[53] which is common in patients with DS (*see* below). It should be noted, however, that rigorously defined specific 'epileptiform' abnormalities (generalised spikes or polyspike and slow wave abnormalities) are very rare (approximately 3 in 1000) in healthy individuals.[54,55] The EEG is just one factor that must be weighed up in making a diagnosis of epilepsy which ultimately rests on clinical judgement.

Video EEG telemetry

The gold-standard investigation for seizure disorders is long-term monitoring with video EEG (vEEG) telemetry. The patient is admitted to hospital with the aim of catching a seizure (ideally more than one) on both video and EEG, allowing the semiology of the seizure to be observed and providing an ictal EEG recording. The critical EEG findings[7] include ictal epileptiform discharges (which may be obscured or even mimicked by movement artefact) and post-ictal slowing of the background rhythm. An important sign that excludes organic causes of unconsciousness is the presence of an intact alpha rhythm (a neurophysiological correlate of alertness most prominent when the patient's eyes are closed) in an unresponsive patient. Aside from practical considerations (vEEG telemetry is an expensive investigation and is not widely available) there are also some important clinical limitations. Firstly, the ictal scalp EEG is often normal in simple partial seizures (in which consciousness is preserved)[56,57] and in frontal lobe seizures.[47,48] As already discussed, frontal lobe seizures are particularly problematic as they may include bizarre motor and behavioural manifestations and are often mistaken for DS. In these cases the video recording will often be extremely useful. A further helpful point is that frontal lobe seizures commonly arise from sleep and the ictal EEG will demonstrate this clearly even if there are no other electrographic signs of epilepsy. Although patients with DS often report seizures in sleep, when they are captured on telemetry they are inevitably preceded by waking,[3] which again can be documented electrographically. A more common problem concerns patients with seizures occurring so infrequently that they are unlikely to have an episode during telemetry. Patients with more than one type of seizure also require special attention. Because DS and ES often occur in the same patient, care must be taken to ensure that a representative example of each seizure type has been captured. Occasionally patients with epilepsy may have a DS for the first time in their lives on a telemetry unit, perhaps brought on by the stress of admission to hospital and 'performance anxiety' secondary to a perceived pressure to have an attack.[58] Thus, where possible someone who has witnessed the patient's seizures should be shown the video (with the patient's consent) to verify that the recorded attack is characteristic of the patient's habitual seizures.

Ambulatory EEG[59] may be conducted as an outpatient but suffers from the disadvantage of having no video-documented semiology to correlate with the EEG. Asking a patient's carer to video seizures may also be very helpful with the accepted limitation that the first few seconds after seizure-onset will usually be missed. In an attempt to reduce the need for long and costly telemetry several investigators have explored the possibility of provoking seizures through suggestion while obtaining video and EEG recordings. Using procedures such as intravenous infusion of saline up to 90% of patients will have a DS[60,61] but these methods remain controversial because of ethical concerns about the use of placebo. Most recently, however, McGonigal and colleagues[62] combined simple suggestion with activation stimuli used routinely in EEG testing (photic stimulation and hyperventilation) and fully disclosed the aims of the procedure to patients. Sixty-six percent of patients experienced a DS provoked in this way compared with 33% in a control group who received identical activation stimuli but without suggestion. In these settings, because of very occasional false positive results in patients with epilepsy,[63,64] it is particularly important to have a witness confirm the provoked seizure as habitual.

Serum prolactin

Serum prolactin[65] rises to levels greater than 500 IU/ml in over 90% of patients following a tonic-clonic seizure and 60% of patients following a complex partial seizure. Simple partial seizures are not followed by a rise in serum prolactin and prolactin levels may be normal after prolonged status epilepticus. Blood must be taken between 20 and 30 minutes after the seizure and compared with a baseline sample. The test is, however, used less and less in specialist centres as false positive results have now been demonstrated in syncope[66] and DS.[67] Thus, whilst a normal post-ictal prolactin may be helpful diagnostically if the seizure was tonic-clonic in semiology, an elevated post-ictal prolactin is non-specific.

Psychiatric assessment of patients with DS

Conscious/unconscious symptom generation

As we have seen, after organic diagnoses have been excluded and a primary psychiatric disorder that has been mistaken for epilepsy ruled out, the diagnostic possibilities are DS and factitious disorder. The distinction made between DS and factitious disorder in psychiatric classification systems implies a dichotomy between what is conscious and what is not. In practice the distinction may be difficult to make and a definite diagnosis of factitious disorder ultimately depends on the patient confessing their intent to deceive. The notion of unconscious symptom generation remains controversial[68] and a more valid way of conceiving the problem might be as a continuum with unconscious motivation at one end, conscious simulation at the other and a large grey area in between, with 'self-deception' lying somewhere in the middle.

Most authorities suggest that the majority of patients are unconscious of any wilful component to their seizures and factitious disorder is held to be rare.[37,65] However, many find this hard to accept. Three points in favour of the symptoms being unconscious are worth considering, although none is by any means conclusive:

1 The majority of patients are compliant with anti-epileptic medication, often for several years and to the point of toxicity, until the correct diagnosis is made.
2 When admitted for EEG telemetry the majority of patients have a seizure within what they must surely perceive to be an intensively monitored setting.
3 DS are generally a poor imitation of epilepsy. In fact, factitious disorder will often be suspected whenever one of these three conditions is not met.

Psychiatric formulation: epidemiological consideration, comorbidity and risk factors for DS

Psychiatric assessment should aim to identify putative risk factors for DS that may help the patient understand why they have the disorder and may direct psychological and other approaches to treatment. What follows is an account of the demographic characteristics of DS and possible predisposing and maintaining factors identified in the literature.

Approximately three quarters of patients are women.[7,9,36,69] Seizures usually begin in the late teens or early twenties but there is a wide range.[7,9,36] Patients in lower socioeconomic groups and with less educational achievement are probably over-represented, although not in comparison with patients with epilepsy.[69]

A history of previous medically unexplained symptoms is present in up to 80% of patients.[7,36,41,70] In some cases symptoms will have attracted a medical diagnosis even though objective evidence of pathology is lacking. The recently reported association of a diagnosis of asthma in patients with DS may be an example of this.[36,71] In addition to a history suggestive of somatisation, there is a high rate of psychiatric comorbidity. Maladaptive personality features of a borderline type are common,[72] often in the form of trait accentuations rather than personality disorder per se.[73,74] Related to this, patients with DS show less adaptive coping styles.[75,76] Comorbid anxiety disorders and depression have been widely reported,[36] but prevalence rates vary between studies and have often not been strikingly greater than observed in patients with epilepsy in those studies that have used a control group.[72,73,77]

The prevalence of abnormal personality in these patients suggests adverse experiences occurring in childhood or adolescence at a time when personality attributes are developing, and the risk factor to have attracted most attention in the literature is a history of childhood abusive experiences. Although there have been negative findings,[78,79] a number of large studies in which abuse has been carefully defined have demonstrated higher rates of reported abuse in patients with DS compared with epileptic controls and unselected psychiatric patients.[69,80,81] Traumatic, abusive experiences in adulthood have also been implicated.[81] Other traumatic experiences or situations that foster low self-esteem, for example bullying at school or unrecognised learning difficulties,[82] may be over-represented but have not been studied in adults with DS.

There is evidence that adverse life events are more common in the year preceding onset of DS,[72] but triggers for initial seizures are often not apparent. Adverse family interactions[83–85] may serve as both predisposing and maintaining factors for DS. A pattern of avoidant behaviour, often exacerbated by carers' overprotective reactions, is a relatively under-recognised maintaining factor but readily apparent on history taking in the form of an agoraphobic pattern of avoidance, ostensibly for fear of having a seizure in an embarrassing or vulnerable setting.[84] Finally, for some patients the psychological and social advantages inherent to a medical sick role are undoubtedly important maintaining factors.[9,68,86] Such advantages include both an avoidance of responsibility and positive benefits such as the caring response elicited in others.

It should be noted that DS share many possible aetiological factors with other somatoform disorders. The paroxysmal nature of the symptoms, however, give this disorder a unique quality that creates special difficulties for diagnosis but also raises specific treatment approaches.

Treatment

Explaining the diagnosis to patients

Treatment begins with an explanation of diagnosis. This must be handled openly but sensitively: if it is not, the patient is likely to reject the diagnosis, decline treatment and go elsewhere for more investigations; a disaster in terms of time and expense, both for the patient and medical services.[87,88]

Presenting the diagnosis of dissociative seizures

In discussing the diagnosis with the patient the following points should be covered:

1 reasons for concluding they don't have epilepsy
2 what they do have (describe dissociation)
3 emphasise they are not suspected of 'putting on' the attacks
4 they are not 'mad'
5 triggering 'stresses' may not be immediately apparent
6 relevance of aetiological factors in their case
7 maintaining factors
8 may improve following correct diagnosis
9 caution that AED withdrawal should be gradual
10 describe psychological treatment.

It is important to involve patients'carers in this explanation.

First, a clear explanation must be given of the reasons for concluding that the patient does not have epilepsy. This should cover any aspects of the patient's seizure semiology that are inconsistent with epilepsy and features in their history which make epilepsy less likely (e.g. a failed response to anti-epileptic drugs, lack of risk factors for epilepsy). A thorough explanation of investigation results should follow which, if relevant, must address any non-specific 'abnormalities' that the patient may previously have been told about and the way in which these can be put in context.

A description of what the patient *does* have then follows. Many patients will react unfavourably to the news that no medical explanation has been found and great care should be taken to emphasise that the doctor understands the attacks are real, disabling and that the patient is not suspected of putting them on. A useful approach can be to tell the patient that they have attacks in which their mind or brain 'switches off', involuntarily, and they lose control. It is often helpful to describe the concept of dissociation, explaining that the attacks represent an extreme form of something which is part of everyday experience using examples illustrating selective and divided attention (e.g. reading a book and not hearing your name called, travelling home from work and remembering nothing of the journey). It should be explained that the symptoms are stress-related but that it is usual for the stresses to be difficult to identify. Patients commonly object that the seizures can't be caused by stress as they occur at times when they are relaxed. In this situation it may be helpful to explain that attacks may be triggered by stressful or unpleasant thoughts that the individual is barely aware of (or can't remember) and may have little to do with their immediate circumstances. The concept that thinking may occur on a number of different levels at any one time can be described. Examples of the link between physical symptoms and emotional state (e.g. crying, autonomic symptoms of arousal) and complex involuntary behavioural accompaniments to emotions (e.g. as seen with sudden grief or with rage) may help illustrate some of the physical attributes of seizures. If the patient experiences somatic symptoms of arousal during their seizures[89] the relationship of these features to anxiety can be described and the seizures likened to a 'panic attack without the panic' in which dissociation ('switching off') protects the patient from unpleasant or frightening emotions.

Patients often express a fear that they are being told they are 'mad'. They should be reassured that the condition they have is common and the profile of a typical patient should be described, emphasising the points that apply to them. A link between traumatic experiences in childhood may be made meaningful by explaining that children exposed to abuse, especially if it is repeated, learn to 'switch off' as a way of coping: DS may represent a re-emergence of this once-adaptive response in the face of challenges, stress or perhaps something that reminds the patient of painful memories. Some[87] have recommended raising the subject of abuse as a causal factor even if a history of it has not emerged. However, such an approach risks encouraging 'false memories' and may best be avoided.

A description of maintaining factors is important and is often welcomed by patients who are sceptical about supposed psychological origins of their symptoms. It can be explained that whatever caused the seizures in the first place may remain unknown, but that worry about seizures, including what they are due to, and worry about the consequences of having a seizure may actually make the seizures worse and more frequent.[90] Patients will often relate to the confusion and anxiety engendered by receiving contradictory advice from a succession of doctors and the role this may have in perpetuating attacks. The concept of how avoidant behaviour, often exacerbated by a well-meaning family's protective reactions, acts to reinforce anxiety about attacks[90] may give the patient and their family a rationale for change.

Finally, the patient should be given hope that their problems are treatable. Most patients are delighted to hear they may come off anti-epileptic medication but they should be warned that this must be done gradually for fear of triggering a withdrawal seizure. It is worth emphasising that once confusion about diagnosis is resolved a significant proportion of patients find that this explanation alone leads to a resolution of the attacks over time.[91]

Approaches to treatment

There have been no controlled trials of treatment in DS. The evidence comes from case reports and small treatment series.[80,90,92,93–101] In the small proportion of patients who have significant comorbid depression or anxiety, appropriate pharmacotherapy is indicated. For the majority, however, some form of psychotherapy will be the mainstay of treatment. In patients with learning difficulties operant behavioural programmes using simple reward systems are often helpful.[94,95] The early literature includes a number of compelling descriptions of insight-oriented, dynamic psychotherapeutic approaches in patients with a history of DS and sexual abuse.[98,99] More recent reports have described psycho-educational group therapy[100] and eye movement desensitisation[101] in similar patient groups. Variations of therapy based on psychodynamic, insight-oriented and educational principles are undoubtedly widely practised and believed to be effective but further studies of such interventions are needed.

The paroxysmal nature of the attacks, the occurrence of somatic symptoms of arousal in many patients and the association with agoraphobic avoidant behaviour suggest that techniques developed in Cognitive Behavioural Therapy (CBT) for the treatment of panic disorder might readily be adapted for DS.[90,92] This CBT model also provides a useful rationale for treatment in patients who report no history of past traumatic experiences or who have received psychotherapy for this but continue to have seizures. A recent study involving 20 patients treated with CBT reported a significant reduction in seizures 6 months after treatment ended and, perhaps more importantly, found improvements in work and social outcome.[92] CBT techniques developed for personality disorder may be helpful but these and other techniques require evaluation.[102] A significant proportion (*see* below) of patients continue to have seizures despite intensive and varied treatment. A realistic approach in such cases is to offer long-term follow-up to provide support for the patient and their family, social interventions to improve quality of life despite seizures, and also to limit the cost and morbidity associated with further unnecessary investigations and medical interventions.

Outcome

A recent review of outcome studies[27] found that after a mean follow-up period of 3 years approximately two thirds of patients continued to have DS and more than half remained dependent on social security. Receiving psychiatric treatment has been associated with a positive outcome in some studies, but not in others. A poor prognosis is predicted by a long delay in diagnosis and the presence of psychiatric comorbidity, including personality disorder.

References

1 Leis AA, Ross MA, Summers AK. Psychogenic seizures: ictal characteristics and diagnostic pitfalls. *Neurology*. 1992; **42**: 95–9.

2 Thacker K, Devinsky O, Perrine K, Alper K, Luciano D. Nonepileptic seizures during apparent sleep. *Annals of Neurology* 1993; **33**: 414–18.

3 Smith D, Defalla BA, Chadwick DW. The misdiagnosis of epilepsy and the management of refractory epilepsy in a specialist clinic. *QJM* 1999; **92**: 15–23.

4 Benbadis SR, Allen HW. An estimate of the prevalence of psychogenic non-epileptic seizures. *Seizure* 2000; **9**: 280–1.

5 Kotsopoulos IA, de Krom MC, Kessels AG, *et al*. The diagnosis of epileptic and non-epileptic seizures. *Epilepsy Research* 2003; **57**: 59–67.

6 Reuber M, Fernandez G, Bauer J, Helmstaedter C, Elger CE. Diagnostic delay in psychogenic nonepileptic seizures. *Neurology* 2002; **58**: 493–5.

7 Meierkord H, Will B, Fish D, Shorvon S. The clinical features and prognosis of pseudoseizures diagnosed using video-EEG telemetry. *Neurology* 1991; **41**: 1643–6.

8 Krumholz A, Neidermeyer E. Psychogenic seizures: A clinical study with follow-up data. *Neurology*. 1983; **33**: 498–502.

9 Kristensen O, Alving J. Pseudoseizures – risk factors and prognosis. *Acta Neurol Scand* 1992; **85**: 177–180.

10 Walker MC, Howard RS, Smith SJ, Miller DH, Shorvon SD, Hirsch NP. Diagnosis and treatment of status epilepticus on a neurological intensive care unit. *QJM* 1996; **89**: 913–20.

11 Stone J, Campbell K, Sharma N, Carson A, Warlow CP, Sharpe M. What should we call pseudoseizures? The patient's perspective. *Seizure* 2003; **12**: 568–72.

12 Scull DA. Pseudoseizures or non-epileptic seizures (NES);15 synonyms. *Journal of Neurology, Neurosurgery & Psychiatry*. 1997; **62**: 200.

13 American Psychiatric Association. *Diagnostic and Statistical Manual of Mental Disorders*. 4th edn DSM-IV. Washington DC: American Psychiatric Association, 1994.

14 World Health Organization. *The ICD-10 Classification of Mental and Behavioural Disorders. Clinical Description and Diagnostic Guidelines*. Geneva: World Health Organization, 1992.

15 Martin RC, Gilliam FG, Kilgore M, Faught E, Kuzniecky R. Improved health care resource utilization following video-EEG-confirmed diagnosis of nonepileptic psychogenic seizures. *Seizure* 1998; **7**: 385–90.

16 Cook M. Differential diagnosis of epilepsy. In Shorvorn S, Perucca E, Fish D, Dodson E (eds). *The Treatment of Epilepsy*. 2nd edn. Oxford: Blackwell, 2004: 64–73.

17 Andermann F. Non-epileptic paroxysmal neurologic events. In Gater JR, Rowan AJ (eds). *Non-epileptic Seizures*. 2nd edn. Boston: Butterworth Heinemann, 2000: 51–69.

18 Lempert T, Bauer M, Schmidt D. Syncope: a videometric analysis of 56 episodes of transient cerebral hypoxia. *Ann Neurol*. 1994; **36**: 233–7.

19 Sheldon R, Rose S, Ritchie D, *et al*. Historical criteria that distinguish syncope from seizures. *J Am Coll Cardiol*. 2002; **40**: 142–8.

20 Lempert T. Recognizing syncope: pitfalls and surprises. *J R Soc Med*. 1996; **89**: 372–5.

21 Parker C. Complicated migraine syndromes and migraine variants. *Pediatr Ann*. 1997; **26**: 417–21.

22 Manford MR, Fish DR, Shorvon SD. Startle provoked epileptic seizures: features in 19 patients. *Journal of Neurology, Neurosurgery & Psychiatry*. 1996; **61**: 151–6.

23 Vidailhet M. Paroxysmal dyskinesias as a paradigm of paroxysmal movement disorders. *Curr Opin Neurol.* 2000; **13**: 457–62.

24 Schenck CH, Mahowald MW. Parasomnias. Managing bizarre sleep-related behaviour disorders. *Postgrad Med.* 2000; **107**: 145–56.

25 Alper K, Devinsky O, Perrine K, Vazquez B, Luciano D. Psychiatric classification of nonconversion nonepileptic seizures. *Archives of Neurology.* 1995; **52**: 199–201.

26 Toni C, Cassano GB, Perugi G, Murri L, Mancino M. Psychosensorial and related phenomena in panic disorder and in temporal lobe epilepsy. *Compr Psychiatry* 1996; **37**: 125–33.

27 Reuber M, Elger CE. Psychogenic nonepileptic seizures: Review and update. *Epilepsy & Behavior* 2003; **4**: 205–16.

28 Gulick TA, Spinks IR, King DW. Pseudoseizures: ictal phenomena. *Neurology* 1982; **32**: 24–30.

29 Gates JR, Ramani V, Whalen S, Loewenson R. Ictal characteristics of pseudoseizures. *Archives of Neurology* 1985; **42**: 1183–7.

30 Bazil CW, Walczak TS. Effects of sleep and sleep stage on epileptic and nonepileptic seizures. *Epilepsia* 1997; **38**: 56–62.

31 Desai BT, Porter RJ, Penry JK. Psychogenic seizures. A study of 42 attacks in 6 patients, with intensive monitoring. *Archives of Neurology* 1982; **39**: 202–209.

32 Wilkus RJ, Dodrill CB, Thompson PM. Intensive EEG monitoring and psychological studies of patients with pseudoepileptic seizures. *Epilepsia* 1984; **25**: 100–7.

33 Holmes GL, Sackellares JC, McKiernan J, Ragland M, Dreifuss FE. Evaluation of childhood pseudoseizures using EEG telemetry and video tape monitoring. *J Pediatrics* 1980; **97**: 554–8.

34 Lancman ME, Asconape JJ, Graves S, Gibson PA. Psychogenic seizures in children: long-term analysis of 43 cases. *Journal of Child Neurology* 1994; **9**: 404–7.

35 Luther JS, McNamara JO, Carwile S, Miller P, Hope V. Pseudoepileptic seizures: methods and video analysis to aid diagnosis. *Annals of Neurology* 1982; **12**: 458–462.

36 Bowman ES, Markand ON. Psychodynamics and psychiatric diagnoses of pseudoseizure subjects. *American Journal of Psychiatry* 1996; **153**: 57–63.

37 Betts T, Boden S. Diagnosis, management and prognosis of a group of 128 patients with non-epileptic attack disorder. Part 1. *Seizure* 1992; **1**: 19–26.

38 King DW, Gallagher BB, Murvin AJ, *et al.* Pseudoseizures: diagnostic evaluation. *Neurology* 1982; **32**: 18–23.

39 DeToledo JC, Ramsey RE. Patterns of involvement of facial muscles during epileptic and nonepileptic events: review of 654 events. *Neurology* 1996; **47**: 621–5.

40 Geyer JD, Payne TA, Drury I. The value of pelvic thrusting in the diagnosis of seizures and pseudoseizures. *Neurology* 2000; **54**: 227–9.

41 Lempert T, Schmidt D. Natural history and outcome of psychogenic seizures: a clinical study in 50 patients. *Journal of Neurology* 1990; **237**: 35–8.

42 Bergen D, Ristanovic R. Weeping as a common element of pseudoseizures. *Archives of Neurology* 1993; **50**: 1059–1060.

43 Walczak T, Bogolioubov A. Weeping during psychogenic nonepileptic seizures. *Epilepsia* 1996; **37**: 208–210.

44 Cohen RJ, Suter C. Hysterical seizures: suggestion as a provocative EEG test. *Annals of Neurology.* 1982; **11**: 391–5.

45 Commission on Classification and Terminology of the International League Against Epilepsy. Proposal for revised classification of epilepsies and epileptic syndromes. *Epilepsia* 1989; **30**: 389–99.

46 Moore PM, Baker GA. Non-epileptic attack disorder: a psychological perspective. *Seizure* 1997; **6**: 429–34.

47 Williamson PD, Spencer DD, Spencer SS, Novelly RA, Mattson RH. Complex partial seizures of frontal lobe origin. *Annals of Neurology* 1985; **18**: 497–504.

48 Saygi S, Katz A, Marks DA, Spencer SS. Frontal lobe partial seizures and psychogenic seizures: comparison of clinical and ictal characteristics. *Neurology* 1992; **42**: 1274–7.

49 Henry J, Woodruff GAJ. A diagnostic sign in states of apparent unconsciousness. *Lancet* 1978; **2**: 920–1.

50 Chadwick D. Epilepsy. *Journal of Neurology, Neurosurgery and Psychiatry* 1994; **57**: 264–77.

51 Binnie CD, Prior PF. Electroencephalography. *Journal of Neurology, Neurosurgery and Psychiatry* 1994; **57**: 1308–19.

52 Reuber M, Fernandez G, Bauer J, Singh DD, Elger CE. Interictal EEG abnormalities in patients with psychogenic non-epileptic seizures. *Epilepsia* 2002; **43**: 1013–20.

53 De la Fuente, Tugendhaft P, Mavroudakis N. Electroencephalographic abnormalities in borderline personality disorder. *Psychiatry Research* 1998; **77**: 131–8.

54 Robin JJ, Tolan JD, Arnold JW. Ten-year experience with abnormal EEGs in asymptomatic adult males. *Aviation Space Env Med* 1978; **49**: 732–6.

55 Gregory RP, Oates T, Merry RTG. Electroencephalogram epileptiform abnormalities in candidates for aircrew training. *Electroencephalogr Clin Neurophysiol* 1993; **86**: 75–7.

56 Devinsky O, Kelley K, Porter RJ, Theodore WR. Clinical and electrographic features of simple partial seizures. *Neurology* 1988; **18**: 1347–52.

57 Bare MA, Burnstine TH, Fisher RS, Lesser RP. Electroencephalographic changes during simple partial seizures. *Epilepsia* 1994; **35**: 715–20.

58 Kapur J, Pillai A, Henry TR. Psychogenic elaboration of simple partial seizures. *Epilepsia* 1995; **36**: 1126–30.

59 Cascino GD. Video-EEG monitoring in adults. *Epilepsia* 2002; **43**(suppl 3): 80–93.

60 Slater JD, Brown M, Jacobs W. Induction of pseudoseizures with intravenous saline placebo. *Epilepsia* 1995; **36**: 580–5.

61 Dericioglu N, Saygi S, Ciger A. The value of provocation methods in patients suspected of having non-epileptic seizures. *Seizure* 1999; **8**: 152–6.

62 McGonigal A, Oto M, Russell AJC, Greene J, Duncan R. Outpatient video EEG recording in the diagnosis of non-epilepstic seizures: a randomised controlled trial of simple suggestion techniques. *J Neurol Neurosurg Psychiatry* 2002; **72**: 549–551.

63 Walczak TS, Williams DT, Berten W. Utility and reliability of placebo infusion in the evaluation of patients with seizures. *Neurology* 1994; **44**: 394–9.

64 Barry JJ, Atzman O, Morrell MJ. Discriminating between epileptic and non-epileptic events: the utility of hypnotic seizure induction. *Epilepsia* 2000; **41**: 81–4.

65 Trimble MR. Pseudoseizures. *Neurologic Clinics* 1986; **4**: 531–47.

66 Oribe E, Amini R, Nissenbaum E, Boal B. Serum prolactin concentrations are elevated following syncope. *Neurology* 1996; **47**: 60–62.

67 Alving J. Serum prolactin levels are elevated also after pseudo-epileptic seizures. *Seizure* 1998; **7**: 85–9.

68 Slavney PR. In defense of pseudoseizure. *General Hospital Psychiatry* 1994; **16**: 243–5.

69 Alper K, Devinsky O, Perrine K, Vazquez B, Luciano D. Nonepileptic seizures and childhood sexual and physical abuse. *Neurology* 1993; **43**: 1950–3.

70 Walczak TS, Papacostas S, Williams DT, Scheuer ML, Lebowitz N, Notarfrancesco A. Outcome after diagnosis of psychogenic nonepileptic seizures. *Epilepsia* 1995; **36**: 1131–7.

71 de Wet CJ, Mellers JD, Gardner WN, Toone BK. Pseudoseizures and asthma. *Journal of Neurology, Neurosurgery & Psychiatry* 2003; **74**: 639–41.

72 Binzer M, Stone J, Sharpe M. Recent onset pseudoseizures – clues to aetiology. *Seizure* 2004; **13**: 146–55.

73 Krishnamoorthy ES, Brown RJ, Trimble MR. Personality and psychopathology in nonepileptic attack disorder and epilepsy: a prospective study. *Epilepsy & Behaviour* 2001; **2**: 418–22.

74 Reuber M, Pukrop R, Bauer J, Derfuss R, Elger CE. Multidimensional assessment of personality in patients with psychogenic non-epileptic seizures. *Journal of Neurology, Neurosurgery & Psychiatry* 2004; **75**(5): 743–8.

75 Frances PL, Baker GA, Appleton PL. Stress and avoidance in Pseudoseizures: testing the assumptions. *Epilepsy Research* 1999; **34**: 241–9.

76 Goldstein LH, Drew C, Mellers J, Mitchell-O'Malley S, Oakley DA. Dissociation, hypnotizability, coping styles and health locus of control: characteristics of pseudoseizure patients. *Seizure* 2000; **9**: 314–22.

77 van Merode T, Twellaar M, Kotsopoulos IA, *et al.* Psychological characteristics of patients with newly developed psychogenic seizures. *Journal of Neurology, Neurosurgery & Psychiatry.* 2004; **75**: 1175–7.

78 Jawad SS, Jail N, Clarke EJ, Lewis A, Whitecross S, Richens A. Psychiatric morbidity and psychodynamics of patients with convulsive pseudoseizures. *Seizure* 1995; **4**: 201–6.

79 Tojek TM, Lumley M, Barkley G, Mahr G, Thomas A. Stress and other psychosocial characteristics of patients with psychogenic nonepileptic seizures. *Psychosomatics* 2000; **41**: 221–6.

80 Betts T, Boden S. Diagnosis, management and prognosis of a group of 128 patients with non-epileptic attack disorder. Part 1. Previous childhood sexual abuse in the aetiology of these disorders. *Seizure* 1992; **1**: 27–32.

81 Reilly J, Baker GA, Rhodes J, Salmon P. The association of sexual and physical abuse with somatization: Characteristics of patients presenting with irritable bowel syndrome and non-epileptic attack disorder. *Psychological Medicine* 1999; **29**: 399–406.

82 Silver LB. Conversion disorder with pseudoseizures in adolescence: a stress reaction to unrecognized and untreated learning disabilities. *J Am Acad Child Psychiatry* 1982; **21**: 508–12.

83 Moore PM, Baker GA, McDade G, Chadwick D, Brown S. Epilepsy, pseudoseizures and perceived family characteristics: a controlled study. *Epilepsy Research* 1994; **18**: 75–83.

84 Krawetz P, Fleisher W, Pillay N, Staley D, Arnett J, Maher J. Family functioning in subjects with pseudoseizures and epilepsy. *Journal of Nervous & Mental Disease* 2001; **189**: 38–43.

85 Stanhope N, Goldstein LH, Kuipers E. Expressed emotion in the relatives of people with epileptic or nonepileptic seizures. *Epilepsia* 2003; **44**: 1094–102.

86 Slavney PR. Pseudoseizures, sexual abuse and hermeneutic reasoning. *Comprehensive Psychiatry* 1994; **35**: 471–7.

87 Shen W, Bowman ES, Markand O. Presenting the diagnosis of pseudoseizure. *Neurology* 1990; **40**: 756–9.

88 Carton S, Thompson PJ, Duncan JS. Non-epileptic seizures: patients' understanding and reaction to the diagnosis and impact on outcome. *Seizure* 2003; **12**: 287–94.

89 Vein AM, Djukova GM, Vorobieva OV. Is panic attack a mask of psychogenic seizures? – a comparative analysis of phenomenology of psychogenic seizures and panic attacks. *Functional Neurology* 1994; **9**: 153–9.

90 Chalder T. Non-epileptic attacks: A cognitive behavioural approach in a single case approach with a four-year follow-up. *Clinical Psychology and Psychotherapy* 1996; **3**: 291–7.

91 Farias ST, Thieman C, Alsaadi TM. Psychogenic nonepileptic seizures: acute change in event frequency after presentation of the diagnosis. *Epilepsy & Behavior* 2003; **4**: 424–9.

92 Goldstein LH, Deale AC, Mitchell-O'Malley S, Toone BK, Mellers JDC. An evaluation of cognitive behavioral therapy as a treatment for dissociative seizures. A pilot study. *Cognitive and Behavioral Neurology* 2004; **17**: 41–9.

93 Ramani V, Gumnit RJ. Management of hysterical seizures in epileptic patients. *Arch Neurol* 1982; **39**: 78–81.

94 Montgomery JM, Espie CA. Behavioural management of hysterical pseudoseizures. *Behavioural Psychotherapy* 1986; **14**: 334–340.

95 Lachenmeyer JR, Olsen ME. Behaviour modification in the treatment of pseudoseizures: a case report. *Behavioural Psychotherapy* 1990; **18**: 73–78.

96 Gates JR. Nonepileptic seizures: Classification, coexistence with epilepsy, diagnosis, therapeutic approaches and consensus. *Epilepsy and Behaviour* 2002; **3**: 28–33.

97 Iriarte J, Parra J, Urrestarzu E, Kuyk J. Controversies in the diagnosis and management of psychogenic pseudoseizures. *Epilepsy and Behavour 2003*; **4**: 354–9.

98 Goodwin J, Simms M, Bergman R. Hysterical seizures: a sequel to incest. *American Journal of Orthopsychiatry* 1979; **49**: 698–703.

99 Gross M. Pseudoepilepsy: a study in adolescent hysteria. *American Journal of Psychiatry* 1979; **136**: 210–3.

100 Zaroff CM, Myers L, Bar WB, Luciano D, Devinsky O. Group psychoeducation as treatment for psychological nonepileptic seizures. *Epilepsy and Behaviour* 2004; **5**: 587–92.

101 Chemali Z, Meadows M. The use of eye movement desensitization and reprocessing in the treatment of psychogenic seizures. *Epilepsy and Behaviour* 2004: 784–7.

102 Goldstein LH. Assessment of patients with psychogenic non-epileptic seizures: psychogenic non-epileptic seizures pose a management problem. *Journal of Neurology, Neurosurgery and Psychiatry* 2004; **75**: 667–8.

Chapter Five

The management of epilepsy in women

MD O'Brien and SK Gilmour-White

There are many aspects to the management of epilepsy in women related to their role in reproduction. Some of these need to be considered in adolescents, some are related to pregnancy, concerning both the mother and her infant, and others with the menstrual cycle and the menopause. This review considers contraception, fertility, teratogenicity and the use of folic acid. It also discusses the special investigations in pregnancy, hyperemesis, the effect of pregnancy on the control of epilepsy, the effect of seizures on the fetus, a first fit in pregnancy, pseudoseizures, seizures during delivery, vitamin K, breastfeeding, postpartum maternal epilepsy, hereditary risks, counselling, catamenial epilepsy, the menopause and bone density.

Introduction

There are special problems in the management of women with epilepsy related to their role in reproduction, which start at the menarche and continue until after the menopause. The prevalence of recurrent epilepsy is about 0.5% of the population and nearly half are women. Maternal epilepsy affects three to four per thousand pregnancies, and epilepsy is the commonest neurological problem in pregnancy. The possibility of pregnancy should be considered in any woman of child-bearing age with epilepsy, because treatment is likely to be necessary for a minimum of two years and maybe indefinitely. This certainly applies to any girl over the age of 15. This topic was the subject of a major review in 1999.[1] Patients may only ask about a few of the following topics at any one time, but most will appreciate a discussion of all the potential problems.[2]

Contraception

Q: 'Can I take a contraceptive pill?'

Combined oral contraceptives (COC)

There is no reason why women with epilepsy on anti-epileptic drugs (AEDs) should not take a COC if they wish to do so after a full discussion of the alternatives. COCs achieve contraception by giving a sufficient dose of oestrogen to inhibit ovulation. The induction of P450 hepatic cytochrome enzyme activity by some anti-epileptic drugs (phenytoin, carbamazepine, oxcarbazepine, pheno-barbitone and primidone) increases the rate of metabolism of both oestrogen and progestogen, thereby lowering the blood levels of these drugs, maybe by 50% or more.[3] Topiramate reduces the level of ethinylestradiol by about 30%, but by a different mechanism.[4] Sodium valproate, the benzodiazepines (clobazam and clonazepam), vigabatrin, lamotrigine, gabapentin, tiagabine, levetiracetam and pregabalin do not affect liver enzyme activity.

It is therefore important to know whether a patient is taking an enzyme inducing anti-epileptic drug (EIAED) before prescribing a COC, and to give appropriate advice when prescribing an EIAED to women already on a COC.

In those women taking an EIAED, initiate contraception with COC containing at least 50 mcg of oestrogen and since the usual 7-day pill-free interval weakens the contraceptive effect, it is more reliable to tricycle, that is to take three cycles of preparations containing 50–60 mcg of oestrogen consecutively, with a shorter pill-free interval of four days.[5a] If breakthrough bleeding occurs, it usually settles during the first two to three cycles; if not, contraception cannot be assured and the dose of oestrogen may need to be increased.

There is no suitable 50 mcg preparation available in the UK. Norinyl-1, which contains 50 mcg of mestranol, a prodrug for ethinylestradiol, is not suitable because it is only 75–80% converted, thus providing less than 40 mcg of oestrogen.[5b] It is possible to use a 20 and a 30 mcg pill, but the oestrogens and progestogens should be compatible,[5c] making it easier to use two of the same 30 mcg preparation.

Since the metabolism of both oestrogen and progestogen is affected, the higher doses of oestrogen should be accompanied by higher doses of progestogen. Patients are often concerned about taking a larger dose of hormones, fearing a higher incidence of side effects, but they can be reassured because this larger dose, given in combination with EIAEDs, is comparable to that associated with normal doses. The failure rate of COC with AEDs is about twice that in the general population;[6] some of this is due to inadequate hormone dosage, which is almost entirely preventable. If a women taking an EIAED and the larger dose of oestrogen is switched to a non-enzyme inducing AED, the higher dose of oestrogen should be maintained for a further two cycles.[5d]

COCs may reduce the blood level of lamotrigine by 40–60%,[7,8] so starting a COC in a patient already on lamotrigine may result in poorer control of the epilepsy, or may cause the recurrence of epilepsy in a patient whose epilepsy is under very good control; a small increment in the dose of lamotrigine is all that is required. There is no problem in giving lamotrigine to patients already on a COC, because the dose of lamotrigine is titrated to the patient's needs.

Women taking EIAEDs should use COC containing at least 50 mcg of oestrogen and tricycle with a 4-day pill-free interval. Note that this is an unlicensed indication and such prescriptions are on a 'named patient basis'.

Combined contraceptive patches are also affected by EIAEDs and are not suitable for long-term use by women taking these medications.

The progestogen only preparations

The progestogen only pill (POP)

Progestogens are similarly affected by EIAEDs, aggravating other difficulties associated with this form of contraception, particularly breakthrough bleeding. Women on EIAEDs should take double the usual dose.[5e]

The depot injection

This problem does not apply to the use of medroxyprogesterone acetate (Depo-Provera), whose metabolism is proportional to hepatic blood flow, suggesting a virtually 100% clearance on first pass through the liver, so that enzyme induction has no additional effect and blood levels are not affected.[9,10]

The progestogen implant

EIAEDs affect the three-yearly progestogen implant which contains etonogestrel (Implanon), so an additional daily progestogen pill is necessary,[5f] which rather defeats the object.

Women taking EIAEDs and a POP should consider a change of contraceptive method, otherwise use Cerazette and double the usual dose, but there is no need to change the dose of Depo-Provera or to shorten the interval between injections.

Post-coital contraception: 'the morning after pill'

The efficacy of the morning after pill is also affected by EIAEDs. When using levonogestrel (Levonelle), the first dose should be doubled to two pills (1.5 mg) with a second dose at 12 hours of one pill (750 mcg).[5g]

Intra-uterine contraceptive devices.

Coils which release hormones locally (the Mirena coil) are not affected by enzyme induction, and may be appropriate for some women taking EIAEDs.[11]

Post-partum contraception

COC preparations reduce the secretion of milk, but POPs may be used and should be started three weeks post-partum. If the mother is not breastfeeding, a COC can be used from three weeks. Women taking EIAEDs should follow the protocols outlined above.

Fertility

Q: 'Could my drugs cause infertility?'

Some anti-epileptic drugs may contribute to infertility in women, but women with epilepsy are less fertile than normal. A study of fertility ratios in women with epilepsy showed that the likelihood of pregnancy is considerably less than age matched controls, falling from 0.83 (0.54–1.21) in 15–19 year olds to 0.55 (0.14–1.39) at age 40–44.[12] This effect is likely to be multifactorial, including lowered libido, social and genetic factors, and not necessarily due to medication, though drugs may be a contributory factor. This also applies to sexual dysfunction, which is more common in women with temporal lobe epilepsy, especially if the epileptiform discharges are on the right.[13] Furthermore, it has been estimated that about 8% of menstrual cycles are anovulatory in normal subjects, but it may be as high as a third of all cycles in women with temporal lobe epilepsy,[14,15] particularly if they are taking valproate.[16]

Some anti-epileptic drugs have been associated with polycystic ovaries and the polycystic ovarian syndrome; valproate has been particularly implicated.[17,18] These findings have been disputed.[19,20] It may be that valproate-induced obesity and the consequent increase in peripheral insulin resistance in patients with polycystic ovaries, together with a genetic susceptibility, are factors in the development of the polycystic ovarian syndrome; although polycystic ovaries and hyperandrogenism without hyperinsulinism have been found in some lean patients.[21] A consensus has been suggested for the investigation and management of these patients.[22]

Teratogenicity

Q: 'Will the drugs affect my baby?'

The incidence of all fetal abnormalities in the general population is between 2% and 3%. There maybe a small increased risk of fetal abnormalities in children of mothers with epilepsy who are not on medication, but a recent meta-analysis[23] showed no increased risk and suggested that previous reports showed publication bias. However, there is definitely an increased risk from AEDs. An important adverse factor is the number of these drugs taken concurrently with an odds ratio (OR) of 2.8 (1.1–9.7) for one drug, to 4.2 (1.1–5.1) for polytherapy.[24] Nakane et al.[25] and Samren[26] found that the risk of major fetal abnormality rises from about double the natural risk with one anti-epileptic drug to about six times the risk with four anti-epileptic drugs, but these patients would have less well controlled epilepsy and drug doses are likely to be relatively high.

The fetal AED syndrome.

This has been associated with several AEDs, particularly phenytoin (the fetal hydantoin syndrome) and valproate. The syndromes are not the same for each drug, though there are many similarities. Features of the fetal hydantoin syndrome[27] include microcephaly, hypertelorism, low-set ears, short neck, transverse palmar creases and minor skeletal abnormalities. This syndrome may be partly dose-dependent and partly due to a genetically determined predisposition, which may explain why this condition can occur with quite low doses in some children and does not occur with quite high doses in others. Characteristic features of the valproate syndrome[28] are said to be arched eyebrows, short nose, thin upper lip and broad nasal bridge. Other features include neural tube defects, cleft lip and palate, radial ray defects, congenital heart defects and genitourinary problems, again there is evidence of an hereditary susceptibility.[29] Major abnormalities asscociated with the barbiturates and hydantoins are congenital heart disease and cleft lip and palate; with valproate and carbamazepine are neural tube defects, hypospadias and congenital heart disease. Phenytoin was once thought to be particularly implicated. However, a meta-analysis of the original data in five prospective European studies between 1971 and 1990, with a total of 1379 children and complete data from 1221 has shown an incidence of major defects with phenytoin monotherapy which is comparable to other AEDs (RR 2.2, 0.7–6.7).[30] Preliminary data from current prospective epilepsy and pregnancy registers are showing similar data. It may be that the previously reported high risks were due to polytherapy and the lack of blood level control.

Data from the UK Epilepsy and Pregnancy Register on 3301 reports with 2637 outcomes has shown a major malformation rate (MMR) of 2.4% (0.9–6.0) in the 173 women with epilepsy who were not on medication; it was 3.4% (2.7–4.4) in the 1891 patients on monotherapy and 6.5% (5.0–9.4) in the 573 patients on polytherapy. The monotherapy MMR for carbamazepine (700) was 2.3% (1.4–3.7) and for lamotrigine (390) 2.1% (1.0–4.0). For valproate (572) it was 5.9% (4.3–8.2), so that the MMR for valproate is significantly higher than the other most commonly used AEDs.[31] All pregnancies in women with epilepsy in the United Kingdom should be reported to the UK Epilepsy and Pregnancy Register (*see* details on page 60) as soon as the pregnancy is confirmed, so that accurate data about the effects of AEDs can become available, and this is particularly important for the recently introduced drugs.

The use of valproate in women of childbearing age

The position of valproate in the treatment of these patients therefore needs special consideration. For women with certain types of epilepsy which respond best to valproate, particularly idiopathic generalised epilepsy with absence attacks, myoclonus and photosensitivity, and who have achieved good control with this drug, the risk of recurrence of fits in pregnancy may need to be balanced against the increased risk of fetal abnormality.

The dose effect

In a re-analysis of five prospective studies,[30] valproate was associated with spina bifida in 3.8% of at-risk pregnancies. An interesting feature of this series was that spina bifida did not occur with doses of less than 1000 mg a day (0/54), 6.7% were found with doses of 1–1.5 g a day (2/30) and this was not significantly different from controls, and 37.5% if the dose exceeded 1.5 g a day (3/8). A retrospective study of 2000 pregnancies showed a relative risk (RR) of 1.0 if the dose of valproate was less than 600 mg a day, an RR of 2.2 with doses between 600 and 1000, and a RR of 3.9 (1.4–11.1) if the dose exceeded 1000 mg a day.[26] Mawer *et al.*[32] and Kaneko *et al.*[33] also found that major defects only occurred with doses above 1000 mg. Omtzigt *et al.*[34] have reported that the average daily dose of valproate taken by the mothers of children with spina bifida was 1640 ± 136 mg compared to 941 ± 48 mg in those not affected; but all these studies involve too few patients to be sure that valproate, in doses even as low as 600 mg a day, is associated with a risk comparable to other AEDs.

Samren *et al.*[30] showed some correlation with the size of each dose of valproate to the incidence of neural tube defects. This correlates with the findings in mice[35] that fetal abnormalities are as much associated with peak blood levels as the total daily dose. It may be that the protein binding becomes saturated, allowing free valproate to reach the developing fetal neural tube.

Valproate exposure and developmental delay

There is some evidence that children exposed to valproate in utero show an increased incidence of developmental delay.[36,37] Gaily *et al.*[38] found no effect from in utero exposure to carbamazepine, but a significantly reduced verbal IQ (VIQ) in children exposed to polytherapy with valproate. An independent effect from valproate could not be determined because the results were confounded by low maternal education and polytherapy. Adab *et al.*[39] showed that children exposed to valproate monotherapy had significantly lower VIQ scores when compared to children exposed to carbamazepine and to phenytoin monotherapy, and there was some evidence of a dose effect. Low VIQ was also associated with the occurrence of five or more tonic-clonic seizures during pregnancy and with low maternal IQ. There were higher rates of dysmorphic features in the valproate-exposed children, and these were most common in those with low VIQ scores. Eriksson *et al.*[40] found significantly lower full scale IQ in both mothers taking valproate and in their offspring, compared to those taking carbamazepine and women with epilepsy not taking any medication. These studies all involved retrospective case ascertainment, though a few had prospective outcome measures. The numbers of children were small and the response rate low. A recent Cochrane review[41] concluded that the currently available data is insufficient to draw any definite conclusions, but the trends now emerging from the seven published studies are consistent. The confounding factors probably mean that these figures represent the worst outcome.

The use of valproate should therefore be avoided in women of childbearing age,[42] particularly in the obese, especially in obese adolescents, and in those women with menstrual irregularity. Consider withdrawal of valproate in women who develop obesity and or menstrual irregularity while on valproate.

Serious consideration should be given to changing medication if at all possible for women of childbearing age who are established on valproate, whether or not they are considering pregnancy, since about 50% of pregnancies in these women are unplanned.[43] If changing medication is not appropriate, the risk may be reduced by spreading the dose throughout the day and to changing to Epilim Chrono to avoid peak blood levels. The total daily dose should be below 1 g a day and certainly below 1.5 g a day, so a suitable regime might be Epilim Chrono 300 mg tds. It is not appropriate to reduce the dose and add lamotrigine. The Glaxo-Smith-Kline register[44] (Weil) of 360 patients on lamotrigine monotherapy showed a MMR of 2.8% (1.5–5.2), and 3.1% (1.1–7.4) for lamotrigine in any polytherapy excluding valproate (163), but 10.5% (5.0–20.2) for lamotrigine with valproate (76).

Conclusion

It is advisable for all women with epilepsy taking anti-epileptic drugs and contemplating pregnancy to be on a single drug and that drug should be given in the lowest possible dose. Of the old and well established drugs, carbamazepine has been thought to be the safest, and phenytoin monotherapy appears to be safer than was once thought. The risk of a major malformation is significantly greater with valproate than any of the other commonly used AEDs. Data is lacking about the risks of most of the newer AEDs, although animal experimental data and limited clinical reports suggest that they are no more teratogenic than the older

AEDs, and maybe safer. The UK pregnancy register shows no significant difference in risk of major abnormality for any of the commonly used AEDs, except for valproate; with this exception, parents can be reassured that there is a more than 90% chance that their infant will be entirely normal, and a 95% chance of not having a major malformation.

Folic acid

There is clear evidence that folic acid supplements reduce the risk of neural tube defects (NTDs) in the offspring of women at risk.[45,46] There is some evidence that folic acid supplements reduce the risk of NTDs in women taking EIAEDs.[47] Valproate and carbamazepine are known to be associated with an increased risk of NTDs, estimated at 1.5% and 0.5% respectively. Some anti-epileptic drugs are folate antagonists, but Tomson et al.[48] found no difference in red cell folate in pregnant women on AEDs, mostly phenytoin and carbamazepine, compared to non-epileptic drug free pregnant women or to non-pregnant age matched healthy women. Furthermore there was no correlation between red cell folate concentrations and doses or plasma levels of phenytoin or carbamazepine. Kirke et al.[49] reported a significant association between neural tube defects and early pregnancy red cell folate concentrations, with a risk of 0.8 per 1000 births for those mothers with a red cell folate greater than 400 mcg/l to 6.6 per 1000 for those with concentrations less than 150 mcg/l – an eight-fold difference – and these authors estimated that 400 mcg of folate a day would reduce the incidence of neural tube defects by 48%.

All women on anti-epileptic drugs contemplating pregnancy should be given a folic acid supplement. This should anticipate pregnancy, since neural tube and cardiac defects occur in the first 28 days after conception. Neural tube closure takes place on about day 26, which is often before the woman realises she is pregnant. A folate supplement started after 30 days will have no protective effect against neural tube defects.

The correct advice is therefore to tell patients to start folic acid when they stop contraception. It has been suggested that all women potentially at risk should be given a folate supplement, because less than 50% of pregnancies in these patients are planned;[42] this is the basis for the fortification of food. Folic acid 5 mg od, which has no effect on epilepsy control, is widely recommended,[50] although there is no evidence that this dose is needed or even that it is effective in women taking AEDs. 360 mcg and 400 mcg were used and shown to be effective in two trials;[51,52] 800 mcg in the Hungarian trial[46] and 4 mg in the MRC trial, chosen to avoid the possibility of a negative result from a lower dose;[45] but it is not known for certain whether less than 1 mg/day is sufficient for women on AEDs and it has seemed better to give 5 mg a day to be safe. Lucock[53] has pointed out that more than 4–500 mcg of pteroylmonoglutamate, the form of folate used in supplements, saturates the transformation during absorption to methylfolate, so that larger doses cannot be utilised, which suggests that there is no need to prescribe more than 1 mg a day. Even this dose will produce unmetabolised folic acid in the serum, the long-term effects of which are unknown.[54] However, Wald et al.[55] have constructed a model from published data linking the relationship between serum folate and folate supplementation to the prevalence of neural tube defects according to maternal serum folate levels. This model predicts increasing protection from neural tube defects up to 5 mg/day, which remains the currently recommended dose.[56]

There is some animal experimental evidence[57] and a few case reports which suggest that folic acid may not protect against valproate-induced neural tube defects,[58] which implies that valproate may act partly by a non-folate dependent mechanism.

Investigations during pregnancy

Q: 'Will I need any special tests?'

Anti-epileptic drug blood concentrations should be measured as soon as it is known that a woman is pregnant to establish a baseline; repeated as indicated for those drugs where blood levels are a useful guide to efficacy. Free drug levels, if available, provide more useful information.

All pregnant women on anti-epileptic drugs, particularly valproate and carbamazepine, should have a series of high definition ultrasound scans. Anencephaly can be detected at 11 weeks, neural tube defects at about 16 to 18 weeks, congenital cardiac malformations at 18–20 weeks, and cleft lip and palate at about 20 weeks. Hypospadias and posterior cleft palates are not reliably detectable by ultrasound scanning. An elevated maternal alpha fetoprotein level measured at 18 weeks may indicate a neural tube defect. Women should be advised about these procedures in advance of pregnancy.[59]

Hyperemesis

Q: 'What do I do about my drugs if I have morning sickness?'

'Morning sickness' occurs more commonly in the morning, but it may occur at any time throughout the day. Some AEDs (phenytoin, phenobarbitone) need only be taken once a day and can therefore be taken at night. Most drugs need to be taken twice a day, but the morning dose can be postponed by a few hours to avoid periods of sickness. If nausea and vomiting are severe, an anti-emetic can be taken half an hour before the AED.

The effect of fits on the fetus

Q: 'If I have a fit, will it harm my baby?'

Minor fits have no known effect on the fetus, but major convulsive seizures associated with cyanosis can produce anoxia in the infant. There is some evidence that seizures in early pregnancy are associated with an increase in major malformations.[60] In late pregnancy, if a fit results in a fall, injury to the fetus may occur and could precipitate early labour or miscarriage.

It is very important to maintain AED administration in pregnancy because both fits and drugs can affect outcome. Furthermore, sudden cessation may precipitate status epilepticus, with serious consequences for both mother and child.

The effect of pregnancy on fits

Q: 'Will my fits get worse during pregnancy?'

Pregnancy does not usually have much effect on the control of epilepsy; a survey in 1994[61] showed that about a fifth of patients have increased fits, more than a half remain unaffected and about a quarter have fewer fits, and this does not change significantly during the three trimesters. Fits are more likely to increase in women with poorly controlled epilepsy and women with increased seizures in pregnancy are often found to have subtherapeutic blood levels.[62] Poor compliance may be a factor, requiring discussion and advice. Otherwise it may be necessary to increase the dose during pregnancy, monitoring the AED blood concentration; though it is not usually necessary to do so in well controlled patients.

Although anti-epileptic drug levels tend to fall during pregnancy, this may be partially offset by a rise in the proportion of the free drug due to alterations in protein binding. This is particularly so for those drugs that are highly protein bound, such as phenytoin, valproate and carbamazepine. Pregnancy has a greater effect on anti-epileptic drugs that are metabolised in the liver compared to those that are mostly cleared by renal excretion.

If the dose is altered during pregnancy it is likely to need adjustment after delivery. Lamotrigine poses a particular problem in this respect with a marked increase in clearance rate during pregnancy. Tran *et al.*[63] found this to be >65% between preconception and delivery, so that 11 of 12 women required an increase in dose. Pennell *et al.*,[64] in nine women, found a mean change from baseline in apparent clearance of $92 \pm 110\%$ in the first trimester, $121 \pm 138\%$ in the second and $315 \pm 214\%$ in the third trimester, overall 164%, but with very wide individual variation. Since this effect starts early in pregnancy, the dose

Table 5.1 Amount of protein binding and route of excretion of anti-epileptic drugs

	% protein binding	*Clearance*
tiagabine	96	liver
phenytoin	90	liver
valproate	90	liver
clonazepam	86	liver
carbamazepine	75	liver
lamotrigine	55	liver
phenobarbitone	45	liver/renal
oxcarbazepine	40	liver
topiramate	15	liver
levetiracetam	10	renal
gabapentin	0	renal
vigabatrin	0	renal
pregabalin	0	renal

escalation needs to be started after the first month,[64,65] and may need to be more than doubled by the third trimester.[65] After delivery, Berry[66] found rises of 200–300% within a few weeks. Ohman *et al.*[67] found a median increase of 170% (0–630), so it is important to reduce the dose in the post-partum period.

Patients with poorly controlled epilepsy should be warned that an increase in dosage may be necessary during pregnancy; those with good control can be advised that any change in their medication is unlikely to be necessary, except for women taking lamotrigine.

Management of a first fit in pregnancy

Excluding eclampsia, it is unusual for a first fit to occur during pregnancy without obvious cause. These patients should be investigated because there is a higher incidence of underlying structural lesions; for example, meningiomas and arteriovenous malformations may present in pregnancy because of swelling of the lesion. Other causes include thrombosis, both arterial and venous, and subarachnoid haemorrhage. Patients with toxaemia may present with epilepsy and if this is the cause of fits around the time of delivery, including the immediate postpartum period, epilepsy is unlikely to be an ongoing problem.

Pseudoseizures

It has been estimated that between 10 and 45% of apparently intractable epilepsy is due to pseudoseizures[68] and the majority of these patients are young women. Perhaps 20% of patients with proven pseudoseizures also have epilepsy.[69] These patients can be very difficult to identify and often go misdiagnosed for many years. The clinical features include prolonged fits while awake, pelvic thrusting, eye closure with resistance, lack of postictal confusion or drowsiness and normal investigations. The diagnosis is made by recording a normal EEG during a seizure, which may require telemetry, and the finding of a normal prolactin level after a fit. These patients are notoriously difficult to treat and should be referred to a specialist centre.

Epilepsy during delivery

Q: 'Will there be any problems at birth?'

This question has been identified as a major and often unexpressed concern.

Effect on the mother

There is no increased risk of purely obstetric problems in women with epilepsy,[70] but all pregnant women with epilepsy on anti-epileptic drugs should have their babies delivered in hospital. The increased risk of epilepsy at delivery and in the next 24 hours, said to be about 3% of women at risk,[1] is usually due to failure to take anti-epileptic drugs, lack of sleep or impaired drug absorption. Patients with generalised epilepsy are more likely to have seizures during delivery than patients with partial epilepsy,[71] particularly if the AED levels are barely or sub-therapeutic.[62] The risk of status epilepticus is very small, but carries a high mortality risk for both mother and infant. In 29 such patients identified in the literature,[72] there was a 50% fetal mortality (14/29) and nine maternal deaths. Clobazam may be used prophylactically in women thought to be at particular risk.

Effect on the infant

Some anti-epileptic drugs, particularly primidone, phenobarbitone and the benzodiazepines, are sedating and some infants show withdrawal symptoms from these drugs in the first few days of life. Withdrawal fits are rare, but are said to be most common with phenobarbitone.

Vitamin K

The EIAEDs cause a reduction in vitamin K dependent clotting factors by an effect on the synthesis of Factors 2, 7, 9, 10 and protein C and S. Although giving vitamin K to women in the last few weeks of pregnancy does raise the fetal plasma vitamin K1 concentration appreciably, it remains an order of magnitude lower than maternal levels because of poor placental passage and low concentrations of transport lipoproteins in fetal plasma; so that fetal plasma vitamin K levels are very low in newborn babies.[73] The vitamin K level rises to near normal in about a week in breastfed babies and reaches eight times the normal value in babies fed with vitamin K fortified formula milk.

The risk of bleeding can be divided into three groups:[74]

1 thc early onset bleeds, which occur in the first 24 hours and are nearly always due to medication, including anti-epileptic drugs
2 the classical neonatal bleeding, which occurs in the first week and
3 the late incidence of bleeding between one week and three months, with a peak at two to six weeks.

Intra-cerebral haemorrhage is rare in the first week after the first 24 hours, but occurs in 50% of patients with late bleeding.[75] Intramuscular vitamin K given at birth seems to be almost completely effective in preventing bleeding.[76] Further vitamin K should be given to babies who are exclusively breastfed for more than one month.

Giving intramuscular (IM) vitamin K1 at birth was a standard practice until the report in 1992 of an increase in childhood cancers in babies given IM vitamin K, but not in babies given oral vitamin K or no vitamin K.[77] There is now an extensive literature on this topic; it seems clear that there is no increased risk of solid tumours, but a small increased risk of acute lymphoblastic leukaemia (ALL) cannot be absolutely excluded on the available data.[78–81] Folate supplements may reduce the risk of ALL.[82]

The theoretical risk of bleeding in children born of mothers taking EIAEDs is sufficient for all pregnant women on these medications to take oral phytomenadione (vitamin K1) 20 mg daily for at least one month before delivery to reduce the risk of bleeding in the first 24 hours, and vitamin K1 0.5 mg should be given IM immediately after delivery. Although Kaaja et al.[83] found no increase in the incidence of bleeding in 662 infants of mothers on EIAEDs, compared to 1324 controls, the numbers may have been insufficient to show an effect.

Breastfeeding

Q: 'Will I be able to breastfeed?'

All the anti-epileptic drugs are excreted in breast milk, but for most AEDs only in low concentrations, so there is no reason why mothers on AEDs should not breastfeed, though with caution for phenobarbitone and primidone. The amount of drug received by the infant is very considerably less than the fetus receives during pregnancy. For example, calculations of the largest amount of drug likely to be received daily by a fully breastfed baby, expressed as a percentage of the lowest recommended daily therapeutic dose for an infant, give the following figures: carbamazepine <5%, phenytoin <5%, valproate <3% and phenobarbitone >50%; so that phenobarbitone and primidone may cause drowsiness. Fetal hepatic immaturity results in a considerable increase in the blood half-life of phenobarbitone. In adults the half-life is around 100 hours (75–125), but in the newborn baby it may be more than 200 hours.[84]

There is little or no information about the newer drugs, except lamotrigine, which is excreted in high levels in breast milk (40–80% of maternal levels),[66] and when combined with slow fetal clearance due to hepatic immaturity, infant blood levels may reach 60% (range 47–77) of the maternal blood level,[66] a problem which is compounded if lamotrigine is given with valproate. Topiramate and levetiracetam also reach high levels in breast milk, but this does not seem to produce significant levels in breastfed babies.[85,86]

Breastfeeding should be encouraged in women with epilepsy on all anti-epileptic drugs. New drugs should not be introduced in the postpartum period to women who are breastfeeding or only with great caution; this particularly applies to phenobarbitone, primidone and lamotrigine . If anti-epileptic medication seems to be causing drowsiness in the infant, it may still be possible to breastfeed, alternating with bottle feeding.

Post-partum maternal epilepsy

Q: 'What happens if I have a fit when I am by myself with the baby at home?'

Mothers with uncontrolled major epilepsy should not be left alone with small children. Maternal epilepsy probably presents a greater risk to infants and toddlers than to the fetus. The child could be injured if held by the mother at the start of a fit or if left unattended during the mother's fit. Mothers should be warned of this risk and seek advice about appropriate precautions, for example changing nappies on the floor and only bathing infants when somebody else is present. Mothers with juvenile myoclonic epilepsy may be at particular risk when woken early by their infant.[87]

If the dose of AED was increased during pregnancy, it is likely to need adjustment in the post-partum period; this applies particularly to lamotrigine.[62–64,66,67]

Hereditary risks

Q: 'Will my baby have epilepsy?'

A child inherits its epileptic liability from both parents. The risk depends on the type of epilepsy. There is no significant risk if the mother has partial epilepsy from an acquired lesion. The overall risk of a child of a parent with idiopathic generalised epilepsy having epilepsy before the age of 20, excluding febrile convulsions, is about 4%, compared to 0.5% in the general population. If there is already one sibling who developed epilepsy before the age of 10, the risk rises to approximately 6%, if one parent and a sibling are affected the risk is about 10% and if both parents or one parent and a first degree relative of the other parent have epilepsy, the risk is about 15%.[88] These figures exclude the genetically determined epilepsy syndromes, such as juvenile myoclonic epilepsy and those inherited conditions which may be associated with epilepsy, such as tuberose sclerosis and neurofibromatosis.[89]

If there is a family history of a known inherited epilepsy syndrome or of a condition which has a strong association with epilepsy, the risk is that of the syndrome. Patients should be referred for specialist genetic advice.

Counselling

Women with epilepsy who are contemplating pregnancy should have the diagnosis re-evaluated and if necessary re-investigated. It has been estimated that about 5–10% of these patients do not have epilepsy[87,90] and 7% are found to have a structural lesion.[87] Many are taking unsuitable medication often at inappropriate doses. Reconsideration of the diagnosis may allow withdrawal of anti-epileptic medication. In some circumstances an endocrinology screen may be appropriate.

It is very important that all patients with epilepsy are fully informed about these issues, but not necessarily all at the same time and at the same age. It would be appropriate for paediatricians as well as neurologists and general practitioners, who often look after patients with epilepsy up to the age of 15 or 16, to mention some of these issues and in particular contraception and folic acid. Teratogenicity, ultrasound scanning, and breastfeeding should be discussed with women who are contemplating pregnancy and they should be given the opportunity to discuss any other matters they wish to raise. Women can be reassured that there is a more than 90% chance of having a normal baby. Poor communication is a common problem; many patients may not understand the concept of percent risk. It may help to explain that 5% risk or a 1/20 chance of an abnormal event is a 95% chance of normality. Positively framed information alters the perception of teratogenic risk in pregnant women.[91]

Catamenial epilepsy

Many women report that their attacks occur in relation to their menstrual periods, but there is a problem with definition.[92] If it is to influence management, it is necessary to take a very narrow view and restrict the term to the time from a day before the onset of a period to the first two days of a period. The cycle must also be very regular, so that the next period can be forecasted accurately; otherwise there are no treatment implications. The precise reason for catamenial epilepsy is unknown, but may be related to the fact that oestrogen is softly epileptogenic, whereas progesterone is weakly anti-epileptogenic.[93] The rapid reduction in serum progesterone levels just before a period may make women more susceptible to epilepsy at that time. Changes in fluid balance may also play a part, but giving diuretics starting a week before a period is due is not effective.

It is sometimes appropriate to treat catamenial epilepsy with intermittent treatment in addition to regular medication. However, the patient must show documented diary evidence that the attacks are confined to a few days around the onset of a period and that the periods occur at very regular intervals, so that day one of the next period can be accurately predicted. It may then be reasonable to give an additional anti-epileptic drug starting a few days before a period is due. For practical purposes this needs to be a quick-acting drug which can be given at full dose in addition to the ongoing medication; clobazam[94] is most widely used, clonazepam or acetazolamide are alternatives.

Intermittent treatment without any background anti-epileptic medication is not usually effective, because the fits are often displaced until after the intermittent treatment stops. Hormonal manipulation is usually ineffective and gynaecological procedures are contraindicated.

The menopause and bone density

The menopause tends to occur earlier in women with epilepsy and there is a negative correlation between the age at the menopause and estimated lifetime seizures. For women with a high seizure frequency this is about three to four years.[95] There is often an increase in seizure frequency at the menopause and about a one third reduction in postmenopausal women, particularly in women who had catamenial epilepsy.[96] Hormone replacement therapy may be used if clinically indicated; there is some clinical evidence to support the theoretical risk of an increase in fits due to oestrogen.[2]

AED use is an independent predictor of increased risk of fractures.[97] This increased risk comes from the effect of EIAEDs on vitamin D, added to the natural risk of osteoporosis due to age and postmenopausal status, as well as the increased risk not only from seizures, but also from unsteadiness due to some AEDs.[98] These women should have a bone health screen and be advised accordingly.[99]

Acknowledgements

We are very grateful to Professor Simon Shorvon and Professor John Guillebaud for their helpful suggestions.

References

1 Crawford P, Appleton R, Betts T, *et al.* Best practice guidelines for the management of women with epilepsy. *Seizure* 1999; **8**: 201–17.

2 Crawford P, Lee P. Gender difference in management of epilepsy – what women are hearing. *Seizure* 1999; **8**: 135–9.

3 Patsalos PN, Froscher W, Pisani F, *et al.* The importance of drug interactions in epilepsy therapy. *Epilepsia* 2002; **43**: 365–85.

4 Garnett WR. Clinical pharmacology of topiramate: a review. *Epilepsia* 2000; **41**(suppl 1): 61–5.

5 Guillebaud J. *Contraception: your questions answered.* 4th edn. Churchill Livingstone. 2004. a: p122, b: p128–9, c: p195, d: p130, e: p294, f: p349, g: p472.

6 Morrell MJ. The new antiepileptic drugs and women: Efficacy, reproductive health, pregnancy and fetal outcome. *Epilepsia* 1996; **37**(suppl 6): 34–44.

7 Sabers A, Buchholt JM, Uldall P, *et al.* Lamotrigine plasma levels reduced by oral contraceptives. *Epilepsy Res* 2001; **47**: 151–4.

8 Sabers A, Ohman I, Tomson T. Lamotrigine plasma levels reduced by oral contraceptives. *Epilepsia* 2002; **43**: 47.

9 Pfizer Ltd. Depo-Provera, summary of product characteristics. 2004.

10 Gupta C, Osterman J, Santen R, *et al.* In vivo metabolism of progestins. *J Clin Endocrinol Metab* 1979; **48**: 816–20.

11 Bounds W, Guillebaud J. Observational series on women using contraceptive Mirena concurrently with anti-epileptic and other enzyme-inducing drugs. *J Fam Plann Reprod Health Care.* 2002; **28**: 78–80.

12 Wallace H, Shorvon S, Tallis R. Age specific incidence and prevalence of treated epilepsy in an unselected population of 2 052 922 and age specific fertility rates of women with epilepsy. *Lancet* 1998; **352**: 1970–3.

13 Herzog AG, Coleman AE, Jacobs AR, *et al.* Relationship of sexual dysfunction to epilepsy laterality and reproductive hormone levels in women. *Epilepsy Behav* 2003; **4**: 407–13.

14 Cummings LN, Guidice L, Morrell MJ. Ovulatory function in epilepsy. *Epilepsia* 1995; **36**: 355–9.

15 Bauer J, Burr W, Elger CE. Seizure occurrence during ovulatory and anovulatory cycles in patients with temporal lobe epilepsy. *Eur J Neurol* 1998; **5**: 83–8.

16 Morrell MJ, Guidice L, Flynn KL, *et al.* Predictors of ovulatory failure in women with epilepsy. *Ann Neurol* 2002; **52**: 704–11.

17 Isojarvi JI, Laatikainen TJ, Knip M, *et al.* Polycystic ovaries and hyperandrogenism in women taking valproate for epilepsy. *N Engl J Med* 1993; **329**: 1383–8.

18 Isojarvi JI, Rattya J, Myllyla VV, *et al.* Valproate, lamotrigine and insulin mediated risks in women with epilepsy. *Ann Neurol* 1998; **43**: 446–51.

19 Genton P, Bauer J, Duncan S, *et al.* On the association between valproate and polycystic ovary syndrome. *Epilepsia* 2001; **42**: 295–304.

20 Meo R, Bilo L. Polycystic ovary syndrome and epilepsy: a review of the evidence. *Drugs* 2003; **63**: 1185–227.

21 Isojarvi JI. Reproductive dysfunction in women with epilepsy. *Neurology* 2003; **61**(suppl 2):S27–34.

22 Bauer J, Isojarvi JIT, Herzog AG, *et al.* Reproductive dysfunction in women with epilepsy: recommendations for evaluation and management. *J Neurol Neurosurg Psychiat* 2003; **73**: 121–5.

23 Fried S, Kozer E, Nulman I, *et al.* Malformation rates in children of women with untreated epilepsy: a meta analysis. *Drug Saf* 2004; **27**: 197–202.

24 Holmes LB, Harvey EA, Coull BA, *et al.* The teratogenicity of anticonvulsant drugs. *N Engl J Med* 2001; **344**: 1132–8.

25 Nakane Y, Okuma T, Takahashi R, *et al.* Multi-institutional study on the teratogenicity and fetal toxicity of anti-epileptic drugs. *Epilepsia* 1980; **21**: 663–80.

26 Samren EB, van Duijin CM, Christaens GC, *et al.* Anti-epileptic drug regimes and major congenital abnormalities in the offspring. *Ann Neurol.* 1999; **46**: 739–46.

27 Hanson JW, Smith DW. The fetal hydantoin syndrome. *J Paediatr* 1975; **87**: 285–90.

28 DiLiberti JH, Farndon PA, Dennis NR, *et al.* The fetal valproate syndrome. *Am J Med Genet* 1984; **19**: 473–81.

29 Malm H, Kajante E, Kivirikko S, *et al.* Valproate embryopathy in three sets of siblings: further proof of hereditary susceptibility. *Neurology* 2002; **59**: 630–3.

30 Samren EB, van Duijn CM, Hiilesmaa VK, *et al.* Maternal use of antiepileptic drugs and the risk of major congenital malformations. *Epilepsia* 1997; **38**: 981–90.

31 Morrow JI, Russell AJC, Irwin B, *et al.* The safety of antiepileptic drugs in pregnancy: results of the UK epilepsy and pregnancy register [abstract]. *Epilepsia* 2004; **45**(suppl 3): 57.

32 Mawer G, Clayton-Smith J, Coyle H, *et al.* Outcome of pregnancy in women attending an outpatient epilepsy clinic: adverse features associated with higher doses of sodium valproate. *Seizure* 2002; **11**: 1059–1311.

33 Kaneko S, Batino D, Andermann E, *et al.* Congenital malformations due to antiepileptic drugs. *Epilepsy Res* 1999; **33**: 145–58.

34 Omtzigt JG, Las FJ, Grobbee DE, *et al.* The risk of spina bifida aperta after first trimester exposure to valproate in a prenatal cohort. *Neurology* 1992; **42**(suppl 2): S35–42.

35 Nau H, Zierer R, Spielmann H, *et al.* A new model for embryotoxicity testing: teratogenicity and pharmacokinetics of valproic acid following constant rate administration in the mouse using human drug and metabolite concentrations. *J Life Sci* 1981; **29**: 2803–13.

36 Adab N, Jacoby A, Smith D, *et al.* Additional educational needs in children born to mothers with epilepsy. *J Neurol Neurosurg Psychiat* 2001; **70**: 15–21.

37 Ohtsuka Y, Silver K, Lopes-Cendes I, *et al.* Effect of antiepileptic drugs on psychomotor development in offspring of epileptic mothers [abstract]. *Epilepsia* 1999; **40**(suppl 2): 296.

38 Gaily E, Kantola SE, Hiilesmaa V, *et al.* Normal intelligence in children with prenatal exposure to carbamazepine. *Neurology* 2004; **62**: 28–32.

39 Adab N, Kini U, Vinten J, *et al.* The longer term outcome of children born to mothers with epilepsy. *J Neurol Neurosurg Psychiat* 2004; **75**: 1575–83.

40 Eriksson K, Viinikainen K, Monkkonen A, *et al.* The effects of antiepileptic drug exposure in utero to neurological and cognitive functioning of children of school age [abstract]. *Epilepsia* 2004; **45**(suppl 3): 57.

41 Adab N, Tudur-Smith C, Vinten J, *et al.* Cochrane Database Systematic Review. 2004.

42 Committee on the Safety of Medicines. Sodium valproate and prescribing in pregnancy. Current problems in Pharmacovigilance 2003; **29**: 6.

43 Fairgrieve SD, Jackson M, Jonas P, *et al.* Population based, prospective study of the care of women with epilepsy in pregnancy. *Brit Med J* 2000; **321**: 674–5.

44 Weil JG, Cunningham MC, Williamson RR, *et al.* Eleven year interim results of an international study of pregnancy outcomes following exposure to lamotrigine [abstract]. *Epilepsia* 2004; **45**(suppl 3): 57.

45 MRC Vitamin Study Research Group. Prevention of neural tube defects; results of the Medical Research Council Vitamin Study. *Lancet* 1991; **338**: 132–7.

46 Czeizel AE, Dudas I. Prevention of the first occurrence of neural tube defects by periconceptual multivitamin supplementation. *N Engl J Med* 1992; **327**: 1832–5.

47 Biale Y, Lewenthal M. Effect of folic acid supplementation on congenital malformations due to anticonvulsant drugs. *Eur J Obstet Gynecol Reprod Biol* 1984; **18**: 211–16.

48 Tomson T, Lindbom U, Berg A. Red cell folate levels in pregnant epileptic women. *Eur J Clin Pharmacol* 1995; **48**: 305–8.

49 Kirke PN, Molloy AM, Daly LE, *et al.* Maternal plasma folate and vitamin B12 are independent risk factors for neural tube defects. *Q J Med* 1993; **86**: 703–8.

50 Genetics Committee, Executive and Council of the Society of Obstetricians and Gynaecologists of Canada. The use of folic acid for the prevention of neural tube defects and other congenital anomalies. *J Obstet Gynaecol Can* 2003; **25**: 959–73.

51 Berry RJ, Li Z, Erickson JD, *et al.* Prevention of neural tube defects with folic acid in China. *N Engl J Med* 1999; **341**: 1485–90.

52 Smithells RW, Seller MJ, Harris R. Further experience of vitamin supplementation for prevention of neural tube defect recurrences. *Lancet* 1983; **1**: 1027–31.

53 Lucock M. Is folic acid the ultimate functional food component for disease prevention? *Brit Med J* 2004; **328**: 211–14.

54 Kelly P, McPartlin J, Goggins M, *et al*. Unmetabolised folic acid in serum. *Am J Clin Nutr* 1997; **65**: 1790–5.

55 Wald NJ, Law MR, Morris JK, Wald DS. Quantifying the effect of folic acid. *Lancet* 2001; **358**: 2069–73.

56 British National Formulary. 2004; **48**: 457.

57 Hansen DK, Grafton TF. Lack of attenuation of valproate induced effects by folinic acid in rat embryos in vitro. *Teratology* 1995; **52**: 277–85.

58 Yerby MS. Management issues for women with epilepsy: neural tube defects and folic acid supplementation. *Neurology* 2003; **61**(suppl 2): S23–6.

59 McFayden A, Gledhill J, Whitlow B, *et al*. First trimester ultrasound screening. *Brit Med J* 1998; **317**: 694–5.

60 Samren EB. Maternal epilepsy and major congenital abnormalities. In: *Maternal epilepsy and pregnancy outcome*. MD thesis, Erasmus University, Rotterdam 1998: 77–9.

61 Vidovic MI, Della-Marina BM. Trimestral changes of seizure frequency in pregnant epileptic women. *Acta Medica Croatica*. 1994; **48**: 85–7.

62 Pennell PB. Antiepileptic drug pharmacokinetics during pregnancy and lactation. *Neurology* 2003; **61**(suppl 2): S35–42.

63 Tran TA, Leppik IE, Blesi K, *et al*. Lamotrigine clearance during pregnancy. *Neurology* 2002; **59**: 251–5.

64 Pennell PB, Montgomery JQ, Clements SD, *et al*. Lamotrigine clearance markedly increases during pregnancy [abstract]. *Epilepsia* 2002; **43**(suppl 7): 234–5.

65 Betts T, Greenhill L. Use of lamotrigine monotherapy in women who are pregnant: is dose escalation needed during pregnancy? Poster at the ILEA meeting Liverpool, April, 2001.

66 Berry DJ. The distribution of lamotrigine throughout pregnancy [abstract]. *Ther Drug Monit* 1999; **21**: 450.

67 Ohman I, Vitols S, Tomson T. Lamotrigine in pregnancy: pharmacokinetics during delivery, in the neonate and during lactation. *Epilepsia* 2000; **41**: 709–13.

68 Devinsky O. Patients with refractory seizures. *N Engl J Med* 1999; **340**: 1565–7.

69 Ramsey RE, Cohen A, Brown MC. Coexisting epilepsy and non-epileptic seizures. In: Rowan AJ, Gates JR, eds. *Non-epileptic seizures*. Boston: Butterworth-Heinemann, 1993; pp 47–54.

70 Richmond JR, Krishnamoorthy P, Andermann E, *et al*. Epilepsy and pregnancy: an obstetric perspective. *Am J Obstet Gynecol* 2004; **190**: 371–9.

71 Katz JM, Devinsky O. Primary generalised epilepsy; a risk factor for seizures in labour and delivery. *Seizure* 2003; **12**: 217–19.

72 Terramo K, Hiilesmaa V. Pregnancy and fetal complications in epileptic pregnancies. In: Janz D, Bossi L, Dam M, *et al*., eds. *Epilepsy, pregnancy and the child*. New York: Raven Press, 1982; pp 53–9.

73 Manderbrot L, Guillaumont M, LeClercq M. Placental transfer of vitamin K_1 and its implications in fetal haemostasis. *Thromb Haemost* 1988; **60**: 39–43.

74 Shearer MJ, Vitamin K. *Lancet* 1995; **345**: 229–34.

75 Rennie JM, Kelsall AWL. Vitamin K prophylaxis in the newborn. *Arch Dis Child* 1994; **70**: 248–51.

76 Tin W, Wariyar U, Hey E. Preventing late bleeding in infants with vitamin K deficiency. *Brit Med J* 1998; **316**: 230.

77 Golding J, Greenwood R, Birmingham K, *et al*. Childhood cancer, intramuscular vitamin K and pethidine given during labour. *Brit Med J* 1992; **305**: 341–6.

78 McKinney PA, Juszczak E, Findlay E, *et al*. Case control study of childhood leukaemia and cancer in Scotland: findings for neonatal intramuscular vitamin K. *Brit Med J* 1998; **316**: 173–7.

79 Passmore SJ, Draper G, Brownbill P, *et al.* Case control studies of relation between childhood cancer and neonatal vitamin K administration. *Brit Med J* 1998; **316**: 178–84.

80 Passmore SJ, Draper G, Brownbill P, *et al.* Ecological studies of relation between hospital policies on neonatal vitamin K administration and subsequent occurrence of childhood cancer. *Brit Med J* 1998; **316**: 184–9.

81 Parker L, Cole M, Craft AW, *et al.* Neonatal vitamin K administration and childhood cancer in the north of England. *Brit Med J* 1998; **316**: 184–9.

82 Thompson JR, FitzGerald P, Willoughby LN, *et al.* Maternal folate supplementation in pregnancy and protection against acute lymphoblastic leukaemia in childhood: a case control study. *Lancet* 2001; **358**: 1935–7.

83 Kaaja E, Kaaja R, Matila R, *et al.* Enzyme inducing antiepileptic drugs in pregnancy and the risk of bleeding in the neonate. *Neurology* 2002; **58**: 549–53.

84 Anderson GD. Phenobarbital and other barbiturates. In: Levy RH, Mattson RH, Meldrum BS, *et al.*, eds. *Antiepileptic Drugs.* 5th edn. Philadelphia: Lippincott Williams & Wilkins 2002: 500.

85 Ohman I, Vitolos S, Luef G, *et al.* Topiramate kinetics during delivery, lactation and in the neonate. *Epilepsia* 2002; **43**: 1157–60.

86 Johannessen SI, Helde G, Brodtkorb E. Levetiracetam in pregnancy and lactation [abstract]. *Epilepsia* 2004; **45**(suppl 3): 58.

87 Betts T, Fox C. Proactive preconceptual counselling for women with epilepsy. *Seizure* 1999; **8**: 322–7.

88 Harper PS. *Practical Genetic Counselling.* 6th edn. London: Arnold, 2004: 185.

89 Nashef L. The definitions, aetiologies and diagnosis of epilepsy. In: Shorvon S, Dreifus F, Fish D, *et al.*, eds. *The Treatment of Epilepsy.* London: Blackwell, 1996: 81.

90 Appleton RE, Chadwick D, Sweeney A. Managing the teenager with epilepsy: paediatric to adult care. *Seizure* 1997; **6**: 27–30.

91 Jasper JD, Goel R, Einarson A, *et al.* Effects of framing on teratogenic risk perception in pregnant women. *Lancet* 2001; **358**: 1237–8.

92 Foldary-Schaefer N, Falcone T. Catamenial Epilepsy. *Neurology* 2003; **61**(suppl 2):S2-S15.

93 Klein P, Herzog AG. Hormonal effects on epilepsy in women. *Epilepsia* 1998; **39**(suppl 8): 9–16.

94 Feely M, Gibson J. Intermittent clobazam for catamenial epilepsy. *J Neurol Neurogurg Psychiat* 1984; **47**: 1279–82.

95 Harden CL, Koppel BS, Herzog AG, *et al.* Seizure frequency is associated with age at menopause in women with epilepsy. *Neurology* 2003; **61**: 451–5.

96 Harden CL, Pulver MC, Jacobs AR. The effect of menopause and perimenopause on the course of epilepsy. *Epilepsia* 1999; **40**: 1402–7.

97 Persson HB, Alberts KA, Farahmand BY, *et al.* Risk of extremity fractures in adult outpatients with epilepsy. *Epilepsia* 2002; **43**: 768–72.

98 Harden CL. The menopause and bone density issues for women with epilepsy. *Neurology* 2003; **61**(suppl 2):S16–22.

99 Drezner MK. Treatment of anticonvulsant drug-induced bone disease. *Epilepsy Behav* 2004; **5**(suppl 2): S41–7.

The UK Epilepsy and Pregnancy Register

Department of Neurology (Ward 21), Royal Victoria Hospital, Belfast BT12 6BA
Tel: 0800 389 1248
Fax: 0289 0235 258
Web: www.epilepsyandpregnancy.co.uk

Chapter Six

Approach to the patient with epilepsy in the outpatient department

S Hadjikoutis and PEM Smith

Epilepsy is a common and serious condition (prevalence 750 per 100 000) with adverse social consequences for employment, education and driving, morbidity from seizures and medication, and increased mortality. The diagnosis requires a detailed history including witness account; this is resource-intensive and requires lengthy specialist consultations. Clinicians must distinguish seizures from the two other common causes of blackouts: syncope and psychogenic attacks. Investigations such as electroencephalogram and MR brain scanning help to identify the causes and classification of epilepsy, but alone rarely provide the diagnosis. Treatment with antiepileptic medication is long-term and potentially hazardous; patients should make the decision to start treatment only following informed discussion with an epilepsy specialist. All patients require reliable written information about their condition. In particular they must know the driving regulations, and the impact of seizures on employment, education and leisure pursuits. Women must understand the potential teratogenic effects of their medication. Certain patient groups with special needs benefit from targeted epilepsy services, e.g. learning disabled, children, teenagers and the elderly. People with epilepsy require long-term specialist follow-up. Although currently provided in mainly in secondary care (including nurse-led clinics), improved liaison with primary care should enable improved access to epilepsy services for all patients. Epilepsy clinic teams aim to provide multidisciplinary and long-term care, working closely with primary care and empowering patients towards improved management of their own condition.

Introduction

Epileptology has changed from a 'Cinderella' speciality to arguably the most exciting area of neurology. We now have a range of effective anti-epileptic medications, high quality imaging identifying a structural basis for the majority of adult-onset epilepsy, and an increasing public awareness of epilepsy and its problems. What is still lacking is the number of specialists needed to deliver an essentially clinical and supportive service for a long-term disorder affecting almost 1% of the population. Guidance from the National Institute for Clinical

Excellence (NICE) on the diagnosis and management of the epilepsies[1] offers national standards for epilepsy care and will help to highlight and correct current deficiencies in provision of epilepsy care.

Epilepsy clinics

Epilepsy is the commonest serious neurological condition after stroke (prevalence 750 per 100 000); the workload of its management is potentially huge. However, most patients become seizure-free on medication and can live normal lives, but 30% have continued seizures and/or significant medication side effects; these require regular epilepsy clinic review. Epilepsy incidence is 50 per 100 000 people per year. However, for each person diagnosed with epilepsy, 4–5 people with blackouts must be assessed; thus 250 per 100 000 people require specialist assessment.

Three patient groups attend epilepsy clinics:

- patients for review, usually but not always with epilepsy
- new patients with undiagnosed blackouts (seizure, syncope or psychogenic), who need urgent (within two weeks) specialist assessment
- new patients with an epilepsy diagnosis (not necessarily correct) with particular issues, who need detailed re-appraisal.

History

Diagnosing episodic altered consciousness requires a general medical perspective, an understanding of the differential diagnosis, and knowledge of seizure and epilepsy classification. A suitably experienced clinician must take a detailed history, including a witness account. There is no short-cut, making blackout diagnosis a time-consuming activity. Investigations such as electroencephalogram (EEG) and magnetic resonance (MR) brain scanning can support the clinical diagnosis, but generally the history is crucial. Where there is doubt (this is common), retaking the history is more helpful than repeating tests.

Key components

The history should focus on precipitants (situation and trigger), warning (prodrome), the episode and the symptoms that follow (recovery).

Table 6.1 lists characteristics helpful in distinguishing the common causes of blackouts: syncope, seizures and psychogenic episodes; other possibilities include migraine, transient ischaemic attacks and movement disorders.[2] The clinician must next decide whether the seizure was provoked or unprovoked, the first (single) seizure or part of a recurrent tendency (epilepsy) and its classification (focal or generalised, idiopathic or symptomatic).

Provoked or unprovoked?

Provoked (acute symptomatic) seizures occur with transient cerebral insults. Examples include alcohol withdrawal, drug intoxication, meningitis/encephalitis,

Table 6.1 History points distinguishing syncope, seizures and psychogenic episodes. Note the syncope features here relate to vasovagal syncope: cardiac syncope (even when tachycardia-related) may occur abruptly and without prodrome.

	Syncope	Seizure	Psychogenic episode
Trigger	Common (upright, bathroom, blood)	Rare (flashing lights, hyperventilation)	Common (anger, panic)
Prodrome	Almost always	Common (aura)	Uncommon (anxiety symptoms)
Onset	Gradual	Usually sudden	Often gradual
Duration	1–30 seconds	1–3 minutes	Often prolonged (occasionally hours)
Colour	Very pale	Cyanosed	Usually normal
Convulsions	Common (brief)	Common (prolonged)	Atypical (fighting, pelvic thrusting, erratic movements)
Eyes closed	Often	Less common	Common (resisting eye opening and eye contact)
Incontinence	Uncommon	Common	Uncommon
Lateral tongue bite	Very rare	Common	Very rare (may bite front of tongue or cheek)
Breathing	Quiet	Apnoea (expiration)	Hyperventilation or apnoea (inspiration)
Post-ictal confusion	Rare	Common	Rare
Recovery	Rapid (wakes on floor)	Slow (wakes in ambulance)	Variable (repeated episodes, may be tearful)
Self injury	Rare	Common	Uncommon (carpet burn, wrist injury)

head injury and intracerebral haemorrhage. Long-term anti-epileptic medication is usually not needed for these.

Single seizure or epilepsy?

Most people with epilepsy are diagnosed following a major seizure, but often have had preceding minor events. People may not consider myoclonic jerks, absence seizures, simple or even complex partial seizures to have been epileptic events, and so they go unreported.

Classification

Seizures are either generalised or focal.

- **Primarily generalised seizures** include typical absences (abrupt onset and offset, 3 Hz spike-and-wave on EEG, usually normal intellect), myoclonic jerks and generalised tonic-clonic seizures.
- **Focal (partial-onset) seizures** include déjà vu or epigastric aura of medial temporal lobe epilepsy, head and eye turning (adversive seizure) of frontal lobe epilepsy, or visual aura of occipital epilepsy. Generalised tonic-clonic seizures in adults are usually secondarily generalised.

Epilepsies are classified as generalised or focal (localisation-related) according to the predominant seizure type, but also takes note of the possible underlying cause:

- **Idiopathic epilepsies** typically have age-specific onset (child or adolescent), favourable response to anti-epileptic drugs (AEDs), normal cerebral imaging and a presumed genetic aetiology. Idiopathic generalised epilepsies (e.g. juvenile myoclonic epilepsy) comprise 30% of epilepsies and present with combinations of generalised seizures.

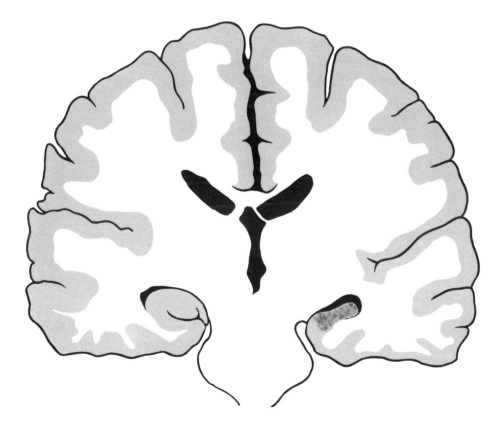

Figure 6.1 Schematic brain section illustrating left-sided mesial temporal sclerosis. Note asymmetry of hippocampi, temporal lobes/cortex and fornices.

- **Symptomatic epilepsies** have a known underlying cause (usually structural), such as mesial temporal sclerosis (*see* Figure 6.1), tumour or cortical dysplasia. They mainly have focal seizures resistant to medication. Cryptogenic epilepsies have a presumed symptomatic cause, but a definite explanation cannot been found (usually normal imaging).

Medication history

This should include:

- current and previous AEDs, including dose, formulation, dates, benefit and adverse effects
- potentially epileptogenic medications, e.g. ciprofloxacin, tramadol, antimalarials
- drugs with important AED interactions, e.g. warfarin, digoxin, oral contraceptive.

Previous medical history

Previous blackout events must be explored in detail and patients asked specifically for any history of absences, myoclonus or photosensitivity. The history should include potential cerebral insults, e.g. premature and/or traumatic birth, febrile seizures, meningitis/encephalitis and head injury. Heart disease (congenital or acquired) may suggest syncope. Depression and anxiety commonly accompany epilepsy, but significant psychiatric history (including abuse and illicit drug dependence) might favour psychogenic seizures.

Family history

The family history should include epilepsy, febrile seizures, syncope and sudden unexpected death. Family histories are notoriously unreliable, incomplete, sometimes deliberately concealed, and may require repeated enquiry or even direct assessment of affected individuals.

Social history

This includes education, employment, driving status, family planning, home situation, sporting interests, use of alcohol and illicit drugs.

Examination

Physical examination contributes surprisingly little to blackout diagnosis.

- **Epilepsy:** Examination includes a search for skin stigmata (neurofibromatosis, tuberous sclerosis), dysmorphic features, body size asymmetry (e.g. nail size), and cerebral bruit. Long-term AEDs may result in tremor, hair loss, weight gain (e.g. sodium valproate, gabapentin), gum hypertrophy, hirsutism, acne, ataxia or absent reflexes (e.g. phenytoin). Patients with focal-onset seizures require examination for visual field defects or long tract signs. Field defects from vigabatrin therapy or temporal lobe epilepsy surgery may have implications for driving, even when seizure-free.

- **Probable syncope:** Cardiovascular examination is essential, particularly the elderly.
- **Psychogenic episodes:** Twenty-five percent of patients with unexplained blackouts have panic disorder and hyperventilation. It can be helpful (to patient and clinician) to provoke the physical symptoms of hyperventilation in the clinic by deep breathing for three minutes. Hyperventilation may also induce typical absences in children. It is worth looking for wrist scars (previous self-harm) and needle marks as predictors of psychogenic episodes.

Investigations

All first seizures must be explained and usually investigated. 'Everyone is allowed one seizure' is nonsense and potentially dangerous. Note, however, that normal EEG and brain scan does not exclude epilepsy.

EEG can help to distinguish generalised from focal epilepsies (*see* Figure 6.2), support an epilepsy syndrome diagnosis and localise the focus of partial seizures. However, it is normal in about 60% of people following a single seizure and in about 40% with epilepsy. EEGs are at their most useful soon after the seizure and

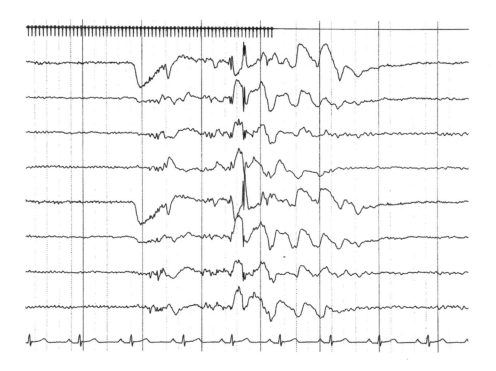

Figure 6.2(a)   EEGs showing (a) generalised spike and wave activity and (b) left temporal epileptic focus. On each tracing right-sided leads are the upper four tracings, left-sided leads the lower four.

before AEDs are prescribed. EEGs are used to support clinical suspicion rather than as the sole means of making the diagnosis of epilepsy. Uncritical interpretation of EEG by those unaware of its limitations presents dangers of erroneous diagnosis of epilepsy, unnecessary restrictions, stigma and long-term treatment. Prolonged video-EEG, however, may capture typical attacks and is particularly helpful in distinguishing epileptic from non-epileptic attacks.

Brain imaging is indicated for spontaneous seizures either of presumed focal onset (aura, focal signs or EEG focus) or refractory to medical treatment. Spontaneous seizures arising in adults are mostly focal and so all should be considered for cerebral imaging. MRI is the modality of choice because computed tomography (CT) scanning often misses epilepsy causes such as mesial temporal sclerosis (*see* Figure 6.1), cortical dysplasia, cavernoma and benign temporal lobe tumours, e.g. ganglioglioma, dysembryoplastic neuroepithelial tumour.[3]

Electrocardiogram (ECG): 12-lead ECG is indicated following all undiagnosed blackouts, especially suspected syncope and in the elderly. Rare cardiac causes of syncope (long QT, Brugada syndrome) mimic epilepsy and can induce sudden death.[4] Investigation of suspected syncope follows standard guidelines,[5] and includes echocardiogram, exercise testing, head-up tilt table testing and 24 hour ECG. Suspected cardiogenic syncope requires urgent cardiology referral.

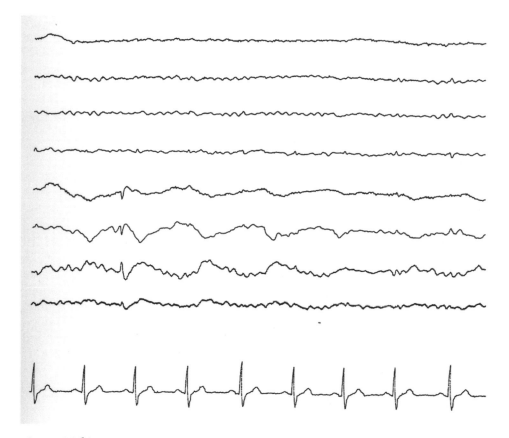

Figure 6.2(b)

Management

Starting medication

AEDs are considered usually following more than one spontaneous epileptic seizure. The MESS study[6] compared immediate with delayed treatment following single seizures and early epilepsy, and showed that 14 patients were randomised to treatment to prevent one patient relapsing by two years. Long-term medication is therefore usually withheld following a single seizure. However, highly epileptogenic causes, such as glioma, justify AEDs after a single event.

AED treatment is usually long-term, requiring informed discussion with an epilepsy specialist. Short-term AED trials are rarely justified. The patient must balance the seizure morbidity (including the small risk of sudden unexpected death (SUDEP))[7] against the consequences, inconvenience and the adverse effects for that individual (including potential teratogenicity).

Choosing medication

The 2004 England and Wales NICE guidelines on the use of new antiepileptic medications[8] advise initially either carbamazepine (focal seizures) or sodium valproate (focal or generalised seizures). Women of childbearing potential (including girls requiring AED into their childbearing years) should probably not be prescribed valproate as first-line owing to teratogenicity.[9] Lamotrigine appears a safer alternative.[10] Alternative monotherapy should be tried before considering polytherapy.[11] Vigabatrin is no longer started (except in babies with West syndrome) because of problems with permanent visual field constriction. The role of other newer drugs (gabapentin, levetiracetam, oxcarbazepine, pregabalin, tiagabine, topiramate) will become clearer following SANAD,[12] a large randomised controlled study comparing first-line monotherapy with new and conventional AEDs.

Stopping medication

Seizure-free patients require detailed discussion before stopping AEDs. In children it is usual to try after two years seizure-free. In adults, continued seizure freedom for driving and employment often justifies the inconvenience of continued medication; many adults therefore remain on medication whilst seizure-free for years. Women wishing to conceive naturally wish to stop AEDs (see below), and often do so without consulting their doctor.[13] Overall, 40% of adults seizure-free for two years will relapse.[14] The risk is highest with previous tonic-clonic or myoclonic seizures, seizures after starting medication, needing more than one AED, and in those with abnormal EEGs.[15] The greater likelihood of seizures in the months following withdrawal[16] is reflected in the UK Driver and Vehicle Licensing Agency's (DVLA) advice to stop driving from the start of AED withdrawal until six months after its completion.

Surgery

Symptomatic epilepsies, e.g. from mesial temporal sclerosis, are commonly resistant to AEDs and justify consideration of surgery.[17] Epilepsy surgery is generally underused in the UK.[18] The detailed preparation for surgery (prolonged and sometimes invasive video EEG monitoring, sodium amytal testing) is available in only a few centres. Potentially curative procedures include removal of proven epileptogenic lesions including temporal lobectomy for mesial temporal sclerosis; palliative procedures include multiple subpial transection, corpus callosotomy, and hemispherectomy in patients with severe symptomatic epilepsies.[19] Vagus nerve stimulation is an option for adults and children[20] with resistant epilepsy.

Special situations

Refractory epilepsy

Refractory focal epilepsy demands a detailed search for structural pathology. Not all MR scans are equal in their quality of data acquisition or reporting (ideally brain MRI should include high definition, thin-sliced images, with fluid attenuated inversion recovery (FLAIR) sequences, and reported by a neuroradiologist); repeat imaging may be necessary. Poor treatment compliance may cause apparently refractory epilepsy. Furthermore, 15% of patients with 'refractory epilepsy' have only psychogenic seizures.[21] Patients who have not responded to two first-line AEDs therefore require careful diagnostic review. The epilepsy classification must also be reviewed since certain AEDs beneficial to focal epilepsies (e.g. carbamazepine, gabapentin) may be ineffective, and even worsen absences, myoclonus and photosensitivity.

Learning disability

A third of patients with severe learning disability have epilepsy. Such consultations can be very challenging. Again the history is crucial and so a carer who knows the patient well must accompany the patient. As far as practical, the conversation should be directed at the patient rather than carers. Close liaison with the community learning disabilities team is essential.

Children and teenagers

Epilepsy in children is a major sub-speciality, not covered by this review. Teenagers with epilepsy can benefit from combined consultations with adult and paediatric specialists to address their complex medical and social problems.[22]

Elderly

Blackout management in the elderly is complicated for several reasons. Patients often live alone (no witness account), may have poor recall of events, and have other medical problems with pre-existing polypharmacy. Most importantly, both epilepsy and syncope are commoner in the elderly, but syncope presenting in old age requires urgent cardiological evaluation. Cerebrovascular disease is closely linked to elderly-onset epilepsy; such patients require consideration of antiplatelet and statin therapy, as well as AED.[23] There is little evidence to support any particular AED in the elderly; in general, AEDs with renal excretion and fewer interactions are preferred.

Pregnancy

Young women need clear information upon which to base treatment and lifestyle decisions (*see* below). However, for women already pregnant, teratogenicity advice comes too late. Epilepsy nurse input into antenatal clinics help management of epilepsy in pregnancy (around 0.5% of all pregnancies). Combined neurologist and obstetrician clinics are useful for complicated cases.

Syncope

Syncope affects 22% of the population[24] and presents potentially an enormous problem. Although only a few are referred to specialists (mainly cardiologists), syncope is still the commonest diagnosis among new referrals to an epilepsy clinic. Epilepsy specialists must therefore work closely with cardiologists, preferably in a joint 'blackout' clinic.

Psychogenic attacks

The scarcity of local liaison psychiatry services means that patients with psychogenic seizures are often followed in epilepsy clinics, becoming major users of epilepsy services. Ideally, one specialist should supervise their management (including sustained AED withdrawal) using regular short-interval follow-up and admissions only under that specialist's care. Without this, patients risk admission as 'known epileptic' and having their medication restarted or increased.

Information for patients

Driving

Loss of driving privileges contributes significantly to the social predicament of epilepsy. Many people are told that they cannot drive until seeing the specialist, and eagerly await advice. Following an unprovoked epileptic seizure (or undiagnosed blackout), UK drivers must stop, inform the DVLA[25] and remain seizure-free for a year before regaining their licence. This law applies even to minor seizures including epileptic myoclonic jerks. Provoked seizures, e.g. within a week of head injury, are dealt with individually by the DVLA. For heavy goods and public service licences, drivers must be 10 years seizure-free and off medication.

Lifestyle

People with epilepsy should be encouraged to live normal lives, within sensible limits.

- **Sports and leisure:** The seizure frequency and type influence advice for specific circumstances such as swimming, cycling on busy roads, and isolation sports (e.g. horse riding, hill walking, etc.).
- **Alcohol** may provoke seizures through sleep loss, AED interaction (chronic alcohol intake induces liver enzymes), forgetting medication or inducing

misplaced confidence that AEDs can be omitted. Pragmatic advice is that patients with epilepsy should limit alcohol consumption to four units in 24 hours.

- **Sleep deprivation** is an avoidable cause of lowered seizure threshold, especially in idiopathic generalised epilepsies.
- **Flashing lights:** True photosensitivity is uncommon in adults especially on medication, but many people with epilepsy misguidedly avoid computers, TVs and discos.

Teratogenicity

Women contemplating pregnancy require balanced and reliable information about the teratogenic potential of their medication. Unfortunately, such data are currently lacking and advice is based to an extent upon opinion and conjecture. Nevertheless, prospective observational data from the UK Epilepsy and Pregnancy Register[9] show valproate to be associated with major congenital malformations more than either carbamazepine or lamotrigine. The risks, though multifactorial, relate to AED burden: monotherapy 4–6%, duotherapy 7–8% and polytherapy 15–20%.[26] Furthermore, there are suggestions, awaiting prospective evaluation, of increased neuro-developmental delay among children exposed to AEDs *in utero*.[27] Unfortunately valproate is the AED of first choice for idiopathic generalised epilepsies and so changing drugs to protect unborn children risks compromising seizure control. Also, switching from valproate to lamotrigine is complicated, taking several months. Despite the absence of conclusive proof and the inherent difficulties in researching this area,[28] young women, particularly on valproate, require specialist review to inform decisions about long-term treatment.

Follow-up

Epilepsy, more than many chronic disorders, justifies long-term follow-up. The diagnosis is history-based and too often is made incorrectly, particularly in non-specialist hands.[29] The choice and need for prescribed medications may be inappropriate, and patients may too easily accept medication side effects and unnecessary lifestyle restrictions. Good practice would suggest annual review, including in 'nurse-led' epilepsy specialist clinics, be offered to all patients with epilepsy. Proactive specialist review of those currently managed in the community may also be justified to check diagnoses, optimise clinical management and provide information.[30]

And finally . . .

Patients need opportunities to ask questions. 'What would you like to ask?' induces more response than 'Do you have any questions?' Early follow-up after the initial diagnosis provides the opportunity to discuss concerns after a period of reflection. Written information is also important, including information sheets, details of websites and local support groups. Most powerful is a personalised letter summarising the consultation and giving specific information. Copying the standard clinic letter is a useful alternative.[31]

Patients with chronic conditions are expert in their individual condition[32] since they constantly live with it. Providing individualised verbal and written information and offering specialist nurse telephone contact encourage greater patient involvement in their long-term management.

Conclusion

Epilepsy clinics provide a multidisciplinary focus for the diagnosis and long-term management of patients with recurrent blackouts and epilepsy. The diagnosis is clinical rather than investigation-based, and the emphasis of management is long-term, team-delivered and founded upon a partnership of specialist care with the patient and with primary care, sharing information, supporting and empowering patients, and aiming for their increasing independence.

References

1 National Institute for Clinical Excellence (NICE). Clinical Guideline 20. The epilepsies: the diagnosis and management of the epilepsies in adults and children in primary and secondary care – Full guideline. October 2004. www.nice.org.uk/page.aspx?o=229388 (accessed 28/11/04).

2 Smith PEM. If it's not epilepsy. *J Neurol Neurosurg Psychiatry* 2001; **70**(suppl): 9–14.

3 Recommendation for neuroimaging of patients with epilepsy. Commission of the International League Against Epilepsy. *Epilepsia* 1997; **38**: 1255–56.

4 Brugada A, Geelen P. Some electrocardiographic patterns predicting sudden cardiac death that every doctor should recognise. *Acta Cardiologica* 1997; **6**: 473–84.

5 Brignole M, Alboni P, Benditt D, *et al*. Task Force on Syncope, European Society of Cardiology. Part 2. Diagnostic tests and treatment: summary of recommendations. *Europace* 2001; **3**: 261–8.

6 Marson A, Jacoby A, Johnson A, *et al*. Medical Research Council MESS Study Group. Immediate versus deferred antiepileptic drug treatment for early epilepsy and single seizures: a randomised controlled trial. *Lancet* 2005; **365**: 2007–13.

7 Walczak TS, Leppik IE, D'Amelio M, *et al*. Incidence and risk factors in sudden unexpected death in epilepsy. *Neurology* 2002; **56**: 519–25.

8 NICE guidance (Technology Appraisal) 76 Newer drugs for epilepsy in adults. Issued March 2004 www.nice.org.uk/TA076guidance (accessed 29/11/04).

9 Committee on the Safety of Medicines. Sodium valproate and prescribing in pregnancy. Current problems in pharmacovigilance. Committee on the Safety of Medicines 2003; **29**: 6.

10 Morrow JI, Russell AJC, Irwin B, *et al*. The safety of antiepileptic drugs in pregnancy: results of the UK epilepsy and pregnancy register. *Epilepsia* 2004; **45**(suppl 3): 57(abstract).

11 Lawthom C, Smith PEM. What is the role of polytherapy in the management of epilepsy? In: Roberts RC, ed. Better care for children and adults with epilepsy – a consensus conference. *Journal of the Royal College of Physicians of Edinburgh* 2003; **33**(suppl 11): 22–30.

12 SANAD: A study of standard and new antiepileptic drugs. www.liv.ac.uk/neuroscience/sanad/ (accessed 29/11/04).

13 Williams J, Myson V, Steward S, Jones G, Wilson JF, Smith PEM. Self-discontinuation of antiepileptic medication in pregnancy: detection by hair analysis. *Epilepsia* 2002; **43**: 824–31.

14 Berg AT, Shinnar S. Relapse following discontinuation of antiepileptic drugs: a meta-analysis. *Neurology* 1994; **44**: 601–8.

15 Chadwick DW representing the MRC Antiepileptic Drug Withdrawal Study Group. Does withdrawal of different anti-epileptic drugs have different effects on seizure recurrence? *Brain* 1999; **122**: 441–8.

16 Berg AT. Discontinuing antiepileptic drugs. In: Engel J, Pedley TA, eds. *Epilepsy: A comprehensive text.* New York: Lippincott-Raven, 1997.

17 Spencer SS. When should temporal-lobe epilepsy be treated surgically? *Lancet Neurology* 2002; **1**: 375–382.

18 Elwes RD. Surgery for temporal lobe epilepsy. *BMJ* 2002; **324**: 496–7.

19 Engel J Jr. Surgery for seizures. *N Engl J Med* 1996; **334**: 647–52.

20 NICE Guidance Interventional Procedure 50 Vagus nerve stimulation for refractory epilepsy in children. Issued March 2004. www.nice.org.uk/IPG050publicinfo (accessed 29/11/04).

21 Devinsky O. Patients with refractory seizures. *N Engl J Med* 1999; **340**: 1565–1570.

22 Smith PEM, Wallace S. Taking over epilepsy from the paediatric neurologist. *J Neurol Neurosurg Psychiatry* 2003; **74**(suppl 1): 37–41.

23 Cleary P, Shorvon S, Tallis R. Late-onset seizures as a predictor of subsequent stroke. *Lancet.* 2004; **363**: 1184–6.

24 Chen-Scarabelli C, Scarabelli TM. Neurocardiogenic syncope. *BMJ* 2004; **329**: 336–41.

25 At a glance; a guide for medical practitioners. DVLA Publications, September 2000. www.dvla.gov.uk/at_a_glance/content.htm (accessed 29/11/04).

26 Zahn C. Neurological care of women with epilepsy. *Epilepsia* 2000; **41**(suppl): 26–31.

27 Adab N, Jacoby A, Smith DF, Chadwick DW. Additional educational needs in children born to mothers with epilepsy. *J Neurol Neurosurg Psychiatr* 2001; **70**: 15–21.

28 Dolk H, McElhatton P. Assessing epidemiological evidence for the teratogenic effects of anticonvulsant medications. *J Med Genet* 2002; **39**: 243–4.

29 Smith DF, Defalla BA, Chadwick DW. The misdiagnosis of epilepsy and the management of refractory epilepsy in a specialist clinic. *QJM* 1999; **92**: 15–23.

30 Smith PEM, Leach JP. Epilepsy: Time to review. *QJM* 2003; **96**: 87–9.

31 Smith PEM. Letters to patients: Sending the right message. Personal View. *BMJ* 2002; **324**: 685.

32 Department of Health. *The expert patient: a new approach to chronic disease management for the twenty-first century.* London: Department of Health, 2001. www.ohn.gov.uk/ohn/people/expert.

Part 2

Infectious and para-infectious disease

Chapter Seven

Subacute sclerosing panencephalitis

RK Garg

Subacute sclerosing panencephalitis (SSPE) is a progressive neurological disorder of childhood and early adolescence. It is caused by persistent defective measles virus. Brain biopsies or postmortem histopathological examination show evidence of astrogliosis, neuronal loss, degeneration of dendrites, demyelination, neurofibrillary tangles, and infiltration of inflammatory cells. Patients usually have behavioural changes, myoclonus, dementia, visual disturbances, and pyramidal and extrapyramidal signs. The disease has a gradual progressive course leading to death within 1–3 years. The diagnosis is based upon characteristic clinical manifestations, the presence of characteristic periodic EEG discharges, and demonstration of raised antibody titre against measles in the plasma and cerebrospinal fluid. Treatment for SSPE is still undetermined. A combination of oral isoprinosine (Inosiplex) and intraventricular interferon alfa appears to be the best effective treatment. Patients responding to treatment need to receive it life long. Effective immunisation against measles is the only solution presently available to the problem of this dreaded disease.

Subacute sclerosing panencephalitis (SSPE) is a serious disorder of the central nervous system. It is a slow virus infection caused by defective measles virus (*see* Table 7.1). The term 'subacute sclerosing panencephalitis' has been used since Greenfield suggested it in 1960 to designate a condition due to a persistent infection by a virus involving both grey matter and white matter.[1] In fact, SSPE had originally been described as three different neuropathological entities. In 1933 Dawson, for the first time, described a child with progressive mental deterioration and involuntary movements who, at necropsy, was found to have a dominant involvement of grey matter in which neuronal inclusion bodies were abundant.[2] He suggested the term 'subacute inclusion body encephalitis'. Later Pette and Doring (1939) reported a single case of what they called 'nodular panencephalitis', a disease with equally severe lesions in both grey and white matter.[3] Six years later, Van Bogaert drew attention to the presence of dominant demyelination and glial proliferation in the white matter and suggested the term 'subacute sclerosing leukoencephalitis'.[4] A viral aetiology was suggested by Dawson, but it was Bouteille *et al.*, in 1965, who on electron microscopy demonstrated the presence of viral structures resembling measles virus in the brain.[5] In 1969 measles virus was actually recovered from the brain of a patient with SSPE.[6] Since then a lot of progress has been made towards understanding of this potentially lethal disorder. Various treatment modalities have been tried with little success. In this article all recent information will be reviewed.

Epidemiology

SSPE has been reported from all parts of the world, but in the West it is considered a rare disease with fewer than 10 cases per year reported in the United States.[7] The reported frequency of SSPE in the United States was approximately one per million childhood population from 1960 to 1970.[8] The incidence declined substantially after introduction of an effective measles vaccine. The annual incidence of SSPE is still quite high but variable among developing countries. Saha *et al.* reported an annual incidence of 21 per million population in India,[9] in comparison with 2.4 per million population in the Middle East.[10,11]

Most patients with SSPE have a history of primary measles infection at an early age (<2 years), which is followed, after a latent period of 6–8 years, by the onset of progressive neurological disorder. Children infected with measles under the age of 1 year carry a risk of 16 times greater than those infected at age 5 years or later. Since the incubation period is typically less than a decade, SSPE is commonly a disease of childhood. A higher incidence (male/female ratio 3:1) has been noted in boys, although primary measles infection shows no such sex disparity. The incidence is higher among rural children, children with two or more siblings, and children with mental retardation. It is also more common in children with a lower birth order and in children living in overcrowded environments.[12–15] Aaby *et al.* have suggested that these features (age of exposure, sex, and geography) are indicative of intensive measles exposure as a risk factor.[16] Other factors, also identified as risk factors for SSPE, may modify the course of acute measles infection – for example, a close temporal relationship of measles with another viral infection such as Epstein-Barr virus or parainfluenza type-1 virus.

Widespread immunisation has produced greater than 90% reduction in the incidence of SSPE in developed nations.[17] When the disease occurs in vaccinated children, it is thought to result from a subclinical measles infection that occurred before the age of 1 year, when immunisation is usually begun. There is no evidence to suggest that attenuated vaccine virus is responsible for sporadic cases of SSPE.[1]

Table 7.1 Various neurological complications of measles

Post-measles encephalitis	Develops soon after infection, reflects an autoimmune reaction
Measles inclusion body encephalitis	Develops weeks or months after infection, in patients with defective cell mediated immunities like HIV infection
Subacute sclerosing panencephalitis	Persistent defective measles virus infection
Postinfectious	Acute immune reaction
Transverse myelitis	Rare, acute immune reaction

Pathogenesis

Measles is caused by an RNA virus, which belongs to the marbillivirus subgroup of paramyxoviruses. Despite the long interval between the acute infection and symptoms of SSPE, there is evidence that measles virus infection of brain occurs soon after the acute infection with subsequent spread throughout the brain.[18] Measles virus is thought to reach the brain through infection of cerebral endothelial cells, perhaps during the acute exanthema of measles when other endothelial cells are also infected.[19] Access into the brain by circulating inflammatory cells is also possible.[20] The measles virus particles are pleomorphic, spherical structures having a diameter of 100 to 250 nm and consisting of six proteins. The inner capsid is composed of a coiled helix of RNA and three proteins. The outer envelope consists of a matrix protein bearing two types of short surface glycoprotein projections of peplomers. One peplomer is a conical haemagglutinin (H) and the other a dumbbell-shaped fusion (F) protein. The envelope carries projections of the H and F proteins. The M (matrix) protein sits within the envelope membrane and can interact with cytoplasmic domains of H and F proteins. In contrast to measles virus infection of non-neuronal cells, which is cytopathic and spreads both by extracellular virus and by cell fusion resulting in multinucleated syncytia formation, little extracellular infectious virus can be recovered from brains of SSPE patients unless neuronal tissues are cocultured with fibroblasts.[21] High levels of neutralising antibody are present in the serum and cerebrospinal fluid of SSPE patients; it further suggests that extracellular virus might not be responsible for measles virus spread in the central nervous system.[22]

Recently, a trans-synaptic transmission of virus has been suggested.[23]

Measles virus isolated from specimens of the brains of such patients may interfere with the replication of the wild type of measles virus and may have a clonal origin.[18,24] Numerous alterations in M protein have been described in SSPE because of extensive point mutations in viral genome, possibly resulting in persistent viral infection.[25–30] The type II transmembrane protein H mediates virus cell attachment by binding to the cell surface protein CD46 (it is a measles virus receptor protein, which is, in fact, a complement-regulating protein with isoforms present on neurons),[31] and is an essential cofactor for fusion.[32] Changes in the H and F proteins can also be associated with persistent infection, with M protein remaining relatively unaffected.[33,34] Since all three proteins are associated with viral budding from infected cells and the putative fusion with uninfected cells, the persistent nature of the infection is thought to be due to defects in these two processes.[35] The exact factors and influences that allow the measles infection to persist are unclear, but may include several immunological factors. For example, in tissue culture, the addition of antibodies against measles virus may alter the pattern of viral gene expression.[36] This observation may explain why measles infection at a very early age, when maternal antibodies are still present in the blood of the patient, carries an increased risk of SSPE.[35] There is evidence that persistent measles virus infection can be found throughout the body in patients with SSPE.[37]

Recently studies have suggested that apoptosis of various cell types may contribute to the neuropathogenesis of measles virus infection in the human central nervous system, either as a direct effect of viral infection or of cytokine-mediated responses, resulting in oligodendroglial and neuronal cell death in SSPE.[38,39]

Pathology

Brain biopsy performed in the early stages of SSPE shows mild inflammation of the meninges and brain parenchyma involving cortical and subcortical grey matter as well as white matter. There is often evidence of neuronal degeneration, gliosis, proliferation of astrocytes, perivascular cuffing, lymphocytic and plasma cell infiltration, and demyelination. Viral infection of oligodendrocytes may be responsible for extensive demyelination, which is often present in patients with SSPE.[40] In later stages, gross examination of brain may reveal mild to moderate atrophy of the cerebral cortex. Microscopic examination shows widespread degeneration of neurons and disorganisation of cortical structures. The parieto-occipital region of the brain is most severely affected, subsequently; pathological involvement spreads to the anterior portions of cerebral hemispheres, subcortical structures, brainstem, and spinal cord. Focal or diffuse perivascular infiltrates of lymphocytes, plasma cells, and phagocytes are present in the meninges and in the brain parenchyma. Inclusion bodies are seen within both nucleus and cytoplasm of neurons and glial cells. Cowdry type-A inclusion bodies, consisting of homogeneous eosinophilic material, are diffusely seen in neurons and oligodendroglia in patients with rapidly progressive fatal disease. Other Cowdry type-B inclusion bodies, small and multiple, are almost always present in the brainstem. Subsequent studies have shown that these nuclear inclusions correspond to viral particles and contain viral antigens.[22] Neurofibrillary tangles may also be seen within neurons and oligodendrocytes.[41] In situ hybridisation methods have shown that cells containing tangles often contain the viral genome, suggesting that viral infection causes the formation of tangles.[42] Late in the course of disease it may be difficult find typical areas of inflammation and even inclusion bodies. The histopathological changes are marked with parenchymal necrosis and gliosis.[43] Studies of inflammatory cell infiltrate in brain tissue from patients with SSPE have shown that the perivascular cells are predominantly CD4+ T cells, with B cells seen more frequently in the parenchymal inflammatory infiltrate.[44] Little infectious virus can be recovered from the brain tissue but viral antigen can be identified immunocytochemically and viral genome can be detected by in situ hybridisation method or by polymerase chain reaction amplification method.[22,45,46]

Box 7.1 Ophthalmological abnormalities with SSPE

- Papillo-oedema
- Papillitis
- Optic atrophy
- Macular or perimacular chorioretinitis
- Cortical blindness
- Anton's syndrome (cortical blindness with denial of blindness)

Clinical features

The initial symptoms are usually subtle and include mild intellectual deterioration and behavioural changes without any apparent neurological signs or findings. Parents and teachers may notice progressive deterioration in scholastic performance. As disease advances non-specific manifestations evolve into disturbances in motor function and development of periodic stereotyped myoclonic jerks. Myoclonic jerks initially involve the head and subsequently trunk and limbs. Muscular contraction is followed by 1–2 seconds of relaxation associated with a decrease in muscle action potential or complete electrical silence. The myoclonic jerks do not interfere with consciousness. They are exaggerated by excitement and may disappear during sleep. Myoclonus can present as a difficulty in gait, periodic dropping of the head, and falling. The myoclonus may not be obvious early in the disease but can be elicited by the patient standing with feet together and arms held forward and then watching for periodic dropping of the head, neck, trunk, or arm; these are often concomitant with contraction of facial musculature and slow eye blinks. Patients may, frequently, develop pyramidal and extrapyramidal signs. Few patients may develop ataxia, dystonia, and dyskinesia. Generalised tonic-clonic seizures and partial seizures may also occur.[7,9,47] Ocular and visual manifestations (*see* Box 7.1) are reported in 10–50% of patients, which include cortical blindness, chorioretinitis, and optic atrophy. Visual symptoms are usually concurrent with neurological manifestations but they may precede neurological manifestation by several years.[48,49] Park *et al.*, in a patient presenting with chorioretinitis, have demonstrated numerous filamentous, microtubular, and intranuclear viral inclusions in the nuclear layers of retina consistent with the measles virus.[50]

In advanced stages of the disease, patients become quadriparetic, spasticity increases, and myoclonus may decrease or disappear. There is autonomic failure with loss of thermoregulation leading to marked temperature fluctuations. There is progressive deterioration of sensorium to a comatose state and ultimately the patient becomes vegetative. Decerebrate and decorticate rigidity appear, breathing becomes noisy and irregular. At this stage, patients frequently die due to hyperpyrexia, cardiovascular collapse, or hypothalamic disturbances.[51]

Diagnosis

Once myoclonus is evident the clinical diagnosis is seldom a problem. However, subtle behavioural changes at an early stage of disease are frequently missed by relatives. Many such patients are often treated by a psychiatrist at this stage. In some cases myoclonus is not present; atonia may be present but can be overlooked.[11] At times SSPE may need to be distinguished from various neurodegenerative conditions in which myoclonus and some other progressive neurological disorder are dominant clinical manifestations (Box 7.2). Occasionally, patients with SSPE can present with lateralising neurological signs, partial seizures, or papillo-oedema; these findings can lead to an erroneous diagnosis of an intracranial space occupying lesion.[52] The diagnosis is based upon typical cerebrospinal fluid changes and a characteristic electroencephalography pattern. The diagnosis of SSPE can be reliably established if the patient fulfils three of the five criteria given by Dyken[47] (*see* Table 7.2).

Table 7.2 Diagnostic criteria of SSPE[47]

1. Clinical	Progressive, subacute mental deterioration with typical signs like myoclonus
2. EEG	Periodic, stereotyped, high voltage discharges
3. Cerebrospinal fluid	Raised gammaglobulin or oligoclonal pattern
4. Measles antibodies	Raised titre in serum (>1:256) and/or cerebrospinal fluid (>1:4)
5. Brain biopsy	Suggestive of panencephalitis

Definitive: criteria 5 with three more criteria; probable: three of the five criteria.

Cerebrospinal fluid

Cerebrospinal fluid examination is usually normal. Frequently, it is acellular with normal or a mildly raised protein concentration. The most remarkable feature of the cerebrospinal fluid examination is a markedly raised gammaglobulin level, which is usually greater than 20% of total cerebrospinal fluid protein. Because of the large increase of intrathecal synthesis of IgG, cerebrospinal fluid IgG concentration ranges from 10–54 μg/dl compared with 5–10 μg/dl in normal children.[53,54] In most cases raised levels of locally synthesised gammaglobulins indicate either an infection or other type of inflammatory process within the central nervous system. When the cerebrospinal fluid is examined by agarose gel electrophoresis or isoelectric focussing, an oligoclonal band of immunoglobulins is often observed. The oligoclonal band signifies the production of gammaglobulin of a restricted class and also implies that there are clones of B cells that have differentiated into plasma cells within the central nervous system.[55]

In patients with SSPE most of IgG in the cerebrospinal fluid has been shown to be directed against measles virus, and the oligoclonal bands can be adsorbed by measles virus.[56] So raised titres of antimeasles antibodies in the cerebrospinal fluid are diagnostic of SSPE. Antimeasles antibody titres are also raised in serum. Raised antimeasles antibody titres of 1:256 or greater in serum, and 1:4 or greater in cerebrospinal fluid is considered diagnostic of SSPE. The characteristic ratio of cerebrospinal fluid titre to serum titre ranges from 1:4 to 1:128 (below 200), this ratio is low compared with the normal ratio (1:200–1:500). Serum cerebrospinal fluid ratios are normal for other viral antibodies and for albumin, indicating that the increased amounts of measles antibodies result from synthesis within the central nervous system and that the blood brain barrier is also normal.[57,58] Various serological methods used are complement fixation, haemagglutination inhibition, virus neutralisation, and enzyme-linked immunosorbent assay (ELISA). ELISA is highly sensitive in detecting measles virus specific IgG as well as IgM.[59]

It is possible to make an accurate diagnosis of SSPE by detecting the measles virus genome in the cerebrospinal fluid. Measles virus RNA can be detected by reverse transcription polymerase chain reaction.

Box 7.2   Other neurodegenerative myoclonic conditions

A. Progressive myoclonic epilepsies (early myoclonus and generalised tonic-clonic seizures)

- Unverricht-Lundborg syndrome.
- Myoclonic epilepsy ragged red fibre (MERRF).
- Lafora body disease.
- Neuronal ceroid lipofuscinoses.
- Sialidoses.
- Hereditary dentatorubralpallidoluysian atrophy.

B. Progressive myoclonic encephalopathies (where myoclonus is generally overshadowed by other clinical manifestations)

- GM2 gangliosidosis.
- Non-ketotic hyperglycinaemia.
- Niemann-Pick disease.
- Juvenile Huntington's disease.
- Alzheimer's disease.
- Creutzfeldt-Jakob disease.

C. Progressive myoclonic ataxias (seizures are either absent or late)

- Spinocerebellar degeneration.
- Wilson's disease.
- Coeliac disease.
- Whipple's disease.

Electroencephalography

Early in the course of the disease, the electroencephalogram (EEG) may be normal or show only moderate, non-specific generalised slowing. The typical EEG pattern is usually seen in myoclonic phase and is virtually diagnostic. The EEG picture is characterised by periodic complexes consisting of bilaterally symmetrical, synchronous, high voltage (200–500 mv) bursts of polyphasic, stereotyped delta waves. Waveforms remain identical in any given lead. These periodic complexes repeat at fairly regular 4–10 second intervals and have 1:1 relationship with myoclonic jerks (*see* Figure 7.1). Frequently there is shortening of the interval between periodic complexes with progression of the disease.[60] The periodic complexes of SSPE first appear during sleep, when they are not accompanied by myoclonic spasms. Often these periodic complexes can be brought out when the patient is awake, if diazepam is administered intravenously during the routine electroencephalographic recording. Late in the course of disease, the EEG may become increasingly disorganised and show high amplitudes and random dysrhythmic slowing. In terminal stages the amplitude of waveforms may fall.

In addition to type I periodic electroencephalographic complexes just described, few other forms of periodic complexes have also been recognised.[11] These various types of periodic complexes have been shown to have some association with the prognosis of the disease. Type II abnormalities are characterised by periodic giant

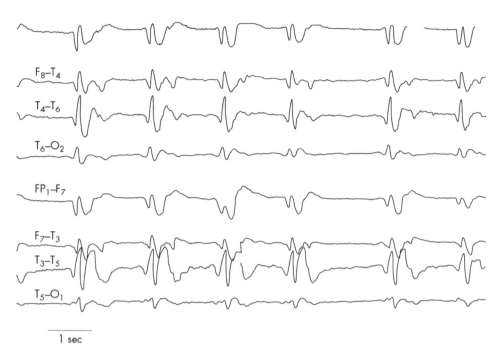

F_8-T_4

T_4-T_6

T_6-O_2

FP_1-F_7

F_7-T_3

T_3-T_5

T_5-O_1

1 sec

Figure 7.1 EEG showing a periodic pattern with slow wave complexes recurring at intervals of 4–6 seconds.

delta waves intermixed with rapid spikes as fast activity. In this pattern of periodic complexes, EEG background is usually slow. The type III periodic complexes pattern is characterised by long spike-wave discharges interrupted by giant delta waves. Yakub demonstrated that video-split EEG monitoring is a more sensitive technique for early diagnosis and detection of atonia or myoclonus,[11] which are time-related to EEG periodic complexes. He further observed that type III periodic complexes were associated with the worst outcome, while patients with type II periodic complexes had the best outcome. In this study outcome was determined by the rate of progression of disease.

Neuroimaging

Neuroimaging has a limited role in the early diagnosis of SSPE. Computed tomography of brain is normal in early stages of disease, in later stages it shows small ventricles and obliteration of hemispheric sulci and interhemispheric fissure due to diffuse cerebral oedema. Generalised or focal cerebral atrophy and ex vacuo ventricular dilatation can be seen after a very prolonged course, but sometimes computed tomograms are normal as late as five years after the onset of the disease. Low attenuation areas in the cortex and basal ganglion have also been observed.[61]

Magnetic resonance imaging (MRI) is more sensitive in detecting white matter abnormalities. Early changes are ill defined high signal intensity areas on T2-weighted images (*see* Figure 7.2), more commonly seen in the occipital sub-cortical white matter than in the frontal region. In most of the cases the grey matter is spared even in advanced clinical and MRI stages. However, Tuncay *et al.* observed early involvement of grey matter.[62] In this study, early lesions were dominantly involving grey matter and subcortical white matter. These lesions were asymmetrical and had a predilection for the posterior parts of cerebral hemispheres (*see* Figure 7.3). Later, high signal changes in deep white matter and severe cerebral atrophy were observed. Parenchymal lesions were significantly correlated with the duration of disease. Though mass effect and contrast enhancement of lesions are not usual features of SSPE, some authors have

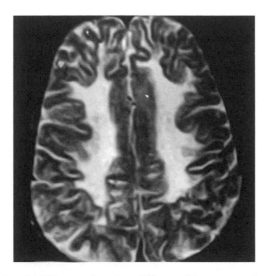

Figure 7.2 T2-weighted MRI scan showing diffuse white matter demyelination in an 8 year old boy with SSPE.

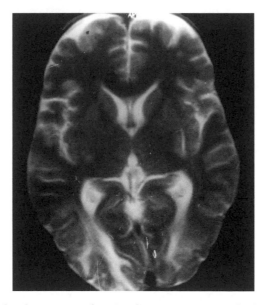

Figure 7.3 T2-weighted MRI scan showing hyperintensity in the both occipital regions (*see* case report).

reported mild mass effect and contrast enhancement in few patients, especially in the early stages of the disease.[63]

Brismar *et al*. have developed a staging system based on neuroimaging findings for SSPE that reflects the degree of white matter changes and atrophy.[64] However, the radiological staging of this SSPE is not always exactly correlated with its clinical manifestations. Even so, sequential MRI may be useful for following the course of the disease.[64]

Brain biopsy

Brain biopsy is seldom required to establish the diagnosis of SSPE. When performed, it will often show the typical histopathological findings described earlier. Examination of frozen sections by immunofluorescence technique may demonstrate the presence of measles virus antigens. Reverse transcription polymerase chain reaction can detect various regions of the measles virus RNA in frozen and even paraffin-embedded brain tissue specimens of patients with SSPE. Nucleic acid hybridisation techniques have also been used to demonstrate the measles virus genome.

SSPE in adults

SSPE, being a disorder of childhood and adolescence, may not be readily recognised when a patient presents later in the life. Approximately 50 cases of SSPE have been reported in those over 18 years of age. Patients with adult onset SSPE present at a mean age of 25.4 years (range 20–35 years). A higher proportion of adult patients have either negative or an undocumented history of prior measles infection in childhood. Visual manifestations, especially cortical blindness, are the commonest mode of clinical presentation. The disease apparently has a more aggressive course in adults and the disease is rapidly progressive in the majority of patients.[65] In a preliminary study, Gokcil *et al*. observed that treatment with oral isoprinosine plus interferon alfa is effective for adult onset SSPE.[66]

SSPE and pregnancy

SSPE can rapidly progress during pregnancy. It has been suggested that the relative older age of presentation, and unusually rapid neurological deterioration, are partially due to immunological and hormonal alterations of pregnancy. In several reported cases, the disease was associated with the death of the child in utero, or in the immediate peripartum period.[67] Thiel *et al*. reported a 20 year old woman who delivered a healthy infant by caesarean section in the 28th gestational week.[68] Serum analysis of the infant revealed slowly diminishing IgG measles virus antibody titres. After six months, the maternal measles antibodies were no longer detectable in the child's serum. Cortical blindness has been reported as the most common presenting manifestation of SSPE even in pregnancy. Characteristic myoclonus may not be apparent; the clinical picture resembles that of eclampsia (*see* case report below).

Acute fulminant SSPE

Most of the patients with SSPE survive for 1–3 years after diagnosis, with a mean survival of about 18 months. In acute fulminant SSPE the disease rapidly evolves leading to death within three months of the diagnosis. In the series of Risk and Haddad, approximately 10% of patients had such a fulminant course.[51] In rapidly evolving SSPE various stages of disease cannot be recognised. The exact mechanism producing an acute fulminant course is not known. Several factors such as exposure to measles at an early age, viral virulence, impaired host defence mechanisms, and concurrent infections with other viruses have been suggested as responsible for producing a rapid course of the disease.[69–71]

Treatment

No adequate therapy is currently available for the treatment of SSPE. Observations of some non-randomised trials suggest that certain antiviral drugs and immunomodulator agents can prolong life if long-term treatment is given (Box 7.3). The issue of the success of treatment is frequently complicated by an extremely variable natural course as a few patients may have very prolonged spontaneous remissions.[51,72,73]

Box 7.3 Drugs used in the treatment of SSPE

- Amantadine
- Cimetidine
- Corticosteroids
- Interferon alfa
- Interferon beta
- Isoprinosine (Inosiplex)
- Intravenous immunoglobulin
- Ribavirin

Combination of intraventricular interferon alfa plus oral isoprinosine is the best effective treatment available.

Isoprinosine (Inosiplex)

Isoprinosine is an antiviral drug, which acts by activating the body's immunological system against measles virus. This drug increases the number of CD4+ lymphocytes, augments natural killer cells function, potentiates the function of interferons, and increases the production of interleukin-1 and interleukin-2. Treatment with isoprinosine remains controversial because of conflicting results.[74] Few uncontrolled studies have reported that isoprinosine prolongs the survival and produces clinical improvement in some patients.[75,76] Nunes *et al.* observed good results combining trihexyphenidyl and isoprinosine in controlling myoclonus refractory to sodium valproate.[77] This drug is administered in daily doses of 100 mg/kg/day and without major side effects. Recurrence of symptoms has been reported frequently; treatment needs to be continued even after apparent remission, possibly for life. Uric acid levels should be monitored, because isoprinosine can cause hyperuricaemia and renal stones.[35]

Interferon alfa

The pathophysiology of natural remissions and relapses in SSPE is unknown. The stable state may depend on a balance between viral replication and the body's immune response, as the state of the immune system has a role in producing remission. The cerebrospinal fluid interferon levels are found to be low in patients with SSPE. Exogenous administration of interferons possibly suppresses viral replication and augments the immune system of the body. Interferon alfa was initially given by the intravenous and intrathecal routes with questionable effect. Panitch et al. were the first to use the drug by the intraventricular route with the help of an Ommaya reservoir planted subcutaneously and a catheter placed in the frontal horn of the right lateral ventricle under general anaesthesia.[78] In this series, the authors found improvement in all the three patients; two of them, however, relapsed after completion of treatment.

The treatment regimen consists of six week courses of natural interferon alfa, started as 100 000 units/m^2 of body surface area and subsequently increased to 1 million units/m^2 body surface area per day given for five days a week. Courses are repeated up to six times, at 2–6 months intervals.

At present, combined treatment of oral isoprinosine and intraventricular interferon alfa appears to be a more effective treatment for SSPE.[79–81] Gokcil et al., in their recent article, reviewed 53 patients who had been treated by intraventricular interferon alfa with or without oral isoprinosine; 30 (59%) of these patients showed significant stabilisation or improvement.[66] They also reported better efficacy with a combination of oral isoprinosine and intraventricular interferon alfa even in adult patients with SSPE. Cerebrospinal fluid measles antibody, and renal and hepatic functions, need to be followed up during treatment. The laboratory end point of treatment is the eradication of detectable measles antibody from the cerebrospinal fluid. Systemic (subcutaneous) interferon alfa, in daily doses of up 5 million units, has been used with intrathecal interferon alfa simultaneously to treat peripheral reservoirs of measles virus and lymphoid and glandular tissue.

Side effects of interferon alfa include fever, lethargy, anorexia, and chemical meningitis. At times, treatment needs to be temporarily discontinued because of an increase in liver enzyme levels. Although, most of the patients treated with intraventricular interferon and oral isoprinosine have not shown side effects of a serious nature, prolonged repeated treatments do carry risks of developing meningitis, interferon alfa induced encephalopathy, and upper and lower motor neurone toxicity.[82]

Ribavirin

The antiviral drug ribavirin has been tested in animal models of SSPE and was found effective. Recently, this drug has been used in patients with SSPE. Tomoda et al. used a combined treatment of high dose intraventricular interferon alfa along with intravenous ribavirin in two non-responding cases of SSPE.[83] In both the patients no further progression was noted. In one patient the hypertonicity, bladder incontinence, and dysphagia improved three months after starting the combination treatment. Similarly, efficacy of high doses of ribavirin and intra-ventricular interferon alfa has been noted by Hosoya *et al.* in two patients.[84]

Other drugs used for the treatment of SSPE

Amantadine is an anti-RNA agent that retards the maturation of viruses by not allowing them to replicate. This drug is very well absorbed from the gastro-intestinal tract, and crosses the blood-brain barrier, but the response to treatment in few cases of SSPE is disappointing.[85] Cimetidine, an H^2-receptor antagonist, was used in the treatment of SSPE. Anlar *et al.* did not observe any worsening in seven cimetidine treated patients during a study period of two months, whereas seven patients in the placebo group deteriorated significantly.[86] In isolated reports interferon beta plus Inosiplex,[87] intravenous immunoglobulin,[88] plasmapharesis, and corticosteroids have been tried with variable results. These forms of treatment need more evaluation before they can be considered for regular management of SSPE.

Symptomatic treatment

Good general nursing care is the most important aspect in the management of SSPE. Anticonvulsants, like sodium valproate and clonazepam, are helpful in controlling the myoclonus. If spasticity is marked and affecting nursing care, baclofen and other antispasticity drugs may be used.

Prognosis

SSPE is a progressive disorder and death usually occurs in 1–3 years. Apart from this classical course, a chronic very slowly progressive form, a very fulminant form leading to death in weeks, and a 'stuttering' form of disease with remission and relapses, have been observed. Approximately 5% of the patients can have substantial spontaneous long-term improvement. Santoshkumar and Radhak-rishnan reported a women with SSPE with almost 17 months of progressive neurological deterioration to the extent that she was completely bedridden and incapable of self care.[73] She experienced a substantial spontaneous improvement; during the next seven years the patient became ambulatory and was independent for her daily activities. Grunewald *et al.* recently reported a 35-year-old patient who remained in remission for almost 25 years.[72]

Spontaneous remission may occur during any stage of the disease and last for a variable period of time before eventual relapse occurs. Santoshkumar and Radhakrishnan have noted the factors that may predict spontaneous remission and prolonged survival in SSPE.[73] The age of onset of SSPE less than 12 years, disappearance of periodic complexes, the tendency for normalisation of the background of follow-up EEGs, and a progressive increase in measles antibody titres in cerebrospinal fluid are the factors that appear to be associated with favourable outcome in SSPE. However, these observations need further evalu-ation. The exact mechanisms responsible for spontaneous improvement are not known.

Conclusion

SSPE is a slow virus infection caused by aberrant measles virus. This disease is still common in developing and underdeveloped countries. One of the most important limitations in treatment of SSPE is difficulty in recognising early manifestations of disease, when the inflammatory changes are, possibly, still reversible. Diagnosis is especially problematic in adult patients with SSPE; differential diagnoses are also different. Treatments available are very costly and are available only at a few centres in the world. Moreover, these treatments are not curative and only help in buying time for these patients. The families of patients with SSPE have a lot of physical, psychological, and economical stresses to endure. A great deal of external support is required for these suffering families to cope with these stresses. At present effective measles vaccination seems to be the only solution to the problem of this dreaded neurological disorder (*see* Box 7.4).

Box 7.4   Summary points

- SSPE is a slow virus disease caused by persistent mutant measles virus infection.
- It affects children, it is uncommon after 18 years of age, and the disease has a more aggressive course in adults.
- The disease is very rare in developed countries, but is still common in developing and poor countries.
- Measles vaccine is not associated with an increased risk of SSPE.
- A defective expression of either the matrix, the fusion, or the haemagglutinin proteins of measles virus is responsible for viral persistence in brain cells and its escape by immune surveillance mechanisms.
- Pathological changes involve both white and grey matter. Neurons and oligodendrocytes contain eosinophilic inclusion bodies. Marked gliosis occurs in brain along with perivascular lymphocytes and plasma cell cuffing.
- The disease starts with subtle mental deterioration followed by seizures, dementia, ataxia, stereotyped myoclonus, and visual disturbances, usually leading to a decorticated state, and death after 1–3 years.
- The EEG is characteristic and reveals periodic, stereotyped high voltage discharges occurring every few seconds.
- Cerebrospinal fluid shows raised gammaglobulin with IgG oligoclonal bands.
- Raised measles antibody titre in cerebrospinal fluid and serum is diagnostic.
- No curative treatment is available. Combination of intraventricular interferon plus oral isoprinosine is effective in halting the progression of the disease.
- Relapse is usually a problem even after good initial results.
- An effective measles vaccination is the only solution available to this fatal disease.

An adult patient with SSPE: case report

A 33-year-old previously healthy woman was admitted to the obstetrics ward complaining of blurring of vision during the 24th week of her first pregnancy. In the next three days behavioural changes and disorientation were observed, progressing to a drowsy state. She was transferred to the neurology ward. The patient's history was not suggestive of measles infection during early childhood.

General physical examination revealed pedal oedema and hypertension (160/94 mm Hg); a gynaecological examination disclosed a viable fetus consistent with gestational age. Her neurological evaluation revealed that the patient was drowsy, disoriented to time, place, and person, unable to answer simple questions properly, or count to 10. The patient was unable to perceive even hand movements or a beam of light. Examination of her optic disks revealed no abnormality. Pupils were of normal size and direct and consensual light reflexes were normal. Other cranial nerves were normal. Her gait was mildly ataxic, she had generalised hypertonia, all deep tendon reflexes were exaggerated, and both plantars were extensor. There was no sign of meningeal irritation.

Laboratory workup did not reveal any abnormality in blood and urine. Cranial computed tomography was normal. A possibility of eclamptic encephalopathy was considered and she was treated accordingly. She did not improve and became deeply comatose and developed left-sided hemiparesis in the next few days. On careful observation the patient had periodic stereotyped left-sided hemimyoclonic jerks involving her left shoulder, arm, and leg; she also had subtle hemifacial jerks with simultaneous closure of both the eyes. Brainstem reflexes were normal. She had frequent bouts of hyperpyrexia, tachycardia, hypertension, and irregular breathing. Electroencephalography was performed and revealed diffuse symmetrical slow wave activity. MRI revealed bilateral asymmetrical hyperintensity in T2-weighted images involving both occipital lobes (*see* Figure 7.3). Cerebrospinal fluid examination showed protein 0.6 g/l, glucose 3.2 mmol/l, and 3–4 cells, all mononuclear. Both serum and cerebrospinal fluid were strongly positive for antimeasles IgG antibodies. An assay of antimeasles IgM antibody assay by ELISA was also positive (value 1.857; positive >0.404, Novum kit).

In the next eight weeks the patient's condition remained unchanged. In the 32nd gestational week, spontaneous labour began and a dead fetus was delivered per vagina. Intrauterine death of the fetus was noted just before delivery. The patient's condition remained unchanged on symptomatic treatment. Eventually, decerebrate rigidity appeared, her autonomic instability worsened, she developed severe pulmonary infection, and died.

References

1 Greenfield JG. Encephalitis and encephalomyelitis in England and Wales during last decade. *Brain* 1950; **73**: 141–66.

2 Dawson JR Jr. Cellular inclusions in cerebral lesions of epidemic encephalitis. *Am J Pathol* 1933; **9**: 7–15.

3 Pette H, Doring G. Uber einheimische panencephalomyelitis vom charakter der encephalitis Japonica. *Deutsche Zeitschrift fur Nerven-heilk* 1939; **149**: 7–44.

4 Van Bogaert L. Une leocoencephalite sclerosante subaigue. *J Neurol Neurosurg Psychiatry* 1945; **8**: 101–20.

5 Bouteille M, Fontaine C, Vedrenne CL, *et al.* Sur un cas d'encephalite subaiguea inclusions. Etude anatomoclinique et ultra structurale. *Rev Neurol (Paris)* 1965; **113**: 454–8.

6 Horta-Barbosa L, Fuccillo DA, Sever JL, *et al.* Subacute sclerosing panencephalitis: isolation of measles virus from a brain biopsy. *Nature* 1969; **221**: 974.

7 Swoveland PT, Johnson KP. Subaute sclerosing panencephalitis and other paramyxovirus infections. In: Mckendall RR, ed. *Handbook of clinical neurology.* Vol 12(56). Virus diseases. Amsterdam: North Holland Publishing Company, 1989: 417–37.

8 Jabbour JT, Duenas DA, Sever JL, *et al.* Epidemiology of subacute sclerosing panencephalitis (SSPE): report of the SSPE registry. *JAMA* 1972; **220**: 959–62.

9 Saha V, John TJ, Mukundan P, *et al.* High incidence of subacute sclerosing panencephalitis in South India. *Epidemiol Infect* 1990; **104**: 151–6.

10 Radhakrishnan K, Thacker AK, Maloo JC, *et al.* Descriptive epidemiology of some rare neurological diseases in Benghazi, Libya. *Neuroepidemiology* 1988; **7**: 159–64.

11 Yakub BA. Subacute sclerosing panencephalitis (SSPE): early diagnosis, prognostic factors and natural history. *J Neurol Sci* 1996; **139**: 227–34.

12 Halsey NA, Modlin JF, Jabbour JT, *et al.* Risk factors in subacute sclerosing panencephalitis: a case-control study. *Am J Epidemiol* 1980; **111**: 415–24.

13 Miller C, Farrington CP, Harbert K. The epidemiology of subacute sclerosing panencephalitis in England and Wales 1970–1989. *Am J Epidemiol* 1992; **21**: 998–1006.

14 Zilber N, Kahana E. Environmental risk factors for subacute sclerosing panencephalitis (SSPE). *Acta Neurol Scand* 1998; **98**: 49–54.

15 Modlin JR, Halsey NA, Eddins DL, *et al.* Epidemiology of subacute sclerosing panencephalitis. *J Pediatr* 1979; **94**: 231–6.

16 Aaby P, Bukh J, Lisse IM, *et al.* Risk factors in subacute sclerosing panencephaltis: age- and sex-dependent host reactions or intensive exposure. *Rev Infect Dis* 1984; **6**: 239–50.

17 Dyken PR, Cunningham SC, Ward LC. Changing character of subacute sclerosing panencephalitis in the United States. *Pediatr Neurol* 1989; **5**: 339–41.

18 Baczko K, Lampe J, Liebert UG, *et al.* Clonal expansion of hypermutated measles virus in a SSPE brain. *Virology* 1993; **197**: 188–95.

19 Kirk J, Zhou A-L, McQuaid, S, *et al.* Cerebral endothelial cell infection by measles virus in subacute sclerosing panencephalitis: ultrastructural and in situ hybridization evidence. *Neuropathol Appl Neurobiol* 1991; **17**: 289–97.

20 McQuaid S, Kirk, Zhou A-L, *et al.* Measles virus infection of cells in perivascular infiltrates in the brain in subacute sclerosing panencephalitis; confirmation by non-radioactive in situ hybridization, immunocytochemistry and electron microscopy. *Acta Neuropathol (Berl)* 1993:**85**: 154–8.

21 Katz M. Clinical spectrum of measles. *Curr Top Microbiol Immunol* 1995; **191**: 1–12.

22 Scully RE, Mark EJ, McNeely BU. Case records of the Massachusetts General Hospital, case 25–1986. *N Engl J Med* 1986; **314**: 1689–700.

23 Lawrence DMP, Patterson CE, Gales TL, *et al.* Measles virus spread between neurons requires cell contact but not CD46 expression, syncytium formation, or extracellular virus production. *J Virol* 2000; **74**: 1908–18.

24 Hirano A. Subacute sclerosis panencephalitis virus dominantly interferes with replication of wild-type measles virus in a mixed infection: implication for viral persistence. *J Virol* 1992; **66**: 1891–8.

25 Carter MJ, Willcocks MM, ter Meulen V. Defective translation of measles virus matrix protein in a subacute sclerosing panencephalitis cell line. *Nature* 1983; **305**: 153–5.

26 Cattaneo R, Schmid A, Speilhofer P, *et al.* Mutated and hypermutated genes of persistent measles virus which caused lethal human brain diseases. *Virology* 1989; **173**: 415–25.

27 Ballart I, Huber M, Schmid A, *et al.* Functional and nonfunctional measles virus matrix genes from lethal human brain infection. *J Virol* 1991; **65**: 3161–6.

28 Hirano A, Ayata M, Wang AH, *et al*. Functional analysis of matrix proteins expressed from cloned genes of measles virus variants that cause subacute sclerosing panencephalitis reveals a common defect in nucleocapsid binding. *J Virol* 1993; **67**: 1848–53.

29 Sidhu MS, Crowley J, Lowenthal A, *et al*. Defective measles virus in human subacute sclerosing panencephalitis brain. *Virology* 1994:**202**: 631–41.

30 Billeter MA, Cattaneo R, Spielhofer P, *et al*. Generation and properties of measles virus mutations typically associated with subacute sclerosing panencephalitis. *Ann NY Acad Sci* 1994; **724**: 367–77.

31 Dorig RE, Marcil A, Chopra A, *et al*. The human CD[46] molecule is a receptor for measles virus (Edmonston strain). *Cell* 1993; **75**: 295–305.

32 Cattaneo R, Rose JK. Cell fusion by the envelope glycoproteins of persistent measles viruses, which caused lethal human brain disease. *J Virol* 1993; **67**: 1493–502.

33 Schmid A, Spielhofer P, Cattaneo R, *et al*. Subacute sclerosing panencephalitis is typically characterized by alterations in the fusion protein cytoplasmic domain of the persisting measles virus. *Virology* 1992; **188**: 910–15.

34 Cathomen J, Naim HY, Cattaneo R. Measles viruses with altered envelop protein cytoplasmic tails gain cell fusion competence. *J Virol* 1998; **72**: 1224–34.

35 Gascon GG, Frosch MP. Case records of the Massachusetts General Hospital: case 15–1998. *N Engl J Med* 1998; **338**: 1448–56.

36 Fujinami RS, Oldstone MB. Antiviral antibody reacting on the plasma membrane alters measles virus expression inside the cell. *Nature* 1979; **279**: 529–30.

37 Brown HR, Goller NL, Rudelli RD, *et al*. Post-mortem detection of measles virus in non-neural tissues in subacute sclerosing panencephalitis. *Ann Neurol* 1989; **26**: 263–8.

38 Anlar B, Soylemezoglu F, Elibol B, *et al*. Apoptosis in brain biopsies of subacute sclerosing panencephalitis patients. *Neuropediatrics* 1999; **30**: 239–42.

39 McQuaid S, McMahon J, Herron B, *et al*. Apoptosis in measles virus-infected human central nervous system tissues. *Neuropathol Appl Neurobiol* 1997; **23**: 218–24.

40 Allen IV, McQuaid S, McMahon J, *et al*. The significance of measles virus antigen and genome distribution in the CNS in SSPE for mechanisms of viral spread and demyelination. *J Neuropathol Exp Neurol* 1996; **55**: 471–80.

41 Ikeda K, Akiyama H, Kondo H, *et al*. Numerous glial fibrillary tangles in oligodendroglia in cases of subacute sclerosing panencephalitis with neurofibrillary tangles. *Neurosci Lett* 1995; **194**: 133–5.

42 McQuaid S, Allen IV, McMahon J, *et al*. Association of measles virus with neuro-fibrillary tangles in subacute sclerosing panencephalitis: a combined in situ hybridization and immunocytochemical investigation. *Neuropathol Appl Neurobiol* 1994; **20**: 103–10.

43 Ohya T, Martinez AJ, Jabbour JT, *et al*. Subacute sclerosing panencephalitis: correlation of clinical, neurophysiologic and neurophathologic findings. *Neurology* 1974; **24**: 211–18.

44 Nagano I, Nakamura S, Yoshioka M, *et al*. Immunocytochemical analysis of the cellular infiltrate in brain lesions in subacute sclerosing panencephalitis. *Neurology* 1991; **41**: 1639–42.

45 Norrby E, Kristensson K. Measles virus in the brain. *Brain Res Bull* 1997; **44**: 213–20.

46 Katayama Y, Kohso K, Nishimura A, *et al*. Detection of measles virus mRNA from autopsied human tissues. *J Clin Microbiol* 1998; **36**: 299–301.

47 Dyken PR. Subacute sclerosing panencephalitis. *Neurol Clin* 1985; **3**: 179–95.

48 Green SH, Wirtschafter J. Ophthalmoscopic findings in subacute sclerosing panencephalitis. *Br J Ophthalmol* 1973; **57**: 780–7.

49 Caruso JM, Robbins-Tien D, Brown W, *et al*. Atypical chorioretinitis as the very first presentation of subacute sclerosing panencephalitis. *Neurology* 1997; **48**(suppl):A286–A7 (abstract).

50 Park DW, Boldt HC, Messicotte SJ, *et al*. Subacute sclerosing panencephalitis manifesting as viral retinitis: clinical and histopathologic findings. *Am J Ophthalmol* 1997; **123**: 533–42.

51 Risk WS, Haddad FS. The variable natural history of subacute sclerosing panencephalitis: a study of 118 cases from the Middle East. *Arch Neurol* 1979; **56**: 610–14.

52 Dimova P, Bojinova V. Subacute sclerosing panencephalitis with atypical onset: clinical, computed tomography and magnetic resonance imaging correlations. *J Child Neurol* 2000; **15**: 258–60.

53 Mehta PD, Kane A, Thormer M. Quantification of measles virus specific immunoglobulins in serum, CSF and brain extract from patients with subacute sclerosing panencephalitis. *J Immunol* 1977; **118**: 2254–61.

54 Tourtellote WW, Ma BI, Brandes DB, *et al*. Quantification of de novo central nervous system IgG measles antibody synthesis in SSPE. *Ann Neurol* 1981; **9**: 551–6.

55 Reiber H, Lange P. Quantification of virus specific antibodies in cerebrospinal fluid and serum: sensitive and specific detection of antibody synthesis in brain. *Clin Chem* 1991; **37**: 1153–60.

56 Mehta PD, Thormar H, Kulcyzcki J, *et al*. Immune response in subacute sclerosing panencephalitis. *Ann NY Acad Sci* 1994; **724**: 378–84.

57 Salmi AA, Norrby E, Panelius M. Identification of different measles virus specific antibodies in serum and cerebrospinal fluid from patients with subacute sclerosing panencephalitis and multiple sclerosis. *Infection and Immunity* 1972; **6**: 248–54.

58 Abdelnoor AM, Dhip-Jalbut SS, Haddad FS. Different virus antibodies in serum and cerebro-spinal fluid of patients suffering from subacute sclerosing panencephalitis. *J Neuroimmunol* 1982; **2**: 27–34.

59 Lakshmi V, Malathy Y, Rao RR. Serodiagnosis of subacute sclerosing panencephalitis by enzyme linked immunosorbent assay. *Indian J Pediatr* 1993; **60**: 37–41.

60 Kuroiwa Y, Celesia G. Clinical significance of periodic EEG patterns. *Arch Neurol* 1980; **37**: 15–20.

61 Modi GH, Campbell BP. Subacute sclerosing panencephalitis. Changes on CT scan during acute relapse. *Neuroradiology* 1989; **31**: 433–4.

62 Tuncay R, Akman-Demir G, Gokygit A, *et al*. MRI in subacute sclerosing panencephalitis. *Neuroradiology* 1996; **38**: 636–40.

63 Anlar B, Saatci I, Kose G, *et al*. MRI findings in subacute sclerosing panencephalitis. *Neurology* 1996; **47**: 1278–83.

64 Brismar J, Gascon GG, von Steyern KV, *et al*. Subacute sclerosing panencephalitis: evaluation with CT and MR. *AJNR Am J Neuroradiol* 1996; **17**: 761–72.

65 Singer C, Lang AE, Suchowersky O. Adult-onset subacute sclerosing panencephalitis: case reports and review of literature. *Mov Disord* 1997; **12**: 342–53.

66 Gokcil Z, Odabasi Z, Demirkaya S, *et al*. α-Interferon and isoprinosine in adult-onset subacute sclerosing panencephalitis. *J Neurol Sci* 1999; **162**: 62–4.

67 Wirguin I, Steiner I, Kidron D, *et al*. Fulminant subacute sclerosing panencephalitis in association with pregnancy. *Arch Neurol* 1988; **45**: 1324–5.

68 Thiel A, Nau R, Fischer F, *et al*. Healthy infant delivered by a mother with subacute sclerosing panencephalitis during pregnancy. *Neurology* 1996; **46**: 1604.

69 PeBenito R, Naqvi SH, Arca MM, *et al*. Fulminating subacute sclerosing panencephalitis: case report and literature review. *Clin Pediatr (Phila)* 1997; **36**: 149–54.

70 Alexander M, Singh S, Gnanamuthu C, *et al*. Subacute sclerosing panencephalitis: CT and MR imaging in a rapidly progressive case. *Neurology India* 1999; **47**: 304–7.

71 Gokcil Z, Odabasi Z, Aksu A, *et al*. Acute fulminant SSPE. Clinical and EEG features. *Clin Electroencephalogr* 1998; **9**: 43–8.

72 Grunewald T, Lampe J, Weissbrich B, *et al*. A 35-year old bricklayer with hemi-myoclonic jerks. *Lancet* 1998; **351**: 1926.

73 Santoshkumar B, Radhakrishnan K. Substantial spontenous long-term remission in subacute sclerosing panencephalitis (SSPE). *J Neurol Sci* 1998; **154**: 83–8.

74 Campoli-Richards DM, Sorkin EM, Heel RC. Inosine pranobex: a preliminary review of its pharmacodynamic and pharmakinetic properties and therapeutic efficacy. *Drugs* 1986; **32**: 383–424.

75 Jones CE, Dyken PR, Huttenlocher PR, *et al*. Inosiplex therapy in subacute sclerosing panencephalitis. *Lancet* 1982; **i**: 1034–7.

76 Haddad FS, Risk WS. Inosiplex treatment in 18 patients with SSPE. A controlled study. *Ann Neurol* 1980; **7**: 185–8.

77 Nunes ML, da-Costa JC, da-Silva LF. Trihexyphenidyl and isoprinosine in the treatment of subacute sclerosing panencephalitis. *Pediatr Neurol* 1995; **13**: 153–6.

78 Panitch HS, Gomez-Plascencia J, Noris FS, *et al*. Subacute sclerosing panencephalitis remission after treatment with interferon. *Neurology* 1986; **36**: 562–6.

79 Gascon G, Yamanis S, Crowell J, *et al*. Combined oral isoprinosine-intraventricular alpha-interferon therapy for subacute sclerosing panencephalitis. *Brain Dev* 1993; **15**: 346–55.

80 Anlar B, Yalaz K, Oktem F, *et al*. Long-term follow-up of patients with subacute sclerosing panencephalitis treated with intraventricular alpha-inteferon. *Neurology* 1997; **48**: 526–8.

81 Cianchetti C, Marrosu MG, Muntoni F, *et al*. Intraventricular alpha-inteferon in subacute sclerosing panencephalitis. *Neurology* 1998; **50**: 315–16.

82 Cianchetti C, Fratta AL, Muntovi F, *et al*. Toxic effect of intraventricular interferon-alpha in subacute sclerosing panencephalitis. *Ital J Neurol Sci* 1994; **15**: 153–5.

83 Tomoda A, Shiraishi S, Hosoya M, *et al*. Combined treatment with interferon-alpha and ribavirin for subacute sclerosing panencephalitis. *Pediatr Neurol* 2001; **24**: 54–9.

84 Hosoya M, Shigeta S, Mori S, *et al*. High-dose intravenous ribavirin therapy for subacute sclerosing panencephalitis. *Antimicrob Agents Chemother* 2001; **45**: 943–55.

85 Robertson WC Jr, Clark DB, Karkesbery WR. Review of 32 cases of subacute sclerosing panencephalitis: effect of amantadine on natural course of disease. *Ann Neurol* 1980; **8**: 422–5.

86 Anlar B, Gucuyener K, Imir T, *et al*. Cimetidine as an immuno-modulator in subacute sclerosing panencephalitis. A double blind placebo-controlled study. *Pediatr Infect Dis J* 1993; **12**: 578–81.

87 Anlar B, Yalaz K, Kose G, *et al*. Beta-interferon plus inosiplex in the treatment of subacute sclerosing panencephalitis. *J Child Neurol* 1998; **13**: 557–9.

88 Gurer YK, Kukner S, Sarica B. Intravenous gamma-globulin treatment in a patient with subacute sclerosing panencephalitis. *Pediatr Neurol* 1996; **14**: 72–4.

Chapter Eight

Tuberculosis of the central nervous system

RK Garg

Tuberculous involvement of the brain and spinal cord are common neurological disorders in developing countries and have recently shown a resurgence in developed ones. Tuberculous meningitis is an important manifestation and is associated with high morbidity and mortality. Diagnosis is based on clinical features, cerebrospinal fluid changes, and imaging characteristics. Bacteriological confirmation is not possible in all cases and serological tests do not have sufficient sensitivity and specificity. The polymerase chain reaction shows promise for the future. Appropriate chemotherapeutic agents should be administered as early as possible, although there is no unanimity concerning chemotherapeutic regimens or optimal duration of treatment. The patient's clinical stage at presentation is the most important prognostic factor. The role of corticosteroids is controversial but they should be administered to all patients presenting in stage III. Surgical procedures are directed at management of the hydrocephalus. Focal lesions, intracranial tuberculomas, and tuberculous abscesses, are usually located in cerebral or cerebellar hemispheres, uncommonly in brainstem and very rarely in the spinal cord. They do not usually require surgical intervention and respond well to antituberculous treatment, along with corticosteroids.

Tuberculosis remains a major global problem and a public health issue of considerable magnitude. In recent times, there has been a resurgence of tuberculosis in both developing and developed countries. Several risk factors have been observed for this serious phenomenon. These include the increasing prevalence of HIV infection, overcrowding in the urban population and in abnormal communities (such as prisons, concentration camps, refugee colonies), poor nutritional status, appearance of drug-resistant strains of tuberculosis, ineffective tuberculosis control programmes, and an increase in migration from countries where tuberculosis is prevalent to the developed world. The incidence of tuberculosis varies from 9 cases per 100 000 population per year in the US to 110–165 cases per 100 000 population in the developing countries of Asia and Africa.[1–3]

Tuberculous involvement of the central nervous system (CNS) is an important and serious type of extra-pulmonary involvement. It has been estimated that approximately 10% of all patients with tuberculosis have CNS involvement.[4]

The incidence of CNS tuberculosis is directly proportional to the prevalence of tuberculous infection in general. In developing countries CNS tuberculosis is a disease of younger age group, usually childhood.[5]

Classification

It is extremely difficult to classify the varied manifestations of CNS tuberculosis. The classification given in Box 8.1 includes all well-accepted forms.

Pathogenesis of CNS tuberculosis

Most tuberculous infections of the CNS are caused by *Mycobacterium tuberculosis*. Less frequently, other mycobacteria may be involved. It is believed that the bacilli reach the CNS by the haematogenous route secondary to disease elsewhere in the body. Rich and McCordock,[6] on the basis of their clinical and experimental observations, suggested that CNS tuberculosis develops in two stages. Initially small tuberculous lesions (Rich's foci) develop in the CNS, either during the stage of bacteraemia of the primary tuberculous infection or shortly afterwards. These initial tuberculous lesions may be in the meninges, the subpial or subependymal surface of the brain or the spinal cord, and may remain dormant for years after initial infection. Later, rupture or growth of one or more of these small tuberculous lesions produces development of various types of CNS tuberculosis.[6,7] The specific stimulus for rupture or growth of Rich's foci is not known, although immunological mechanisms are believed to play an important role. Rupture into the subarachnoid space or into the ventricular system results in meningitis. The type and extent of lesions that result from the discharge of tuberculous bacilli into the cerebrospinal fluid (CSF) depend upon the number and virulence of the bacilli, and the immune response of the host. Infrequently, infection spreads to the CNS from a site of tuberculous otitis or calvarial osteitis. A study of immunological parameters showed a correlation between the development of tuberculous meningitis in children and significantly lower numbers of CD4 T-lymphocyte counts when compared with children who had primary pulmonary complex only.[8] The pathogenesis of localised brain lesions is also thought to involve haematogenous spread from a primary focus in the lung (which is visible on the chest radiograph in only 30% of cases). It has been suggested that with a sizeable inoculation or in the absence of an adequate cell-mediated immunity, the parenchymal cerebral tuberculous foci may develop into tuberculoma or tuberculous brain abscess.[9]

Tuberculous meningitis

Pathology

In tuberculous meningitis there is a thick, gelatinous exudate around the sylvian fissures, basal cisterns, brainstem, and cerebellum. Hydrocephalus may occur as a consequence of obstruction of the basal cisterns, outflow of the fourth ventricle, or occlusion of the cerebral aqueduct. Hydrocephalus frequently develops in children and is associated with a poor prognosis. The brain tissue immediately underlying the tuberculous exudate shows various degrees of oedema, perivascular infiltration, and a microglial reaction, a process known as 'border zone reaction'. The basal exudates of tuberculosis are usually more severe in the vicinity of the circle of Willis, and produce a vasculitis-like syndrome. Inflammatory changes in the vessel wall may be seen, and the lumen of these vessels may be narrowed or occluded by thrombus formation. The vessels at the base of the brain are most severely affected, including the internal carotid artery, proximal middle cerebral artery, and perforating vessels of the basal ganglion. Cerebral infarctions are most common around the sylvian fissure and in the basal ganglion. In the majority of patients the location of infarction is in the distribution of medial striate and thalamoperforating arteries. Haemorrhagic transformation of infarcted tissue is not unusual.[5,10–12]

Box 8.1   Classification of CNS tuberculosis

Intracranial
- tuberculous meningitis (TBM)
- TBM with miliary tuberculosis
- tuberculous encephalopathy
- tuberculous vasculopathy
- space-occupying lesions: tuberculoma (single or multiple); multiple small tuberculoma with miliary tuberculosis; tuberculous abscess

Spinal
- Pott's spine and Pott's paraplegia
- tuberculous arachnoiditis (myeloradiculopathy)
- non-osseous spinal tuberculoma
- spinal meningitis

Box 8.2   Diagnostic features of tuberculous meningitis[13]

Clinical
- fever and headache (for more than 14 days)
- vomiting
- altered sensorium or focal neurological deficit

CSF
- pleocytosis (more than 20 cells, more than 60% lymphocytes)
- increased proteins (more than 100 mg/dl)
- low sugar (less than 60% of corresponding blood sugar)
- India ink studies and microscopy for malignant cells should be negative

Imaging
- exudates in basal cisterns or in sylvian fissure hydrocephalus
- infarcts (basal ganglionic)
- gyral enhancement
- tuberculoma formation

Evidence of tuberculosis elsewhere

Clinical features

In most patients with tuberculous meningitis there is a history of vague ill health lasting 2–8 weeks prior to the development of meningeal irritation. These non-specific symptoms include malaise, anorexia, fatigue, fever, myalgias, and head-ache. The prodromal symptoms in infants include irritability, drowsiness, poor feeding, and abdominal pain. Eventually, the headache worsens and becomes continuous. Neck stiffness is reported by about 25% of patients, but meningismus is detected in a higher number of patients at the time of examination. Bulging fontanelles develop in infants, who become increasingly irritable. Nausea, vomiting and altered sensorium may develop. Continuous low-grade pyrexia is typically present in about 80% of patients. A prior history of tuberculosis is present in approximately 50% of children with tuberculous meningitis and 10% of adult patients.[5,10,13]

Cranial nerve palsies occur in 20–30% of patients and may be the presenting manifestation of tuberculous meningitis. The sixth cranial nerve is most commonly affected. Vision loss due to optic nerve involvement may occasionally be a dominant and presenting illness. Optochiasmatic arachnoiditis, third ventricular compression of optic chiasma (if hydrocephalus develops), optic nerve granu-loma, and ethambutol toxicity are possible factors for vision loss in these patients. Ophthalmoscopic examination may reveal papilloedema. Funduscopy may reveal choroid tubercles, yellow lesions with indistinct borders present either singly or in clusters. These choroid tubercles are more frequent with tuberculous meningitis associated with miliary tuberculosis and are virtually pathognomonic of tubercu-lous aetiology, although they are present in only 10% of patients in whom the meningitis is not associated with miliary involvement.[7,12]

Hemiplegia may occur at the onset of the disease or at a later stage. Quad-riplegia secondary to bilateral infarction or severe cerebral oedema is less common and occurs only at an advanced stage in a few patients. At times, abnormal movements may dominate the clinical picture. Choreiform or hemi-ballistic movements, athetosis, generalised tremors, myoclonic jerks, and ataxia have been observed, more commonly in children than in adults. Seizures, either focal or generalised, may occur during acute illness or months after treatment.[7]

As the disease progresses, increasing evidence of cerebral dysfunction sets in. Apathy and irritability tend to progress to increasing lethargy, confusion, stupor and coma. The terminal illness is characterised by deep coma, decerebrate or decorticate rigidity, and spasm.

Diagnosis

The abnormalities found in CSF of untreated patients with tuberculous meningitis are well described. Usually, there is a predominant lymphocytic reaction (60–400 white cells per ml) with raised protein levels (0.8–4 g/l). In the early stages of infection, a significant number of polymorphonuclear cells may be observed, but over the course of several days to weeks they are typically replaced by lymphocytes. There is a gradual decrease in the sugar concentration of the CSF, which is usually less than 50% of serum glucose concentration; the values may range between 18–45 mg/dl.[5,7,10,12,13] Definitive diagnosis of tuberculous menin-gitis depends upon the detection of the tubercle bacilli in the CSF, either by smear examination or by bacterial culture. It has been claimed that if large volumes of CSF are carefully examined the organism can be found in over 90% of centrifuged CSF specimens (*see* Box 8.3), the highest detection rates being achieved in ventricular fluid. With repeated examinations of sequential CSF examinations Kennedy and Fallon[14] reported tubercle bacilli in 87% of patients. In other series especially from developing countries bacteriological confirmation of the diagnosis could be achieved in as few as 10% of the cases.[5] Culture of the CSF for tubercle bacilli are not always positive. Rates of positivity for clinically diagnosed cases range from 25% to 70%. It requires several weeks before culture is positive for mycobacterium bacilli.

Because of frequent difficulty in detecting tubercle bacilli in smears or cultures of CSF, a number of tests have been developed to establish an early and definitive diagnosis.[15] In the past, radioactive bromide partition testing and identification of components of the mycobacterial cell wall (eg, tuberculostearic acid) have been reported to have a sensitivity and specificity over 90%. However, the clinical utility of these has not been found to be satisfactory. Antibodies against tubercle bacilli can be detected with enzyme-linked immunosorbent assay (ELISA) with variable success. The latex particle agglutination test, which allows the rapid detection of tubercle bacillus antigen in CSF, has been reported to be a simple and specific test.[16] The intradermal tuberculin skin test is helpful when positive. The test may, however, be falsely negative even in the absence of immunosuppression and in association with a positive reaction to common antigens used to determine anergy (e.g. *Candida* and mumps). The tuberculin skin test has been reported to be negative initially in 50–70% of cases and often becomes positive during therapy. The best method for diagnosing mycobacterial infection, however, is the polymerase chain reaction, in which cDNA probes are used to identify mycobacterial RNA or DNA sequences in CSF. This test is highly sensitive and specific in the diagnosis of tuberculous meningitis.[17]

Box 8.3   Methods to increase mycobacterial yield of CSF smear examination[18]

- examine the deposit on centrifugation of a 10 ml CSF sample
- examine the deposit for at least 30 min
- examine several CSF samples over a few days

Imaging

Computed tomography (CT) or magnetic resonance imaging (MRI) of the brain may reveal thickening and intense enhancement of meninges, especially in basilar regions. Ventricular enlargement is present in a majority of patients. The degree of hydrocephalus correlates with the duration of the disease. Infarcts are another characteristic imaging feature (*see* Figures 8.1 and 8.2) of tuberculous meningitis.[13] The reported frequency of infarcts demonstrated by CT varies from 20.5% to 38%, however, in general, the incidence of infarction is significantly higher on MRI than on CT. In addition, a large number of infarcts are seen to be haemorrhagic in nature on MRI, a finding not well documented on CT scan. The

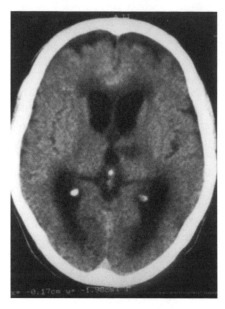

Figure 8.1 Contrast-enhanced CT of brain showing hydrocephalus and a right thalamic infarct.

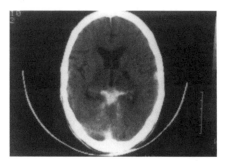

Figure 8.2 Contrast-enhanced cranial CT of a patient with tuberculous meningitis. Thick basilar exudate and an infarct in right thalamic region is seen.

majority of infarcts are seen in thalamic, basal ganglion, and internal capsule regions.[7] Thick basilar exudates appear as intensely enhancing areas in the basal cisterns (spider-leg appearance) (Figure 8.2) and in the sylvian fissures.[13] Tuberculomas are infrequently seen on CT or MRI of patients with tuberculous meningitis. Davis *et al.*[19] found tuberculomas in 16% of patients with culture-positive or presumptive tuberculous meningitis. Multiple small intracranial tuberculoma are frequent when tuberculous meningitis is part of miliary tuberculosis[20,21] (Box 8.4; Figure 8.3). The carotid or MR angiogram shows changes in vessels of the circle of Willis. These changes include uniform narrowing of large segments, small segmental narrowing, irregular beaded appearance and complete occlusion.[22] These vascular changes are due to either vasculitis or mechanical compression by the basilar exudate.

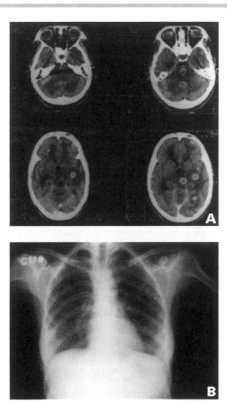

Figure 8.3 (A) Contrast-enhanced CT of brain showing multiple tuberculomas in a patient with tuberculous meningitis; (B) chest X-ray showing miliary shadows.

Tuberculous encephalopathy

Tuberculous encephalopathy, a syndrome exclusively present in infants and children, has been described by Udani and Dastur[23] in Indian children with pulmonary tuberculosis. The characteristic features of this entity are the development of a diffuse cerebral disorder in the form of convulsions, stupor and coma without signs of meningeal irritation or focal neurological deficit. CSF is largely normal or may show a slight increase in proteins and cells. Pathologically, there is diffuse oedema of cerebral white matter with loss of neurons in grey matter. A picture resembling haemorrhagic leukoencephalopathy or a post-infectious demyelinating encephalomyelitis may be observed.[11,23]

Intracranial tuberculoma

Tuberculomas are firm, avascular, spherical granulomatous masses, measuring about 2–8 cm in diameter. They are well limited from surrounding brain tissue which is compressed around the lesion and shows oedema and gliosis. The inside of these masses may contain necrotic areas composed of caseous material, occasionally thick and purulent, in which tubercle bacilli can be demonstrated. Intracranial tuberculomas can occur at any age. In developing countries young adults and children are predominantly affected while in developed countries they are more common in older patients. The symptoms produced by tuberculoma are related to their location. Low-grade fever, headache, vomiting, seizures, focal neurological deficit, and papilloedema are characteristic clinical features of supratentorial tuberculomas. Intratentorial tuberculomas are more common in children and may present with brainstem syndromes, cerebellar manifestations, and multiple cranial nerve palsies.[24-26]

On CT, tuberculomas are characterised as low or high-density and rounded or lobulated masses and show intense homogenous or ring enhancement after contrast administration. They have an irregular wall of varying thickness. Moderate to marked perilesional oedema is frequently present. Tuberculomas may be single or multiple and are more common in frontal and parietal lobes, usually in parasagittal areas. On CT, the 'target sign', a central calcification or nidus surrounded by a ring that enhances after contrast administration, is considered pathognomonic of tuberculoma.[27] In developing countries like India, tuberculomas are frequently confused with cysticercus granuloma. Rajshekhar *et al.*[28] used CT features to differentiate between these two conditions after establishing definite diagnoses by stereotactic brain biopsy. On CT scanning, tuberculoma measure more than 20 mm in diameter, are frequently irregular in outline, and are always associated with marked cerebral oedema (leading to midline shift) and progressive focal neurological deficit. The MRI features of tuberculoma depend on whether the lesion is non-caseating, caseating with a solid centre, or caseating with a liquid centre. The non-caseating granulomas are hypointense on T1-weighted images and hyperintense on T2-weighted images; after contrast administration the lesion usually shows homogenous enhancement. The second type of tuberculoma are hypointense or isointense on T1-weighted images and also on T2-weighted image. After contrast administration there is ring enhancement. These types of granuloma have variable degree of perilesional oedema. The tuberculoma with central liquefaction of the caseous material appears centrally hypointense on T1 and hyperintense on T2-weighted images with a peripheral hypointense ring which represents the capsule of tuberculoma (*see* Figures 8.4 and 8.5). Images after contrast administration show ring enhancement.[22] Stereotactic diagnostic biopsy can help in establishing an accurate diagnosis.[25]

Box 8.4 Case report: disseminated tuberculosis

A 30-year-old woman presented with headache, vomiting and fever (104°F) of 6 days duration. She was conscious, oriented and attentive, and had bilateral lateral rectus palsy along with bilateral papilloedema. Left plantar was extensor. Neck rigidity and Kernig's sign were present. Other systemic and general examinations were normal. All haematological and serum biochemical parameters, including liver function tests, were normal. Chest X-ray showed miliary shadows in both lungs (Figure 8.3B). CSF revealed elevated opening pressure, proteins 248 mg/dl, sugar 34 mg/dl (corresponding blood sugar was 98 mg/dl); 204 cells/ml, 15% polymorphs rest lymphocytes. CT head showed multiple small enhancing lesions in brain parenchyma (Figure 8.3A). The patient was given antituberculous treatment and corticosteroids. She showed significant improvement in all her symptoms after 15 days.

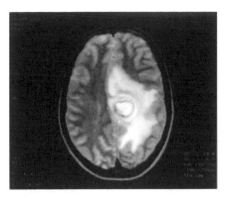

Figure 8.4 T2-weighted MRI of brain showing a large caseating tuberculoma in the parasagittal area of the left parietal lobe.

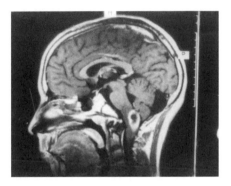

Figure 8.5 Sagittal T2-weighted cranial MRI showing a caseating tuberculoma in the medulla oblongata.

Intracranial tuberculous abscess

Tuberculous brain abscess is a condition distinct from CNS tuberculoma. In developing countries tuberculous abscesses have been reported in 4% to 7.5% of patients with CNS tuberculosis. The histopathological diagnosis of tuberculous brain abscess depends on the following criteria: microscopic evidence of pus in the abscess cavity, microscopic changes in the abscess wall, and isolation of *M tuberculosis*.[11,29] Abscesses are usually solitary and larger and progress much more rapidly than tuberculomas. CT and MRI pictures of a tuberculous abscess show a granuloma with a liquid centre, however, they are much larger and frequently multiloculated and with marked surrounding oedema. Clinical features include partial seizures, focal neurological deficit, and raised intracranial tension.[29] Surgical exploration and drainage of pus may produce excellent long-term results.

Pott's spine and Pott's paraplegia

It is estimated that involvement of the spine occurs in less than 1% of patients with tuberculosis. It is a leading cause of paraplegia in developing nations (*see* Box

8.5). Infection in the vertebral bodies usually starts in cancellous bone adjacent to an intervertebral disc or anteriorly under the periosteum of the vertebral body; the neural arch is rarely affected. Vertebral destruction leads to collapse of the body of the vertebra along with anterior wedging. Spinal cord compression in Pott's spine is mainly caused by pressure from a paraspinal abscess which is retropharyngeal in the cervical region (*see* Figure 8.6), and spindle shaped in thoracic (*see* Figure 8.7) and thoracolumbar regions. Neurological deficits may also result from dural invasion by granulation tissue and compression from the debris of sequestrated bone, a destroyed intervertebral disc, or a dislocated vertebra. Rarely, vascular insufficiency in the territory of the anterior spinal artery has also been suggested. Neurological involvement can occur at any stage of Pott's spine and even years later, when there has been apparent healing, because of stretching of the cord in the deformed spinal canal. The thoracic spine is involved in about 65% of cases, and the lumbar, cervical and thoracolumbar spine in about 20%, 10%, and 5%, respectively. The atlanto-axial region may also be involved in less than 1% of cases. Males are affected more often than females in most series, and the disease generally affects young persons.[30–32]

Typically, there is a history of local pain, tenderness over the affected spine or even overlying bony deformity in the form of gibbus. Paravertebral abscess may be palpated on the back of a number of patients. These patients usually have acute or subacute, progressive, spastic type of sensorimotor paraparesis. The incidence of paraparesis in patients with Pott's spine varies from 27% to 47%. Conventional spinal X-rays are usually adequate to demonstrate the destruction of adjacent vertebral bodies and intervening disc spaces. However, superior investigative modalities used for the diagnosis of Pott's paraplegia include myelography (*see* Figure 8.7), CT scan (*see* Figure 8.8), MRI (*see* Figure 8.9), and CT-guided needle biopsy. These help to define precisely the level of spinal involvement, amount of bone destroyed, morphology and extent of the paravertebral abscess and cord compression. Vidyasagar and Murthy,[32] who used only plain radiography, myelography, and CT scan, showed that myelography gave the best indication for spinal cord compression even when other superior investigative facilities were available. They found CT-guided needle biopsy to be very useful in establishing the aetiological diagnosis in their cases, picking up unexpected tumour metastases in several cases. A combination of surgical decompression and treatment with antituberculous drugs is needed for the majority of patients with Pott's paraplegia. A period of 12 months of postoperative antituberculous therapy is adequate.[30–33]

Box 8.5   Causes of parapalegia in CNS tuberculosis

- Pott's paraplegia
- non-osseous compressive myelopathies (tuberculoma): extradural, intradural, extramedullary, intramedullary
- transverse myelitis
- spinal meningitis
- spinal tuberculous abscess
- tuberculous arachnoiditis (myeloradiculopathy)
- syrinx formation

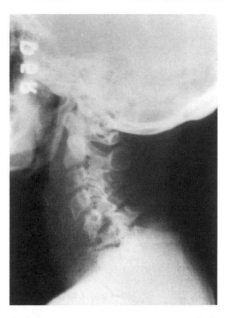

Figure 8.6 X-ray of cervical spine showing retropharyngeal abscess along with destruction of C6–7 vertebra.

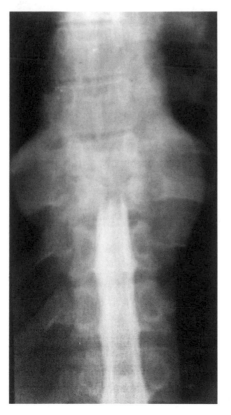

Figure 8.7 A lumbar myelogram showing spinal block at the level of T9 vertebra. A fusiform paravertebral swelling and destruction of T8 and T9 vertebra are also seen.

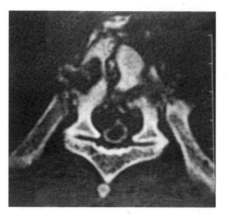

Figure 8.8 CT-myelogram showing extensive destruction of T9 vertebra, a paraspinal abscess producing spinal block.

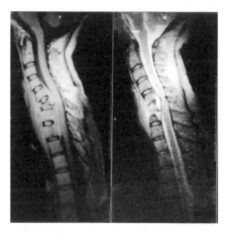

Figure 8.9 Sagittal T1-weighted MRI of two patients showing vertebral collapse of C6 and 7 vertebra along with posterior wedging and paraspinal abscess compressing the spinal cord.

Non-osseous spinal cord tuberculosis

Non-osseous spinal cord tuberculosis can occur in the form of tuberculomas. Dastur[34] reviewed 74 cases of tuberculous paraplegia without evidence of Pott's disease and observed that extradural tuberculomas occured in 64% while arachnoid lesions without dural involvement, and subdural/extramedullary lesions occured in 8% of patients in each group. Intramedullary tuberculomas are extremely rarely reported, reports from developing countries have also been sporadic. The clinical features are indistinguishable from those of any extra-medullary or intramedullary tumour, although acute worsening may occur. Intramedullary lesions are frequently located in the thoracic region. More than one site in the spinal cord may also be affected. One case with conus medullaris syndrome has been described. Non-osseous spinal cord tuberculomas may increase in size while the patient is on antituberculous therapy. MRI is the investigation of choice for these lesions.[34–37]

Spinal tuberculous meningitis

A predominantly spinal form of tuberculous meningitis may result from rupture of Rich's focus into the spinal arachnoid space rather than the basal meninges. The acute form presents with fever, headache, and radiating root pains, accompanied by myelopathy. The chronic form, usually localised to a few segments, presents with progressive spinal cord compression and may suggest a spinal cord tumour. The characterisic MRI features include CSF loculation and obliteration of the spinal subarachnoid space with loss of outline of spinal cord in the cervicothoracic region and matting of nerve roots in the lumbar region. Spinal forms of tuberculous meningitis may be associated with syrinx formation.[11,22,38]

Tuberculous arachnoiditis

Tuberculous arachnoiditis is a relatively common cause of myeloradiculopathy in countries where tuberculosis is endemic. The inflammatory exudate surrounds, but does not infiltrate, the spinal cord and nerve roots. Frequently, there is vascular involvement with periarteritis and occlusion of small vessels. Neuronal structures are damaged by direct compression as well as by ischaemia. The changes of arachnoiditis may be focal, multifocal, or diffuse. In tuberculous arachnoiditis features of spinal cord or nerve root involvement may predominate but most often there is a mixed picture. Frequently, there is clinical evidence of multifocal radiculomyelopathy, but even when meningeal involvement is widespread, symptoms may arise from a single level. The hallmark of diagnosis is the characteristic myelographic picture, showing poor flow of contrast material with multiple irregular filling defects, cyst formation, and sometimes spinal block. Rarely, myelography may be normal. The CSF changes are those of a chronic meningitis, frequently CSF sugar concentration is normal. Occasionally lumbar tap may be dry. These patients need adequate antituberculous treatment for at least one year. The role of corticosteroids is uncertain, but there are several reports of apparently marked improvement following corticosteroid administration. If the patient does not respond to medical treatment, surgery may be required.[38,39]

CNS tuberculosis in HIV-infected persons

Mycobacterium tuberculosis and atypical tubercle bacilli *Mycobacterium avium intracellulare* infection have been described as uncommon CNS manifestations of AIDS. The clinical spectrum of CNS tuberculosis with HIV infection includes meningitis, cerebral abscesses, and tuberculomas. CNS involvement occurs in 10–20% of patients with AIDS-related tuberculosis, and in these patients mortality is high. HIV-infected intravenous drug abusers are, in particular, at high risk of developing focal CNS tuberculosis. Clinical features, including imaging characteristics, are similar to those seen in patients without HIV infection (*see* Box 8.6). In patients with *M avium intracellulare* infection, single or multiple mass lesions appear to be more than twice as common as meningitis. Every effort should be made to establish the correct diagnosis as most types of CNS tuberculosis in HIV-infected patients are responsive to treatment.[29,40,41]

Box 8.6 CNS tuberculosis in AIDS: features

- CNS involvement in 10–20% of AIDS-related tuberculosis
- high mortality rate
- increased risk of tuberculous meningitis
- granulomas are less common than meningitis
- intravenous drugs abusers are at higher risk
- does not appear to alter the clinical course, response to therapy or prognosis
- infection with atypical mycobacteria is common

Treatment of CNS tuberculosis

In contrast to the rapid advances in the management of pulmonary tuberculosis, there have been only a few clinical studies in patients with CNS tuberculosis, including tuberculous meningitis. There is currently no consensus about the form of chemotherapy or optimal duration of treatment.

Penetration of antituberculous drugs into CSF

There is some evidence that the majority of current antituberculous drugs penetrate into the CSF. In the presence of meningeal inflammation, the CSF concentrations of these drugs are at least equal to or higher than those in non-inflamed meninges; intrathecal administration of these drugs is therefore not indicated. Isoniazid diffuses readily into the CSF in the presence or absence of meningeal inflammation. The CSF concentrations obtained are approximately 20–90% of serum levels. Levels of isoniazid in the CSF are lower in fast acetylators of the drug. Rifampicin achieves high serum levels after oral administration, and CSF levels are approximately 20% of serum in the presence of meningeal inflammation. Little or no ethambutol is detectable in the CSF of persons with normal meninges. However, in patients with meningeal inflammation, the ethambutol level approaches 10–50% of serum levels. Similarly, streptomycin is not detectable in normal meninges, while in patients with meningitis CSF levels may reach up to 20% of serum concentrations. Pyrazinamide, ethionamide and cycloserine penetrate well into the CSF, both in patients with meningeal inflammation, and in those with normal meninges.[42,43]

Treatment regimens

The Centers for Disease Control recommend[44] that treatment is started with isoniazid (10–20 mg/kg/day up to 300 mg), rifampicin (10–20 mg/kg/day, up to 600 mg/day) and pyrazinamide (15–30 mg/kg/day, up to 2 g a day). Patients should be monitored for hepatotoxicity from rifampicin or isoniazid which is seen in up to 20% of patients. Ethambutol or streptomycin may be added if the response is not satisfactory. The duration of therapy should be at least 6 months and in some instances up to 12 months' treatment is required. The World Health Organization (WHO)[18] put CNS tuberculosis under TB treatment Category 1, and recommend initial phase therapy (for 2 months) with streptomycin, isoniazid, rifampicin, and pyrazinamide, followed by a 7-month continuation phase with isoniazid and rifampicin. However, a number of other studies report varying experiences with short-course (6 months) treatment. As the emergence of neurological deficit has been seen in some of these studies, a minimum of 12 months of treatment would be worthwhile.[10] A similar drug regimen has been recommended for all forms of CNS tuberculosis. The optimal regimens for the treatment of CNS tuberculosis due to atypical mycobacteria in persons with HIV infection have not been finally established, although a four-drug regimen is needed to treat *M avium intracellulare* infection. Current recommendations include using azithromycin (500–100 mg/day) and clarithromycin (500 to 1000 mg/day) in combination with ethambutol (15 mg/kg/day) or clofazimine (100 mg/day). Alternative regimens include the use of ciprofloxacin and rifampicin. A significant increase in the frequency of adverse reactions to antituberculous therapy has been observed in patients with HIV infection.[7,45,46]

Role of corticosteroids

One of the controversial aspects of treatment of tuberculous meningitis is the use of corticosteroids.[47] The response to steroids may be dramatic with rapid clearing of sensorium, regression of abnomalities of CSF, defervescence, and relief of headache.[7] It was believed that corticosteroids had no place in the management of tuberculous meningitis because the drug did not alter the clinical outcome. However, more recent studies have shown that corticosteroids improved both survival rate and neurological outcome in patients with tuberculous meningitis.[47–49] Schoeman *et al.* confirmed the useful role of corticosteroids in young children. They observed that, in addition to survival, corticosteroids significantly improved intellectual outcome and enhanced resolution of the basal exudates and intracranial tuberculoma were shown by serial CT scanning. Prednisolone treatment (60 mg/day in adults and 1–3 mg/kg/day in children) is suggested in patients with tuberculous meningitis with one or more of the indications listed in Box 8.7. The dosage may reduced by 50% in the second and third week and then be tapered gradually over the next 4 weeks. There is no need for intrathecal corticosteroids.[47] The main argument against using corticosteroids is that they decrease meningeal inflammation and, in turn, can affect CSF penetration of antituberculous drugs. In a clinical trial[50] in which eight patients were treated with isoniazid, rifampicin, streptomycin, and pyrazinamide, in combination with corticosteroids (dexamethasone, 5 mg intravenously hourly during the first week, followed by oral prednisolone, 60 mg daily), the use of corticosteroids did not reduce the CSF concentration of any of the antituberculous drugs.[48]

Paradoxical worsening

It has been observed frequently that intracranial tuberculomas appear or paradoxically increase in size while patients are being treated for tuberculous meningitis. These lesions are usually discovered accidentally when follow-up CT scan is performed routinely or when new neurological signs develop during the course of antituberculous therapy.[51,52] A recent study[48] noted that about 8% of patients developed asymptomatic tuberculoma during the first month of treatment. Concomitant steroid therapy probably has a preventive role against these focal lesions. Paradoxical enlargement has also been observed in isolated intracranial tuberculoma while the patient was on antituberculous therapy. However, with continued treatment, eventual resolution of these tuberculoma occurs.[51,52]

Box 8.7 Indications for corticosteroids in tuberculous meningitis

- altered sensorium
- focal neurological deficit
- spinal fluid pressure in excess of 300 mmH$_2$O
- spinal block (CSF protein > 400 mg/dl)
- presence of tuberculomas
- basal exudates

Surgery

Surgical procedures in patients with tuberculous meningitis are primarily directed to the treatment of hydrocephalus.[47] Serial lumbar punctures, together with diuretics and osmotic agents, are useful as a temporary measure to relieve elevated intracranial pressure, thus probably preventing the progression of hydrocephalus. If these temporary steps fail, ventriculo-peritoneal or ventricu-loatrial shunting may relieve the signs and symptoms of hydrocephalus, and may bring considerable improvement in sensorium and neurological deficit. Shunts in these individuals may require revision because the high protein content of CSF causes blockage. As it is generally agreed that shunts can safely be inserted even in the presence of active disease, early shunting with drug therapy may offer the best therapeutic outcome.[7,12]

Intracranial tuberculomas that act as single space-occupying lesions with midline shifts and increased intracranial pressure, and that fail to respond to chemotherapy should be surgically removed. If the tuberculoma is totally removed, about 80% of patients will enjoy long-term recovery, particularly if they were treated in the early stage of the disease.[25,26]

Prognosis and sequelae

The single most important determinant of outcome, for both survival and sequelae, is the stage of tuberculous meningitis[47,53] at which treatment has been started (*see* Box 8.8). If treatment is started in stage I, mortality and morbidity is very low, while in stage III almost 50% of patients die, and those who recover may have some form of neurological deficit (*see* Box 8.9).[47] About 20% to 30% of survivors manifest a variety of neurological sequelae, the most important of which are mental retardation, psychiatric disorders, seizures, blindness, deafness, ophthalmoplegia, and hemiparesis. Endocrinopathies may become evident months or year after recovery. The endocrinopathies are most probably due to progressive damage of either the hypothalamus itself or adjacent basal cisterns. Obesity, hypogonadism, Frolich syndrome, sexual precocity, diabetes inspidus, and growth retardation have been reported. Intracranial calcification develops in 20% to 48% of patients with tuberculous meningitis, usually becoming detectable 2–3 years after the onset of the disease.[5,54]

Conclusion

Box 8.8   MRC staging of tuberculous meningitis[53]

Stage I: prodromal phase with no definite neurological symptoms

Stage II: signs of meningeal irritation with slight or no clouding of sensorium and minor (cranial nerve palsies), or no neurological deficit

Stage III: severe clouding of sensorium, convulsions, focal neurological deficit and involuntary movements

---

Box 8.9   Worst prognostic factors for tuberculous meningitis

Most important
Stage III (mortality 50–70%)

Others
• extreme of ages
• malnutrition
• presence of miliary disease
• presence of underlying debilitating disease, e.g. alcoholism
• hydrocephalus
• focal neurological deficit
• low CSF glucose levels
• markedly elevated CSF protein

The varied manifestations of CNS tuberculosis, a common neurological disorder in developing countries, have now become relevant for other parts of the world, as the whole spectrum of these disorders is now being reported worldwide. The increasing problem of drug resistance has added a new challenge. The early recognition and timely treatment of the disease is critical if the considerable mortality and morbidity associated with the condition is to be prevented.

References

1 Snider DE Jr, Roper WL. The new tuberculosis. *N Engl J Med* 1992; **226**: 703–5.
2 Harries AD. Tuberculosis and human immunodeficiency virus infection in developing countries. *Lancet* 1990; **335**: 387–90.
3 Raviglione MC, Snider DE, Kochi A. Global epidemiology of tuberculosis. Morbidity and mortality of a world wide epidemic. *JAMA* 1995; **273**: 220–6.
4 Wood M, Anderson M. Chronic meningitis. In: *Neurological infections; major problems in Neurology*. vol 16. Philadelphia: WB Saunders, 1998: 169–248.
5 Molavi A, LeFrock JL. Tuberculous meningitis. *Med Clin North Am* 1985; **69**: 315–31.
6 Rich AR, McCordock HA. Pathogenesis of tubercular meningitis. *Bull John Hopkins Hosp* 1933; **52**: 5–13.

7 Berger JR. Tuberculous meningitis. *Curr Opin Neurol* 1994; **7**: 191–200.

8 Rajajee S, Narayanan PR. Immunological spectrum of childhood tuberculosis. *J Trop Pediatr* 1992; **21**: 490–6.

9 Sheller JR, Des Prez RM. CNS tuberculosis. *Neurol Clin* 1986; **4**: 143–58.

10 Newton RW. Tuberculous meningitis. *Arch Dis Child* 1994; **70**: 364–6.

11 Dastur DK, Manghani DK, Udani PM. Pathology and pathogenetic mechanisms in neuro tuberculosis. *Radiol Clin North Am* 1995; **33**: 733–52.

12 Leonard JM, Des Prez RM. Tuberculous meningitis. *Infect Dis Clin North Am* 1990; **4**: 769–87.

13 Ahuja GK, Mohan KK, Prasad K, Behari M. Diagnostic criteria for tuberculous meningitis and their validation. *Tubercle Lung Dis* 1994; **75**: 149–52.

14 Kennedy DH, Fallon RJ. Tuberculous meningitis. *JAMA* 1979; **241**: 264–8.

15 Daniel TD. New approaches to the rapid diagnosis of tuberculous meningitis. *J Infect Dis* 1987; **155**: 599–607.

16 Krambovitis E, McIllmurray MB, Lock PE, Hendrickse W, Holzel H. Rapid diagnosis of tuberculous meningitis by latex particle agglutination. *Lancet* 1984; **2**: 1229–31.

17 Nguyen LN, Fox LFF, Pham LD, Kuijper S, Kolk AHJ. The potential contribution of polymerase chain reaction to the diagnosis of tuberculous meningitis. *Arch Neurol* 1996; **53**: 771–6.

18 Harries A, Maher D. *TB: a clinical manual for South East Asia*. Geneva: World Health Organization, 1997.

19 Davis LE, Rastogi KR, Lambert LC, Skipper BJ. Tuberculous meningitis in the south-west United States: a community based study. *Neurology* 1993; **43**: 1775–8.

20 Eide FF, Gean AD, So IT. Clinical and radiographic findings in disseminated tuberculosis of the brain. *Neurology* 1993; **43**: 1427–9.

21 Gee GT, Bazan III C, Jinkins JR. Miliary tuberculosis involving the brain: MR findings. *AJR* 1992; **159**: 1075–6.

22 Jinkins JR, Gupta R, Chang KH, Rodriguez-Carbajal J. MR imaging of central nervous system tuberculosis. *Radiol Clin North Am* 1995; **33**: 771–86.

23 Udani PM, Dastur DK. Tuberculous encephalopathy with and without meningitis: clinical features and pathological correlations. *J Neurol Sci* 1970; **10**: 541–61.

24 Talamas O, Del Brutto OH, Garcia-Ramos G. Brainstem tuberculoma. *Arch Neurol* 1989; **46**: 529–35.

25 Rajshekhar V, Chandy MJ. Tuberculomas presenting as isolated intrinsic brain stem masses. *Br J Neurosurg* 1997; **11**: 127–33.

26 Vengsarkar US, Pisipati RP, Parekh B, Panchal VG, Shetty MN. Intracranial tuberculoma and CT scan. *J Neurosurg* 1986; **64**: 568–74.

27 Van Dyk A. CT of intracranial tuberculomas with special reference to the 'target sign'. *Neuroradiology* 1988; **30**: 329.

28 Rajshekhar V, Haran RP, Prakash SG, Chandy MJ. Differentiating solitary small cysticercus granulomas and tuberculomas in patients with epilepsy: clinical and computed tomographic criteria. *J Neurosurg* 1993; **78**: 402–7.

29 Farrar DJ, Flanigan TP, Gordon NM, Gold RL, Rich JD. Tuberculous brain abscess in patient with HIV infection: case report and review. *Am J Med* 1997; **102**: 297–301.

30 Razai AR, Lee M, Cooper PR, Errico TJ, Koslow M. Modern management of spinal tuberculosis. *Neurosurgery* 1995; **36**: 87–98.

31 Nussbaum ES, Rockswold GL, Bergman TA, Erickson DL, Seljeskog EL. Spinal tuberculosis: a diagnostic and management challenge. *J Neurosurg* 1995; **83**: 243–7.

32 Vidyasagar C, Murthy HKRS. Management of tuberculosis of the spine with neurological complications. *Ann J Coll Surg Engl* 1994; **76**: 80–4.

33 Miller JD. Pott's paraplegia to day. *Lancet* 1995; **340**: 264.

34 Dastur HM. Diagnosis and neurosurgical treatment of tuberculous diseases of the CNS. *Neurosurg Rev* 1983; **6**: 111–19.

35 Mantzoros CS, Brown PD, Dembry L. Extraosseous epidural tuberculoma. Case report and review. *Clin Infect Dis* 1993; **17**: 1032–6.

36 Garg RK, Karak B, Misra S. Acute paraparesis with tuberculous meningitis. *Postgrad Med J* 1998; **74**: 269–71.

37 Gero B, Sze G, Sharif H. MR imaging of intradural inflammatory disease of spine. *Am J Neuroradiol* 1991; **12**: 1009–19.

38 Wadia NH. Radiculomyelopathy associated with spinal meningitis (arachnoiditis) with special reference to spinal tuberculous variety. In: Spillane JD, ed, *Tropical neurology*. London: Oxford University Press, 1973: 63–72.

39 Wadia NH, Dastur DK. Spinal meningitides with radiculomyelopathy. Part I: Clinical and radiological features. *J Neurol Sci* 1969; **8**: 239–60.

40 Berenguer J, Moreno S, Laguna F, *et al*. Tuberculous meningitis in patients infected with human immunodeficiency virus. *N Engl J Med* 1992; **326**: 668–72.

41 Dube MP, Holtom PD, Larsen RA. Tuberculous meningitis in patients with and without human immunodeficiency virus infection. *Am J Med* 1992; **93**: 520–4.

42 Donald PR, Gent WL, Seifart HI, Lamprecht JH, Parkin DP. Cerebrospinal fluid isoniazid concentrations in children with tuberculous meningitis: the influence of dosage and acetylation status. *Pediatrics* 1992; **89**: 247–50.

43 Ellard GA, Humphries MJ, Allen BW. Cerebrospinal fluid drug concentrations and the treatment of tuberculous meningitis. *Am Rev Resp Dis* 1993; **148**: 650–5.

44 Snider DE, Rieder HL, Combs D, Bloch AD, Hayden CH. Tuberculosis in children. *Pediatr Infect Dis J* 1988; **7**: 271–8.

45 Kemper CA, Meng TC, Nussbaum J, *et al*. Treatment of mycobacterium avium complex bacteremia in AIDS with a four drug regimen: rifampin, ethambutol, clofazimine and ciprofloxacin. *Ann Intern Med* 1992; **116**: 466–72.

46 Small PM. Schecter GF, Goodman PC, Sande MA, Chaisson RE, Hopewell PC. Treatment of tuberculosis in patients with advanced human immunodeficiency virus infection. *N Engl J Med* 1991; **324**: 289–94.

47 Holdiness MR. Management of tuberculous meninglitis. *Drugs* 1990; **39**: 224–33.

48 Schoeman JF, Vanzyl LF, Laubscher JA, Donald PR. Effect of corticosteroids on intracranial pressure, computed tomographic findings, and clinical outcome in young children with tuberculous meningitis. *Pediatrics* 1997; **99**: 226–31.

49 Kumarvelu S, Prasad K, Khosla A, Behari M, Ahuja GK. Randomized controlled trial of dexamethasone in tuberculous meningitis. *Tubercle Lung Dis* 1994; **75**: 203–7.

50 Kaojarern S, Supmonchai K, Phuapradit P, Mokkhavesa C, Krittiyanunt S. Effects of steroids on cerebrospinal fluid penetration of antituberculous drugs in tuberculous meningitis. *Clin Pharmacol Ther* 1991; **49**: 6–12.

51 Teoh R, Humhrie MJ, O'Mahoney G. Symptomatic intracranial tuberculomas developing during treatment of tuberculosis. a report of 10 patients and review of literature. *Q J Med* 1987; **63**: 449–53.

52 Pauranik A, Behari M, Maheshwari MC. Appearance of tuberculoma during treatment of tuberculous meningitis. *Jpn J Med* 1987; **26**: 332.

53 Medical Research Council. Streptomycin in tuberculosis trials committee. Streptomycin treatment of tuberculous meningitis. *Lancet* 1948; **i**: 582–96.

54 Wallace RC, Burton EM, Barrett FF, Leggiadro RJ, Gerald BE, Lasater OE. Intracranial tuberculosis in children: CT appearance and clinical outcome. *Pediatr Radiol* 1991; **21**: 241–6.

Chapter Nine

Diagnosis and treatment of viral encephalitis

A Chaudhuri and PGE Kennedy

Acute encephalitis constitutes a medical emergency. In most cases, the presence of focal neurological signs and focal seizures will distinguish encephalitis from encephalopathy. Acute disseminated encephalomyelitis is a non-infective inflammatory encephalitis that may require to be treated with steroids. Acute infective encephalitis is usually viral. Herpes simplex encephalitis (HSE) is the commonest sporadic acute viral encephalitis in the Western world. Magnetic resonance imaging of brain is the investigation of choice in HSE and the diagnosis may be confirmed by the polymerase chain reaction test for the virus in the cerebrospinal fluid. In this article, we review the diagnosis, investigations, and management of acute encephalitis. With few exceptions (for example, aciclovir for HSE), no specific therapy is available for most forms of viral encephalitis. Mortality and morbidity may be high and long-term sequelae are known among survivors. The emergence of unusual forms of zoonotic encephalitis has posed an important public health problem. Vaccination and vector control measures are useful preventive strategies in certain arboviral and zoonotic encephalitis. However, we need better antiviral therapy to meet the challenge of acute viral encephalitis more effectively.

The diagnosis of acute encephalitis is suspected in a febrile patient who presents with altered consciousness and signs of diffuse cerebral dysfunction. Worldwide, infection of the central nervous system is the commonest cause of acute encephalitis. Herpes simplex virus (HSV), varicella zoster virus (VZV), Epstein-Barr virus (EBV), mumps, measles, and enteroviruses are responsible for most cases of acute viral encephalitis among immunocompetent individuals in the United Kingdom. In a large Finnish study reported recently, VZV was found to be the commonest virus associated with encephalitis as well as meningitis and myelitis, comprising 29% of all confirmed or probable aetiological agents while HSV and enteroviruses accounted for 11% each and influenza A virus 7% of the cases.[1]

Tuberculosis, rickettsial diseases, and human African trypanosomiasis are important non-viral causes of meningoencephalitis but will not be covered in this article. Acute disseminated encephalomyelitis (ADEM) and its more severe form, acute haemorrhagic leucoencephalitis (AHLE) represent non-infective central nervous system inflammatory diseases. Non-inflammatory diffuse brain dysfunction is termed encephalopathy; metabolic dysfunction and intoxications are its best examples.

In encephalitis, a degree of leptomeningeal inflammation is invariably present and the clinical symptoms reflect both diffuse and focal cerebral pathology as well as meningitis (fever, headache, and signs of meningism). The degree of altered consciousness is a measure of the severity of acute encephalitis and may range from drowsiness to coma. Seizures, both focal and generalised, are common. In contrast to aseptic viral meningitis, neuropsychiatric symptoms often predominate in encephalitis, for example, anomia, hallucinations, psychosis, personality changes, and agitation. Acute encephalitis constitutes a neurological emergency and it is imperative that appropriate treatment is started as soon as possible based on the likely clinical diagnosis (*see* Box 9.1).

Establishing the diagnosis

Encephalopathy

The presence of fever in itself is not sufficient to make a diagnosis of infective encephalitis since encephalopathy may be precipitated by systemic infections or sepsis without cerebral inflammation (septic encephalopathy). Cerebral malaria is considered to be an example of infective encephalopathy rather than true encephalitis since the neurological symptoms of cerebral malaria result from brain hypoxemia and metabolic complications (hypoglycaemia and acidosis) due to the heavy parasitaemia of the red blood cells by *Plasmodium falciparum* leading to capillary occlusion.[2]

Patients with neuroleptic malignant syndrome have fever, altered consciousness, and nuchal rigidity and may present even after the offending neuroleptic has been withdrawn.[3] Traumatic brain injury and ongoing epileptic seizures must be excluded before making a diagnosis of acute encephalitis. Seizures are generalised in encephalopathy, although focal seizures and focal neurological deficit may rarely occur (for example, hypoglycaemic encephalopathy and hemiplegia). Clues must be sought to distinguish encephalitis from encephalopathy and Box 9.4 summarises a number of features that may help to make this distinction.[4,5] However, this distinction may not always be possible on clinical grounds.

Box 9.1 Clinical diagnosis

Acute or subacute onset global cerebral dysfunction: three diagnostic categories
- Infective encephalitis (typically viral; *see* Box 9.2).
- Encephalopathy (typically metabolic or toxic; *see* Box 9.3).
- Acute disseminated encephalomyelitis (ADEM).

The physician addresses three important questions:
- How likely is the diagnosis of encephalitis?
- What could be the cause of encephalitis?
- Which is the best treatment plan for the patient with encephalitis?

Box 9.2   Causes of infectious meningoencephalitis

Viral

DNA viruses: herpes simplex virus (HSV1, HSV2), other herpes viruses (HHV6, EBV, VZV, cytomegalovirus), and adenovirus (for example, serotypes 1, 6, 7, 12, 32).

RNA viruses: influenza virus (serotype A), enterovirus (for example, serotypes 9, 71), poliovirus, measles, rubella, mumps, rabies, arboviruses (for example, Japanese B encephalitis, La Crosse strain of California virus, St Louis encephalitis virus, West Nile encephalitis virus, lymphocytic choriomeningitis virus, Eastern, Western, and Venezuelan equine encephalitis viruses), reovirus (Colorado tick fever virus), and retrovirus (HIV).

Bacterial

Mycobacterium tuberculosis, Mycoplasma pneumoniae, Listeria monocytogenes, Borrelia burgdorferi (Lyme disease), *Tropheryma whippeli* (Whipple's disease), *Bartonella henselae* (cat scratch fever), leptospira, brucella (particularly *Brucella melitensis*), legionella, *Salmonella typhi* (typhoid fever), nocardia, actinomyces, *Treponema pallidum* (meningovascular syphilis), and all causes of bacterial (pyogenic) meningitis.

Rickettsial

Rickettsia rickettsii (Rocky Mountain spotted fever), *Rickettsia typhi* (endemic typhus), *Rickettsia prowazekii* (epidemic typhus), *Coxiella burnetii* (Q fever), *Erlichia chaffeensis* (human monocytic erlichiosis).

Fungal

Cryptococcosis, coccidioidomycosis, histoplasmosis, North American blastomycosis, candidiasis.

Parasitic

Human African trypanosomiasis, *Toxoplasma gondii, Nagleria fowleri, Echinococcus granulosus*, schistosomiasis.

Acute disseminated encephalomyelitis (ADEM)

ADEM is characterised by focal neurological signs and a rapidly progressive course in a usually apyrexial patient, usually with a history of febrile illness or immunisation preceding the neurological syndrome by days or weeks (post-infectious or postvaccinal encephalomyelitis). ADEM may be distinguished from infective encephalitis by the younger age of the patient, prodromal history of vaccination or infection, absence of fever at the onset of symptoms, and the presence of multifocal neurological signs affecting optic nerves, brain, spinal cord, and peripheral nerve roots. A syndrome of isolated acute ataxia due to post-infectious meningocerebellitis in children (acute ataxia of childhood) is commonly associated with VZV infection (chickenpox). Acute childhood cerebellar syndrome has also been reported after enterovirus, EBV, mycoplasma and, rarely, after HSV infection. This syndrome is relatively abrupt in onset and may be associated with confusion and corticospinal signs in addition to the cerebellar symptoms (gait ataxia, limb ataxia, dysarthria, and nystagmus).[6] In the latter cases, neuroimaging is usually normal and the cerebrospinal fluid typically shows a mild pleocytosis with raised protein. Despite some ambiguity as to whether the acute cerebellar syndrome is infectious or postinfectious, it is currently held to be a benign variant of ADEM. Early treatment of ADEM with large doses of steroids (intravenous injections of methylprednisolone at a dose of 500 mg daily for 5–7 days in adults) may possibly improve the outcome of severe ADEM, although few controlled trials of steroid therapy in ADEM have been undertaken.[7]

Box 9.3   Common causes of encephalopathy

- Anoxic/ischaemic.
- Metabolic.
- Nutritional deficiency.
- Toxic.
- Systemic infections
- Critical illness.
- Malignant hypertension.
- Mitochondrial cytopathy (Reye's and MELAS syndromes).
- Hashimoto's encephalopathy.
- Paraneoplastic.
- Neuroleptic malignant syndrome.
- Traumatic brain injury.
- Epileptic (non-convulsive status).

Box 9.4   Helpful diagnostic pointers for encephalopathy

- Absence of fever, headache, and meningism.
- Steady deterioration of mental status.
- Absence of focal neurological signs or focal seizures (except hypoglycaemia).
- Characteristic biochemical abnormalities in blood and urine.
- No peripheral leucocytosis.
- Normal cerebrospinal fluid.
- Diffuse slowing in electroencephalography.
- Normal magnetic resonance imaging.

Infective encephalitis

The diagnosis of infective encephalitis should be based on positive evidence and not by exclusion. Infective encephalitis may be the obvious diagnosis in a patient presenting with an abrupt history of fever and headache progressing to declining mental status with development of focal neurological symptoms and focal seizures. However, establishing the diagnosis of central nervous system infection can be difficult. Because herpes simplex encephalitis (HSE) is the most common cause of sporadic acute viral encephalitis, it is now a common practice to start treatment with aciclovir once a diagnosis of infective encephalitis is clinically suspected even if the aetiology of the infective agent is unknown. However, there is no therapeutic benefit from the use of aciclovir in non-herpetic encephalitis.

Establishing the cause of infective encephalitis

This requires a careful and systematic assessment of the patient (*see* Box 9.5).

Box 9.5   Evaluation of a patient with infective encephalitis

History
- Geographic and seasonal factors.
- Foreign travel or migration history.
- Contact with animals (for example, farm house) or insect bites.
- Immune status.
- Occupation.

Clinical signs
- General: skin and mucous membrane, lymph nodes.
- Neurological: focal cortical, brain stem, autonomic signs.

Investigations
- Blood (biochemical and haematological), chest radiography.
- Electroencephalography.
- Computed tomography, magnetic resonance imaging of head (with contrast).
- Single photon emission computed tomography (SPECT, optional, depending on availability).
- Cerebrospinal fluid: cells, biochemistry, and molecular diagnostic tests (polymerase chain reaction).
- Brain biopsy (in a very few selected cases).

History

A detailed history needs to be taken from the relatives since a patient with encephalitis is likely to be confused, disorientated, delirious, or comatose. Both the geographical distribution and seasonal occurrence may offer important clues.[4]

Japanese encephalitis is endemic in the Asian countries and often exhibits a seasonal pattern with cases peaking at the rainy season. Occasionally farm animal diseases might indicate a possible risk of viral encephalitis in the community because animals act as reservoirs for certain types of viruses causing encephalitis in humans. The 1999 outbreak of West Nile virus encephalitis in New York[8] was preceded by the death of city birds due to avian encephalitis. Four weeks after the outbreak of human encephalitis, specimens obtained from a Chilean flamingo in a nearby zoo identified the flavivirus as the cause of the West Nile virus encephalitis affecting both birds and humans.[9] Emerging infections due to the Nipah virus and the avian influenza viruses had also posed potentially serious risk of encephalitis in specific geographical areas.[10]

It is essential that a history should always be sought for recent foreign travel, insect or animal bites, and possible contact with individuals suffering from infectious diseases. The underlying medical condition is also relevant since immunosuppressed individuals are more susceptible to certain specific infective encephalitis, for example, listeriosis, cryptococcus, and cytomegalovirus. Cyto-megalovirus encephalitis is common in HIV-infected patients, particularly in neonates.[11] The mode of onset and progression of the viral illness may provide valuable clues to the aetiology, for example, biphasic course of the enterovirus infection.[12] Neurological complications of viral haemorrhagic fevers are often caused by aseptic meningitis and intracerebral bleed. Rabies is an example of a zoonotic encephalitis that presents with very distinctive clinical symptoms (hydrophobia and aerophobia), or rarely, as an ascending paralysis simulating Guillain-Barré syndrome.[13] Early neurological symptoms of human African trypanosomiasis (irritability, sleep disorder, changes in personality) are indis-tinguishable from viral encephalitis and may be associated with deep hyper-aesthesia of the soft tissues, especially in Europeans.[14] Important clues may also be provided by the occupational history, for example, Lyme disease or Kyanasur Forest disease in a forestry worker inhabiting an appropriate geographical area.

Clinical signs

General examination

Skin rashes are common in rickettsial fever, varicella zoster and Colorado tick fever. Parotitis often occurs with mumps and erythema nodosum may be associated with granulomatous infections (tuberculosis and histoplasmosis). Mucous membrane lesions are common in herpes virus infections. Concurrent or prodromal upper respiratory tract infecion is characteristic of influenza virus and mycoplasma.

Neurological examination

Neurological signs in acute encephalitis do not reliably identify the underlying aetiology despite the propensity of certain neurotropic viruses to affect specific focal areas of the central nervous system. The most commonly reported focal abnormalities are hemiparesis, aphasia, ataxia, pyramidal signs (brisk tendon reflexes and extensor plantar responses), cranial nerve deficits (oculomotor and facial), involuntary movements (myoclonus and tremors), and partial seizures. The evolution of the clinical signs will depend on the virus, the age, and the immune status of the patient. In general, the very young and the very old have the most serious clinical manifestations of encephalitis. A constellation of frontotemporal signs with aphasia, personality change, and focal seizures is characteristic of HSE. The presence of multifocal lower motor neurone signs in a febrile patient might indicate poliomyelitis. Symptoms of autonomic or hypothalamic dysfunction may also be seen in acute encephalitis. These include loss of temperature and vasomotor control (dysautonomia), diabetes insipidus, and the syndrome of inappropriate secretion of antidiuretic hormone.

Investigations

General

Relative lymphocytosis in the peripheral blood is common in viral encephalitis. Leukopenia and thrombocytopenia are characteristic of rickettsial infections and viral haemorrhagic fevers. The most sensitive and specific test for cerebral malaria is the peripheral blood film and both thick and thin peripheral smears are necessary. Peripheral blood monocytes may reveal the characteristic cytoplasmic inclusions in patients with human monocytic ehrlichiosis, 10% of whom are known to develop a meningoencephalitic syndrome.[15] Chest radiography is also advisable in all patients with acute encephalitis. Characteristic changes on chest radiography may point to the possibility of mycoplasma, legionella, or tuberculous infections.

Electroencephalography (EEG)

EEG is strongly recommended in any suspected case of acute encephalitis since it may help in distinguishing focal encephalitis from generalised encephalopathy. In the latter, EEG shows diffuse, bihemispheric slow wave forms, for example, triphasic slow waves in hepatic encephalopathy. EEG is invariably abnormal in HSE, though earlier the changes may be non-specific (slowing) with more characteristic changes (2–3 Hz periodic lateralised epileptiform discharges originating from the temporal lobes) limited to about half the cases in the later stages.

Neuroimaging

Brain imaging is now an established practice in patients with suspected acute encephalitis and usually precedes any other specific investigations. Magnetic resonance imaging is the cranial imaging of choice in acute encephalitis, although it may be simpler to obtain a computed tomogram quickly and easily in restless patients. Characteristic neuroimaging changes may offer clues as to the specific infective aetiologies – for example, frontotemporal changes in HSE and thalamic haemorrhage in Japanese encephalitis. Small haemorrhagic changes and pathognomonic lesions in the limbic system in HSE are visualised better on magnetic resonance imaging than on computed tomography.[16] Meningeal and gyral enhancement after Gd-DTPA administration has been reported in HSE.[17] Changes in magnetic resonance imaging in Eastern equine encephalitis are characterised by disseminated lesions in the brainstem and basal ganglia.

Box 9.6   Neuroimaging and EEG in acute encephalitis

Neuroimaging
- Magnetic resonance imaging is the imaging of choice and should be considered as an emergency.
- Magnetic resonance imaging appearances may be diagnostic (HSE, Eastern equine encephalitis, Japanese encephalitis).

- Computed tomography is the logical choice if on-site magnetic resonance imaging facility is not available or patient is restless.
- Cerebral SPECT scanning (HmPAO) is an optional test for suspected HSE and may have prognostic value.

EEG
- May help in the differential diagnosis of encephalitis v encephalopathy.
- Some EEG changes may be relatively specific (for example, periodic lateralised epileptiform discharges (PLEDS) in HSE or triphasic slow waves in hepatic encephalopathy).

Functional neuroimaging

Bitemporal hyperperfusion in the cerebral blood flow study using technetium-labelled hexamethylpropyleneamineoxime (^{99m}Tc-HmPAO) and single photon emission computed tomography (SPECT) may offer supportive evidence favouring the diagnosis of HSE.[18] Temporal lobe hyperperfusion in the ^{99m}TcHmPAO cerebral SPECT scan is a sensitive marker of HSE and the changes often persist beyond clinical recovery.[19] This test may be considered where facilities exist and is of particular value in cases where the symptom onset is relatively subacute because brain magnetic resonance imaging in paraneoplastic limbic encephalitis may mimic changes seen in HSE. An early study of localised $^1H^1$-proton magnetic resonance spectroscopy was promising in assessing the neuronal loss due to HSE.[17]

Cerebrospinal fluid analysis by lumbar puncture

This is an essential part of the investigation of encephalitis and should be the next logical step after neuroimaging provided it is considered safe. While cerebrospinal fluid abnormalities support the diagnosis of a meningoencephalitic syndrome, the changes in the cerebrospinal fluid constituents are often non-specific and may not be helpful in securing a specific aetiological diagnosis in many cases. Cerebrospinal fluid in viral encephalitis typically shows a lymphocytic pleocytosis with normal glucose and normal or mildly raised protein. The cerebrospinal fluid profile in acute viral encephalitis is indistinguishable from aseptic meningitis. Cerebrospinal fluid pleocytosis (>5 lymphocytes/mm^3) is present in >95% cases of acute viral encephalitis.[5,19]

Absence of cerebrospinal fluid lymphocytosis should alert to an alternative aetiology (encephalopathy). A caveat to this is the possibility that the cells in the cerebrospinal fluid might lyse during the storage and transport of the sample if the analysis was delayed. Initial cerebrospinal fluid pleocytosis may be absent in atypical HSE. Patients who are immunocompromised (for example, by cancer chemotherapy or irradiation) often fail to mount an inflammatory response. The cell count in cerebrospinal fluid exceeds 500/mm^3 in 10% cases of acute viral encephalitis.[20]

Box 9.7   Lumbar puncture in acute encephalitis

Essential to confirm the pathology of meningoencephalitis (cerebrospinal fluid lymphocytosis).

Must await neuroimaging (computed tomography/magnetic resonance imaging).

During the procedure
- Measurement of cerebrospinal fluid opening pressure is important.
- Samples must be dispatched immediately for cell counts and morphology.
- Gram stain as well as acid and alcohol fast bacilli (AAFB) stain should be requested routinely.
- Simultaneous blood glucose sample must be collected.

Microbiological tests in cerebrospinal fluid
- Polymerase chain reaction for HSV, VZV, and M tuberculosis.
- Enteroviruses (appropriate cases).
- Polymerase chain reaction for cytomegalovirus and cryptococcal antigen test (especially if immunosuppressed).
- Specific viral antigen and antibody (*see* text).

Lumbar puncture should be delayed
- If computed tomography/magnetic resonance imaging is indicative of raised intracranial pressure.
- If patient has convulsive status epilepticus.
- Soon after a generalised seizure.
- If coagulopathy or severe thrombocytopenia (for example, haemorrhagic fever) is present.

A high cerebrospinal fluid lymphocytosis might indicate tuberculous meningitis, mumps encephalitis, or uncommon viruses – for example, Eastern equine encephalitis, California encephalitis, lymphocytic choriomeningitis virus; atypical lymphocytes in cerebrospinal fluid are occasionally seen in[20] EBV, cytomegalovirus, and rarely in HSV encephalitis. The presence of a higher number of polymorphonuclear leucocytes in the cerebrospinal fluid after first 48 hours indicates bacterial meningitis as the likely aetiology. Other than bacterial meningitis, cerebrospinal fluid polymorphonuclear leucocytosis may be present in ADEM and AHLE, primary amoebic meningoencephaltis due to *Naegleria fowlerii*, and occasionally in enteroviral, echovirus 9, and Eastern equine virus encephalitis. Approximately 20% of patients with acute encephalitis will have an excess of red blood cells (>500/mm^3) in the cerebrospinal fluid in the absence of a traumatic tap.[20] This is typically associated with necrotising and haemorrhagic encephalitis (HSE and AHLE), listerial and primary amoebic meningoencephalitis. Cerebrospinal fluid xanthochromia is more typical of tuberculous meningitis and is rarely seen in HSE. However, presence or absence of red cells or xanthochromia is of virtually no use in discriminating HSE from other causes of acute encephalitis.[21] Any significant reduction in cerebrospinal fluid glucose (as a ratio of the corresponding plasma glucose) is unusual in viral encephalitis.

Cerebrospinal fluid lymphocytic pleocytosis and reduced glucose is highly characteristic of tuberculous meningoencephalitis. A low cerebrospinal fluid glucose is also seen in other bacterial, fungal, parasitic, or neoplastic meningo-encephalitis, occasionally in mumps and lymphocytic choriomeningitis virus encephalitis, and very rarely in the late stages of HSE.[22] Differentiating viral encephalitis from tuberculous meningoencephalitis may be difficult in the endemic areas, especially in children because cerebrospinal fluid lymphocytosis is common in both the conditions and the yield for smear positivity of *M tuberculosis* in the cerebrospinal fluid is low. In this situation, serial samples of cerebrospinal fluid and contrast enhanced neuroimaging (computed tomography/magnetic resonance imaging) may offer the only opportunity to distinguish tuberculous meningoencephalitis from viral encephalitis.

Cerebrospinal fluid virological studies

Measuring anti-HSV antibodies in the cerebrospinal fluid may be diagnostically useful, but detectable cerebrospinal fluid antibody levels usually develop after the first week of the illness. These assays are of little use, therefore, within the first few days of the illness when early diagnosis and treatment are essential.[22] There are several problems with the interpretations of serum and cerebrospinal fluid viral antibodies.[23] These tests take time to perform and a clinician would be best advised not to wait for these results before initiating treatment. Rises in antiviral antibody titres may be non-specific and indicate polyclonal activation due to the infection. Also, raised antiviral antibodies in a single serum sample may reflect persistent viral antibody levels from previous infection, or reactivation rather than a primary infection. Further, precise timing of the paired samples may be difficult; false negative results may occur and do not exclude the diagnosis of infective encephalitis.

More recently, diagnostic polymerase chain reaction for viral DNA amplification technique has significantly facilitated the diagnosis of infective encephalitis. Cerebrospinal fluid polymerase chain reaction is diagnostic for encephalitis due to HSV, VZV, cytomegalovirus, and EBV. There are several advantages of the polymerase chain reaction technique. This technique is exquisitely sensitive for the presence of viral genome in spinal fluid, can be rapidly accomplished (within 6–8 hours), requires only a very small volume of cerebrospinal fluid, and is highly specific for certain viruses – for example, HSV since the primers, if appropriately chosen, will not amplify DNA sequences from other viruses.[22]

Brain biopsy

Isolation of HSV from brain tissue obtained at biopsy was previously considered the gold standard for the diagnosis of HSE. Brain biopsy was a part of all the major treatment trials of HSE conducted by the National Institutes of Allergy and Infectious Diseases Collaborative Antiviral Study Group (NINAID-CASG) in the 1980s.[24,25] In these trials, 1 cm^3 of the brain tissue was obtained from the anterior portion of the involved inferior temporal gyrus by subtemporal craniectomy under general anaesthesia. The sensitivity of the brain biopsy in HSE exceeds 95% with specificity greater than 99%. Brain biopsy in acute encephalitis was routinely advocated during the days when vidarabine was the only therapeutic agent in HSE. The introduction of aciclovir early in the treatment of HSE has largely rendered this policy unnecessary. Presently, brain biopsy in the setting of acute encephalitis may still have to be considered only if the diagnosis of HSE itself is doubtful. Brain biopsy in acute encephalitis may also be considered when surgical decompression is the treatment of choice for raised intracranial pressure refractory to medical management.

Selected syndromes of viral encephalitis

HSE is the commonest acute meningoencephalitis in the Western world[26,27] and will be discussed below because of its clinical importance. Two other types of viral encephalitis will also be briefly covered; the first as a representative example of encephalitis in an immunocompromised host (cytomegalovirus encephalitis) and the other as an emerging zoonotic encephalitis (Nipah virus encephalitis).

Herpes simplex encephalitis

The annual incidence of HSE approximates 2000 cases in the USA alone.[27] HSV-1 accounts for more than 90% of childhood and adult cases of HSE. In contrast, HSV-2 is responsible for most neonatal and occasional adult cases of HSE. Unlike HSV-1, HSV-2 is a common cause of aseptic meningitis (usually in patients with primary genital herpes) and both HSV-1 and HSV-2 have been implicated in patients with recurrent meningitis (Mollaret meningitis).[28] Neonatal HSE results from the disseminated HSV-2 infection in the newborn acquired during the genital passage at the time of delivery. HSE can occur at any time during the year and affects both sexes, children and adults. Pathologically, HSE is an acute necrotising encephalitis with preferential involvement of the frontotemporal, cingulate, and insular cortex.[29] There is no clinical symptom or sign that is specific or sensitive for HSE. A preceding history of labial fever blisters is not necessarily of diagnostic value in HSE.[27] The onset of HSE is usually abrupt, with the clinical course rapidly progressing over several days. Acute anomia and recent memory loss occurs in one fifth of cases.[5] Personality changes may be subtle and easily missed. Seizures are common, usually complex partial, and often with secondary generalisation. Focal neurological deficits such as hemiparesis and aphasia develop when HSE is untreated, and may progress to coma. In a retrospective clinicopathological analysis of 46 cases of HSE, symptoms on admission included a prodromal influenza-like illness (48%), sudden onset of headache, confusion and alteration of conscious level (52%), meningism (65%), aphasia or mutism(46%), deep coma (35%), raised intracranial pressure (33%), focal neurological signs (89%), and seizures occurring in 61% of cases during the course of the illness.[29] One third of cases develop in patients less than 20 years and half of all the cases are seen in patients over 50 years of age.[30]

It is the combination of the clinical features and laboratory findings that establishes the diagnosis of HSE. Peripheral white cell counts may be raised with a shift to the left. About 50% of patients with HSE have focal abnormalities on a noncontrast computed tomogram (reduced attenuation over one or both temporal and/frontal regions) and midline shift in half of those with abnormalities on computed tomography.[29] Computed tomography of the head within the first 4–5 days of symptom onset in HSE may even be normal.[31] Cranial magnetic resonance imaging remains the most sensitive anatomic neuroimaging not only for the early diagnosis but also for defining the distribution of cerebral injury in HSE. The magnetic resonance imaging scan in HSE typically shows early changes of focal oedema in the medial aspects of the temporal lobes, orbital surfaces of the frontal lobes, insular cortex, and cingulate gyrus (*see* Figure 9.1). Magnetic resonance imaging remains the imaging of choice in suspected HSE and should ideally be the first diagnostic step after initial clinical examination. Electro-encephalography is abnormal in practically all cases.[29] Cerebrospinal fluid may show a normal or raised pressure, typically show lymphocytic pleocytosis (10–200 cells/mm^3), normal glucose, and raised protein (0.6 to 6 g/l). In some, cerebrospinal fluid will have red blood cells (10–500 cells/mm^3) and in even fewer cases, borderline hypoglycorrhachia (2–2.5 mmol/l). Cerebrospinal fluid polymerase chain reaction for HSV in experienced laboratories is virtually 100% specific and the sensitivity of this test exceeds 90%.[22] The likelihood of a false negative result for HSV in the cerebrospinal fluid polymerase chain reaction in a case of HSE is extremely low and is usually encountered if the cerebrospinal fluid was collected too early (first 24–48 hours), too late (after 10–14 days), after aciclovir therapy, or if there was a long delay in processing the sample that was stored inappropriately after collection. False negative tests can also occur when haemoglobin or heparin are present in the cerebrospinal fluid assay.[5]

Recently, cases of atypical HSE have been described.[32] These cases are often mild, presenting with a syndrome of febrile encephalopathy in the absence of focal neurological features, initial cerebrospinal fluid pleocytosis or abnormal computed tomography. Mild or atypical HSE is due to infection with either HSV-1 or HSV-2. These cases may be associated with an immunocompromised state or

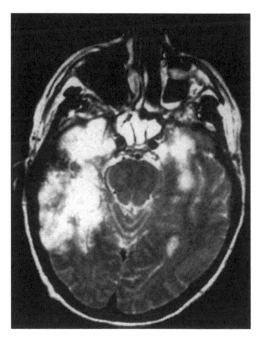

Figure 9.1 T2-weighted magnetic resonance image showing extensive area of increased signal in the right and, to a lesser extent, left temporal lobe in a case of HSE (reproduced with permission from Baringer, 2000). [22]

asymmetric HSV infection affecting predominantly the non-dominant temporal lobe. It is estimated that atypical forms may contribute to 20% of all cases of HSE. These cases also emphasise the importance of performing HSV cerebrospinal fluid polymerase chain reaction study on all patients presenting with febrile encephalopathy even in the absence of cerebrospinal fluid pleocytosis or focal neurological findings.

Box 9.8 Herpes simplex encephalitis

- Commonest cause of non-endemic, acute fatal encephalitis in the Western world.
- High level of clinical suspicion is necessary.
- First central nervous system viral infection to be successfully treated with antiviral therapy.
- One of the first to have routine cerebrospinal fluid polymerase chain reaction diagnosis with high specificity and sensitivity.
- Seen in neonates and adults.
- Abrupt onset with frontotemporal features.
- Treatment initiation on clinical suspicion is required.
- A combination of magnetic resonance imaging, EEG, and cerebrospinal fluid tests is usually diagnostic.
- High mortality and morbidity in untreated patients.
- Milder symptoms in atypical HSE.

Cytomegalovirus encephalitis

Cytomegalovirus encephalitis is rare in normal subjects but is a common encephalitis among the immunosuppressed and neonates. In an autopsy study, 12% of all HIV-infected patients and 2% of transplant recipients had cytomegalovirus encephalitis.[33] In an immunocompetent host, cytomegalovirus encephalitis is usually self-limiting, presenting with a febrile episode and non-specific clinical manifestations of meningoencephalitis (headache, confusion, rarely seizures, dysphasia, and coma). The cerebrospinal fluid shows pleocytosis, mildly raised protein, and normal glucose.[34] Cases of coexisting HSV and cytomegalovirus encephalitis have been reported both in the immunocompetent[35] and immunocompromised[36] hosts. Cytomegalovirus encephalitis is relatively common in HIV-infected patients, usually in the course of systemic cytomegalovirus infection, cytomegalovirus radiculomyeltis, or retinitis. The characteristic neuropathopathology is of ventriculoencephalitis and nearly half of these patients will have coexisting processes due to HIV encephalopathy, toxoplasmic encephalitis, or primary central nervous system lymphoma.

Box 9.9 New emergence of zoonotic encephalitic viruses

- West Nile virus.
- Nipah and Hendra viruses.
- B virus (cercopithecine herpes virus).

The clinical picture of cytomegalovirus encephalitis in an immunosuppressed host is typically dominated by confusion and fatigue with a relatively rapid progression to coma and death. Polymorphonuclear cerebrospinal fluid pleocytosis is only seen in patients with coexisting radiculomyelitis whereas the pleocytosis is predominantly mononuclear and sparse in isolated ventriculoencephalitis. Protein level is relatively high (over 1 g/l) and viral cultures of cerebrospinal fluid are negative in patients with AIDS and cytomegalovirus encephalitis. Sensitivity of cerebrospinal fluid polymerase chain reaction for the detection of cytomegalovirus encephalitis is around 79% with a specificity of 95%.[33] A potential pitfall of polymerase chain reaction as a diagnostic tool for cytomegalovirus encephalitis is that it might be too sensitive, detecting cytomegalovirus in the absence of encephalitis among HIV-infected patients.

Nipah virus encephalitis

Nipah virus encephalitis was first recognised among pig farmers in Malaysia between 1998 and 1999 and subsequently documented among the abattoir workers in Singapore. Cerebrospinal fluid samples from several affected patients yielded a new paramyxovirus (named Nipah virus).[9] This virus was closely related, but not identical, to another animal virus (Hendra virus) that had previously caused disease among horses and three patients in Australia.[37] Nipah virus encephalitis is the first wide scale epizoonotic encephalitis with direct animal-to-human transmission, unlike most other epizoonotic encephalitis (for example, Japanese encephalitis, West Nile virus encephalitis, Eastern equine virus encephalitis), where vectorial transmission is the rule. Over 200 people were affected in Malaysia alone and the cluster outbreak severely disrupted the pig farming industry. The affected pigs died unusually and suddenly. The human illness was characterised by a history of direct contact with pigs in the livestock farm, short incubation period (two weeks), rapidly declining level of consciousness, prominent brain stem dysfunction, and high fatality rates. Distinctive clinical signs included segmental myoclonus, areflexia, hypotonia, and dysautonomia (hypertension and tachycardia). Initial findings in the cerebrospinal fluid were abnormal in 75% of cases, EEG showed diffuse slow waves with focal abnormalities over temporal regions (75%), computed tomograms were normal and magnetic resonance imaging of the brain during the acute phase of illness showed widespread focal lesions in the subcortical and deep white matter.[10]

Treatment of acute viral encephalitis

Where possible, specific treatment must be targeted to the suspected or identified aetiological agent. Antiviral therapy with aciclovir is indicated in HSV encephalitis. Aciclovir is an analogue of 2'-deoxyguanosine and selectively inhibits viral replication. It exerts its antiviral effect after being metabolised to aciclovir triphosphate. Monophosphorylation of aciclovir is the first step in this process and is catalysed by a viral thymidine kinase induced in cells selectively infected by HSV, VZV, or by a phosphotransferase produced by cytomegalovirus.[38] Host enzymes subsequently phosphorylate the monophosphate to diphosphate and triphosphate. Aciclovir triphosphate inhibits the synthesis of viral DNA by competing with a 2'-deoxyguanosine triphosphate as a substrate for viral DNA polymerase. Viral DNA synthesis is arrested once aciclovir (rather than 2'-deoxyguanosine) is inserted into the replicating DNA. The incorporation of aciclovir into viral DNA is an irreversible process and it also inactivates viral DNA polymerase. The potency of aciclovir triphosphate to inhibit HSV-1 DNA polymerase is 30–50 times more than its ability to inhibit human cellular alpha-DNA polymerase.[39] Aciclovir has a relatively short half-life in plasma and more than 80% of aciclovir in circulation is excreted unchanged in urine,[40] thus renal impairment can rapidly precipitate aciclovir toxicity. Studies have consistently confirmed that aciclovir is most effective when given early in the clinical course of HSE before the patient becomes comatose and reduces both mortality and morbidity in treated patients.[26,30,41] The standard dose of aciclovir for HSE is 10 mg/kg three times daily (30 mg/kg/day) for 14 days. The dose for neonatal HSE is 60 mg/kg/day. The duration of treatment is 21 days for immunosuppressed patients. Aciclovir is effective against encephalitis due to HSV-1, HSV-2, and VZV.[38] Doses of aciclovir in VZV encephalitis are similar to HSE.

It has become a common medical practice to initiate aciclovir treatment in every patient with suspected acute infective encephalitis. While this practice is justified and carries the advantage of initiating early treatment of HSE, there are certain potential problems with 'blunderbuss' aciclovir therapy. Despite its remarkable safety, the decision to treat every case that could even remotely be HSE with aciclovir has two potential drawbacks. First and most importantly, giving aciclovir may delay or obscure the actual diagnosis (if not HSE) due to a false sense of security. Thus, diagnosis of other infective encephalitis, ADEM, or non-infective encephalopathies like Reye's syndrome, mitochondrial myopathy, encephalopathy, lactacidosis, stroke (MELAS), or Hashimoto's encephalopathy may be delayed or even missed. Secondly, aciclovir is not completely innocuous and can precipitate a toxic encephalopathy[38] that can confound the diagnosis of acute encephalitis if this has not been made before the treatment was initiated.

Since early aciclovir treatment for HSE is essential, more patients than those actually having HSE will be initiated on this treatment based on clinical suspicion. In an immunocompetent host, evidence of lesions on magnetic resonance imaging affecting any of the temporal or frontobasal lobes supports the diagnosis of HSE and such a patient must be treated with aciclovir for a minimum of 14 days. If aciclovir is started on admission and magnetic resonance imaging of brain is found to be normal, then the treatment should continue until the cerebrospinal fluid polymerase chain reaction results for HSE become available and the treatment withdrawn in cases where this test is negative and an alternative diagnosis has been established. If an alternative diagnosis has not been reached and the cerebrospinal fluid polymerase chain reaction is negative for HSV, then it is our policy to continue aciclovir therapy for 10 days. There has been only a single case of HSE with normal cerebral magnetic resonance imaging in the current literature. In this patient, the diagnosis of HSE was made by polymerase chain reaction from a sample of cerebrospinal fluid obtained on the day of admission but a repeat cerebrospinal fluid polymerase chain reaction after eight days of ongoing aciclovir therapy was negative.[42] Recurrence of HSE has been reported weeks to three months later when the treatment was given for 10 days or less.[5] Reports have indicated that relapse after therapy may be as high as 5% but relapse has not been documented when higher doses were administered for 21 days.[43] Although aciclovir resistance has been reported in mucocutaneous herpes simplex among AIDS patients,[44] the development of aciclovir resistance in HSE has not yet been reported and it is only a theoretical possibility at present.

Box 9.10   Aciclovir treatment in HSE

- Specific and highly effective.
- Safe, but requires dose adjustment for renal function.
- Treatment increases survival likelihood to 65–100% if disease is present for four days or less.[30]
- Dose is 10 mg/kg every eight hours for at least 14 days in an immuno-competent host.

The clinical response of cytomegalovirus encephalitis to antiviral drugs is not known and anecdotal experience suggests it is not dramatic. Aciclovir is ineffective in cytomegalovirus encephalitis. Combination therapy with ganciclovir (5 mg/kg intravenously twice daily) with or without foscarnet (60 mg/kg every eight hours or 90 mg/kg every 12 hours) is currently recommended;[45] cidofovir is a possible alternative. Antiretroviral therapy must be added or continued in HIV-infected patients. Appropriate antibacterial chemotherapy will be required where tuberculous, listerial, ricketssial infections are suspected or diagnosed as the cause of meningoencephalitis. The role of large doses of corticosteroids (dexamethasone or methylprednisolone) in the setting of acute infective encephalitis is debatable. While steroids might be specifically indicated in certain situations such as tuberculous meningoencephalitis or granulomatous angiitis after varicella zoster infection, its efficacy in the setting of acute viral encephalitis is unproven and cannot be generally recommended. A study that had evaluated high dose dexamethasone in Japanese encephalitis found no benefit from steroid therapy.[46]

Supportive therapy for acute encephalitis is an important cornerstone of any treatment strategy. Seizures are controlled with intravenous fosphenytoin. Principles for the medical management of raised intracranial pressure should be followed where clinically indicated. Careful attention must be paid to the maintenance of respiration, cardiac rhythm, fluid balance, prevention of deep vein thrombosis, aspiration pneumonia, and secondary bacterial infections. Since some of the treatments may have specific toxicity (for example, aciclovir is nephrotoxic, raises serum liver enzymes, and can cause thrombocytopenia), appropriate blood counts and biochemical parameters must be closely monitored. Each dose of aciclovir should be given intravenously slowly as an infusion over at least one hour and the dose may require adjustment based on renal function. All cases of acute encephalitis must be hospitalised and should have access to intensive care unit equipped with mechanical ventilators. Isolation for patients with community acquired acute infective encephalitis is not required; rabies encephalitis, however, is an exception. Consideration of isolation should also be given for severely immunosuppressed patients, patients with an exanthematous encephalitis, and those with a potentially contagious viral haemorrhagic fever.

Complications and outcome of acute viral encephalitis

Mortality rates in non-herpes viral encephalitis may range from very low (for example, EBV encephalitis) to very high (for example, Eastern equine encephalitis). Established rabies encephalitis is invariably fatal. Mortality rates in untreated HSE is around 70% and fewer than 3% would return to normal function.[26,27] In a retrospective analysis of patients with a diagnosis of HSE, only 16% of untreated patients had survived.[29] Early diagnosis with aciclovir reduces the mortality of HSE to 20–30%.[25–27] Among the aciclovir treated patients in the NINAID-CASG trials, 26 of the 32 (81%) treated patients survived and serious neurological disability was seen in nearly half of the survivors.[26] Older patients with poor level of consciousness (Glasgow coma scale of 6 or less) had the worst outcome. Young patients (aged 30 years or under) with good neurological function at the time of initiating aciclovir therapy did substantially better (100% survival, over 60% had little or no sequel).[30] Persistent unilateral hyperperfusion in the cerebral SPECT scan is also a poor prognostic marker for recovery.[19]

A number of secondary complications may also arise in the course of an acute viral encephalitis.[12] These are raised intracranial pressure, cerebral infarction, cerebral venous thrombosis, syndrome of inappropriate secretion of antidiuretic hormone, aspiration pneumonia, upper gastrointestinal bleeding, urinary tract infections, and disseminated intravascular coagulopathy. The late sequelae of viral encephalitis largely depend on the age of the patient, aetiology of the encephalitis, and the severity of the clinical episode. Epilepsy, persistent anomia, aphasia, motor deficit, and a chronic amnestic state similar to Korsakoff's psychosis have been known among the survivors of severe HSE. Very rarely, a neuropsychiatric syndrome marked by oral exploratory behaviour (incomplete Kluver-Bucy syndrome) has been anecdotally observed during the early phase of recovery in HSE. Extrapyramidal syndrome (parkinsonism) as a late sequel of viral encephalitis was first recognised after the epidemic of influenza virus encephalitis that was characterised by a somnolent-ophthalmoplegic syndrome and fatigue (encephalitis lethargica or von Economo's disease).[47] Occasional cases of postencephalitic parkinsonism have since been reported after sporadic viral encephalitis, especially after Japanese encephalitis.[48] Nearly a third of all children with Japanese encephalitis will die and up to 75% of the surviving children may be left with major neurological sequelae, including mental retardation, epilepsy, behavioural abnormalities (obsessive-compulsive personality), speech and extrapyramidal (parkinsonian) movement disorders.[49] The syndrome of prolonged and persistent fatigue, myalgia, nervousness, concentration impairment, and post-exertional malaise is well recognised after viral encephalitis (postviral chronic fatigue syndrome).[50]

Conclusions

In all cases of acute encephalitis, appropriate investigations and supportive care form the integral part of the management strategy. The availability of aciclovir, an excellent anti-HSV therapy, has led to early initiation of the treatment with substantial improvement in the clinical outcome of HSE. The outlook of the non-herpes viral encephalitis, for example, Japanese encephalitis, is often less satisfactory. It is yet unknown if the availability of newer antiviral therapy (ribavarin and pleoconaril) will substantially change the natural course of non-herpes viral encephalitis. Some viral encephalitis may be prevented by immunisation (for example, mumps, measles, rubella, Japanese encephalitis, and rabies). Adequate vector control and environmental sanitation are essential to prevent large outbreaks of arboviral encephalitis such as Japanese encephalitis. Cluster outbreaks of West Nile virus encephalitis in New York City[8] and the emergence of zoonotic encephalitis due to Nipah virus in Malyasia[9] continue to signal an important public health principle that any new outbreaks of unusual and fatal diseases in animals may herald related events, maybe new infections, in humans.[51]

Acknowledgement

AC is supported by the Barclay Research Trust held at the University of Glasgow.

References

1 Koskiniemi M, Rantalaiho T, Piiparinen H, *et al.* Infections of the central nervous system of suspected viral origin: a collaborative study from Finland. *J Neurosurg* 2001; 7: 400–8.

2 White NJ, Ho M. The pathophysiology of cerebral malaria. *Adv Parasitol* 1992; **31**: 84–94.

3 Amore M, Ziazzeri N. Neuroleptic malignant syndrome after neuroleptic discontinuation. *Prog Neuropsychopharmacol Biol Psychiatry* 1995; **19**: 1323–34.

4 Davis LE. Acute viral meningitis and encephalitis. In: Kennedy PGE, Johnston RT, eds. *Infections of the nervous system*. London: Butterworths, 1987: 156–76.

5 Davis LE. Diagnosis and treatment of acute encephalitis. *The Neurologist* 2000; **6**: 145–59.

6 Adams RD, Victor M, Ropper AH. *Viral infections of the nervous system. Principles of neurology*. 6th edn. New York: McGraw Hill, 1998: 742–76.

7 Coyle PK. Post-infectious encephalomyelitis. In: Davis LE, Kennedy PGE, eds. *Infectious diseases of the nervous system*. Oxford: Butterworth-Heinemann, 2000: 83–108.

8 Nash D, Mostashari F, Fine A, *et al.* The outbreak of West Nile virus infection in the New York City area in 1999. *N Engl J Med* 2001; **344**: 1807–14.

9 Steele KE, Linn MJ, Schoepp RJ, *et al.* Pathology of fatal West Nile virus encephalitis in native and exotic birds during the 1999 outbreak in New York City. *J Vet Pathol* 2000; **37**: 208–24.

10 Goh KJ, Tan CT, Chew NK, *et al.* Clinical features of Nipah virus encephalitis among pig farmers in Malaysia. *N Engl J Med* 2000; **342**: 1229–35.

11 Tselis A, Lavi E. Cytomegalovirus infection of the adult nervous system. In: Davis LE, Kennedy PGE, eds. *Infectious diseases of the nervous system*. Oxford: Butterworth-Heinemann, 2000: 109–38.

12 Booss J, Esiri MM. *Viral encephalitis. Pathology, diagnosis and management*. Oxford: Blackwell Scientific Publications, 1986.

13 Hemachuda T, Mitrabhakdi E. Rabies. In: Davis LE, Kennedy PGE, eds. *Infectious diseases of the nervous system*. Oxford: Butterworth-Heinemann, 2000: 401–44.

14 Duggan AJ, Hutchington MP. Sleeping sickness in Europeans: a review of 109 cases. *J Trop Med Hyg* 1966; **69**: 124–31.

15 Standaert SM, Clough LA, Schaffner W, *et al.* Neurologic manifestations of human monocytic ehrlichiosis. *Infect Dis Clin Pract* 1998; **7**: 358–62.

16 Schroth G, Gawehn J, Thorn A, *et al.* Early diagnosis of herpes simplex encephalitis by MRI. *Neurology* 1987; **37**: 179–83.

17 Demaerel P, Wilms G, Robberecht W, *et al.* MRI of herpes simplex encephalitis. *Neuroradiology* 1992; **34**: 490–3.

18 Launes J, Nikkinen P, Lindworth L, *et al.* Diagnosis of acute herpes simplex encephalitis by brain perfusion single photon emission computed tomography. *Lancet* 1988; **i**: 1188–90.

19 Launes J, Siren J, Valanne L, *et al.* Unilateral hyperperfusion in brain-perfusion SPECT predicts poor prognosis in acute encephalitis. *Neurology* 1997; **48**: 1347–51.

20 Tyler KL. Aseptic meningitis, viral encephalitis and prion diseases. In: Fauci AS, Braunwald E, Isselbacher KJ, *et al.*, eds. *Harrison's principles of internal medicine.* 14th edn. New York: McGraw Hill, 1998: 2439–51.

21 Whitley RJ, Soong SJ, Linneman C Jr, *et al.* Herpes simplex encephalitis: clinical assessment. *JAMA* 1982; **247**: 317–20.

22 Baringer JR. Herpes simplex virus encephalitis. In: Davis LE, Kennedy PGE, eds. *Infectious diseases of the nervous system.* Oxford: Butterworth-Heinemann, 2000: 139–64.

23 Kennedy PGE. The widening spectrum of infectious neurological disease. *J Neurol Neurosurg Psychiatry* 1990; **53**: 629–32.

24 Whitley RJ, Soong SJ, Dolin R, *et al.* Adenine arabinoside therapy of biopsy-proven herpes simplex encephalitis: National Institute of Allergy and Infectious Diseases Collaborative Antiviral Study. *N Engl J Med* 1977; **297**: 289–94.

25 Whitley RJ, Alford CA, Hirsch MS, *et al.* Vidarabine versus acyclovir therapy in herpes simplex encephalitis. *N Engl J Med* 1986; **314**: 144–9.

26 Whitley RJ. Viral encephalitis. *N Engl J Med* 1990; **323**: 242–50.

27 Johnston RT. *Viral infections of the nervous system.* 2nd edn. Philadelphia: Lippincott-Raven, 1998.

28 DeBasi RL, Tyler KL. Recurrent aseptic meningitis. In: Davis LE, Kennedy PGE, eds. *Infectious diseases of the nervous system.* Oxford: Butterworth-Heinemann, 2000: 445–80.

29 Kennedy PGE. A retrospective analysis of forty-six cases of herpes simplex encephalitis seen in Glasgow between 1962 and 1985. *Q J Med* 1988; **68**: 533–40.

30 Whitley RJ, Gnann JW. Viral encephalitis: familiar infections and emerging pathogens. *Lancet* 2002; **359**: 507–14.

31 Zimmermann RD, Russell EJ, Leeds NE, *et al.* CT in the early diagnosis of herpes simplex encephalitis. *AJR Am J Roentgenol* 1980; **134**: 61–6.

32 Fodor PA, Levin MJ, Weinberg A, *et al.* Atypical herpes simplex virus encephalitis diagnosed by PCR amplification of viral DNA from CSF. *Neurology* 1998; **51**: 554–9.

33 Arribas JR, Storch GA, Clifford DB, *et al.* Cytomegalovirus encephalitis. *Ann Intern Med* 1996; **125**: 577–87.

34 Studahl M, Ricksten A, Sandberg T, *et al.* Cytomegalovirus encephalitis in four immunocompetent patients. *Lancet* 1992; **340**: 1045–6.

35 Yanagisawa N, Toyokura Y, Shiraki H. Double encephalitis with herpes simplex virus and cytomegalovirus in an adult. *Acta Neuropathol (Berl)* 1975; **33**: 153–64.

36 Laskin OL, Stahl-Bayliss CM, Morgello S. Concomitant herpes simplex type 1 and cytomegalovirus ventriculoencephalitis in acquired immunodeficiency syndrome. *Arch Neurol* 1987; **44**: 843–7.

37 Selvey LA, Wells RM, McCormick JG, *et al.* Infection of humans and horses by a newly described morbillivirus. *Med J Aust* 1995; **162**: 642–5.

38 Balfour HH Jr. Antiviral drugs. *N Engl J Med* 1999; **340**: 1255–68.

39 Furman PA, St Clair MH, Spector T. Acyclovir triphosphate is a suicide inactivator of the herpes simplex virus DNA polymerase. *J Biol Chem* 1984; **259**: 9575–9.

40 de Miranda P, Blum MR. Pharmacokinetics of acyclovir after intravenous and oral administration. *J Antimicrob Chemother* 1983; **12**(suppl 3): 29–37.

41 Skoldenberg B, Forsgren M, Alestig K, *et al*. Acyclovir versus vidarabine in herpes simplex encephalitis: randomised multicentre study in consecutive Swedish patients. *Lancet* 1984; **ii**: 707–12.

42 Hollinger P, Matter L, Sturzenegger M. Normal MRI findings in herpes simplex virus encephalitis. *J Neurol* 2000; **247**: 799–801.

43 Ito Y, Kimura H, Yabuta Y, *et al*. Exacerbation of herpes simplex encephalitis after successful treatment with acyclovir. *Clin Infect Dis* 2000; **30**: 185–7.

44 Safrin S, Crumpacker C, Chatis P, *et al*. A controlled trial comparing foscarnet with vidarabine for acyclovir-resistant mucocutaneous herpes simplex in the acquired immunodeficiency syndrome. *N Engl J Med* 1991; **325**: 551–5.

45 Enting R, de Gans J, Reiss P, *et al*. Ganciclovir/foscarnet for cytomegalovirus meningo-encephalitis in AIDS. *Lancet* 1992; **340**: 559–60.

46 Hoke CH Jr, Vaughn DW, Nisalak A, *et al*. Effects of high dose dexamethasone on the outcome of acute Japanese encephalitis. *J Infect Dis* 1992; **165**: 131–6.

47 von Economo C. *Encephalitis lethargica. Its sequelae and treatment* (translated by Newman KO). London: Oxford University Press, 1931.

48 Pradhan S, Pandey N, Shashank S, *et al*. Parkinsonian symptoms due to predominant involvement of substantia nigra in Japanese encephalitis. *Neurology* 1999; **53**: 1781–6.

49 Ravi V, Desai A, Shankar SK, *et al*. Japanese encephalitis. In: Davis LE, Kennedy PGE, eds. *Infectious diseases of the nervous system*. Oxford: Butterworth-Heinemann, 2000: 231–58.

50 Behan PO, Bakheit AMO. Clinical spectrum of post-viral fatigue syndrome. *Br Med Bull* 1991; **47**: 793–808.

51 Tyler KL. West Nile virus encephalitis in America. *N Engl J Med* 2001; **344**: 1858–9.

Chapter 10

Acute disseminated encephalomyelitis

RK Garg

Acute disseminated encephalomyelitis (ADEM) is an acute demyelinating disorder of the central nervous system, and is characterised by multifocal white matter involvement. Diffuse neurological signs along with multifocal lesions in brain and spinal cord characterise the disease. Possibly, a T cell mediated autoimmune response to myelin basic protein, triggered by an infection or vaccination, underlies its pathogenesis. ADEM is a monophasic illness with favourable long-term prognosis. The differentiation of ADEM from a first attack of multiple sclerosis has prognostic and therapeutic implications; this distinction is often difficult. Most patients with ADEM improve with methylprednisolone. If that fails, immunoglobulins, plasmapheresis, or cytotoxic drugs can be given. Recent literature suggests that a significant proportion of patients with ADEM will later develop multiple sclerosis; however, follow-up experience from developing countries does not support this view.

Acute disseminated encephalomyelitis (ADEM) is an acute widespread demyelinating condition, which principally affects brain and spinal cord (*see* Box 10.1). It usually follows an infection or vaccination. The disease is characterised by multifocal white matter lesions on neuroimaging. ADEM is a monophasic disease. Uncommonly ADEM can relapse frequently. If these relapses are thought to represent part of the same acute monophasic illness, the term 'multiphasic ADEM' is used. Any recurrences beyond the first few months of initial clinical illness suggest the presence of a chronic immune process and a diagnosis of multiple sclerosis should be considered. Devic's disease or neuromyelitis optica is characterised by simultaneous attacks of optic neuritis and myelitis with no evidence of involvement of other parts of the central nervous system. Precisely what relationship these distinct entities have with each other is a subject of intense controversy. In the recent past a lot of new information about ADEM and its association with other demyelinating disorders has been made available. In this article all this information will be reviewed.

Epidemiology

The exact incidence of ADEM is not known. In the past ADEM commonly followed common childhood infections (like measles, smallpox, and chickenpox) and was associated with significant mortality and morbidity. Because of significant advances in infectious disease control ADEM in developed countries is now seen most frequently after non-specific upper respiratory tract infections and the aetiological agent remains unknown. In a recent study by Murthy *et al.*, despite vigorous attempts to identify microbial pathogens in 18 patients, only one patient had Epstein-Barr virus isolated as the definite microbial cause of ADEM. Of the other two patients with rotavirus disease, in one patient infection was considered as possibly associated with ADEM. Failure to identify a viral agent suggests that the inciting agents are unusual or cannot be recovered by standard laboratory procedures.[1] In developing and poor countries, because of poor implementation of immunisation programmes, measles and other viral infections are still widely prevalent and account for frequent occurrences of postinfectious demyelinating diseases. ADEM in developing countries is much more frequent than reported.[2] In the past it had been observed that ADEM occurred in one out of 1000 measles infections. ADEM was relatively uncommon after varicella infection and the incidence that had been reported was about one per 10 000 patients. The incidence of ADEM after rubella infection was approximately one per 500 infections. Mortality and major neurological sequelae of ADEM after varicella and rubella infections were much lower in comparison with ADEM after measles infection. ADEM found after measles was associated with mortality rates as high as 25% and 25–40% of survivors were left with permanent neurological sequelae.[3–5] The main bacterial infection, which has been implicated with the occurrence of ADEM, is mycoplasma. Other viral and bacterial infections that have been implicated with ADEM are listed in Box 10.2.

Another common variant of ADEM is that which follows vaccination (post-immunisation encephalomyelitis). This form is clinically indistinguishable from the postinfectious variety except the former more often involves the peripheral nervous system. When rabies vaccine was generated from virus grown in rabbit brain, the rate of neurological complications was estimated to be as high as one in 400 vaccinations. The reported incidence of neuroparalytic complications with the Semple type of antirabies vaccine varied between one per 600 to one per 1575 vaccinations. Such complications are now rare as non-neural tissue based vaccines are being used. An incidence rate of one per 25 000 vaccinations occurred with duck embryo antirabies vaccine, a preparation containing minimal amount of neural tissue. Introduction of the non-neural human diploid cell vaccine has virtually eliminated neuroparalytic complications of rabies vaccinations.[6–11]

When smallpox vaccination was a part of a universal immunisation programme, encephalomyelitis followed one in 4000 vaccinations. Currently, post-immunisation encephalomyelitis is most commonly associated with measles, mumps, and rubella vaccinations. The incidence is 1–2 per million for live measles vaccine immunisations, which is significantly lower than that for postinfectious encephalomyelitis from measles itself. The risk of occurrence of ADEM is 20 times lower after vaccination than ADEM after natural measles virus infection.[2,12,13]

Box 10.1   Acute disseminated encephalomyelitis and related disorders

Acute disseminated encephalomyelitis
- Postinfectious.
- Postvaccinial.

Acute haemorrhagic leucoencephalitis
Restricted form of acute, inflammatory demyelinating diseases
- Transverse myelitis.
- Optic neuritis.
- Cerebellitis.
- Brain stem encephalitis.

Multiphasic form of acute disseminated encephalomyelitis and multiple sclerosis

---

Box 10.2   Preceding infectious illnesses

A. Infections

Viral
- Measles.
- Mumps.
- Influenza A or B.
- Hepatitis A or B.
- Herpes simplex.
- Human herpes virus E.
- Varicella, rubella.
- Epstein-Barr virus.
- Cytomegalovirus.
- HIV.

Others
- Mycoplasma pneumoniae.
- Chlamydia.
- Legionella.
- Campylobacter.
- Streptococcus.

B. Vaccines
- Rabies.
- Diphtheria, tetanus, pertussis.
- Smallpox.
- Measles.
- Japanese B encephalitis.
- Polio.
- Hepatitis B.
- Influenza.

Pathology and pathogenesis

The hallmark of the pathological findings of postinfectious encephalomyelitis is areas of perivenous demyelination and infiltration of lymphocytes and macrophages. Other changes include hyperaemia, endothelial swelling, and vessel wall invasion by inflammatory cells, perivascular oedema, and haemorrhage. These changes are present in the small blood vessels of both white and grey matter. As the lesions become older, the macrophages increase and lymphocytes decrease in number. At a late stage of disease foci of fibrillary fibrosis can also be seen in adjacent brain tissue. Although postinfectious encephalomyelitis typically involves the white matter, lesions in grey matter have also been seen. Basal ganglia, thalamus, and even cortical grey matter may be involved.[14,15]

The pathological findings described in ADEM are very similar to experimental allergic encephalomyelitis (EAE). EAE is an autoimmune encephalomyelitis that can be induced experimentally in susceptible animals by exposing them to a myelin antigen such as myelin basic protein, proteolipid protein, and myelin oligodendrocyte glycoprotein. In complete Freund's adjuvant these myelin antigens can produce a diffuse white matter encephalomyelitis. Myelin basic protein and proteolipid protein are the most encephilitogenic. The existing evidence suggests that ADEM results from a transient autoimmune response against myelin or other autoantigens, possibly, via molecular mimicry or by non-specific activation of an autoreactive T cell clone. Peptides from microbial proteins that have sufficient structural similarity with the host's self peptides can activate autoreactive T cells; this mechanism is referred to as molecular mimicry. EAE, in the Theiler's murine encephalomyelitis model, is initiated by CD4+ T helper cells by infiltrating the central nervous system and subsequently recruiting additional lymphocytes and mononuclear cells to cross the blood-brain barrier, resulting in inflammation and demyelination. CD8+ T cells have also been implicated in a secondary autoimmune response.[16–19] Disease can be transferred to susceptible mice by injection of T cells that recognise myelin-associated protein. Semple antirabies vaccine contains a fair amount of neural antigens that can excite a cross reactive T cell response.[20] Probably genetic susceptibility explains why encephalomyelitic complications develop in only a small minority of patients who have received rabies vaccine prepared from rabbit brain, or have had measles. Of the many candidate polymorphic major histocompatibility complex (MHC) and non-MHC genes, which contribute to disease susceptibility, including those which encode for effector (cytokines and chemokines) or receptor molecules within the immune system, human leucocyte antigen class II genes have the most significant influence.[21]

Acute haemorrhagic leucoencephalitis is a more severe and frequently fatal hyperacute variant of ADEM. The pathological features of acute haemorrhagic leucoencephalitis are similar to that of hyperacute experimental allergic encephalomyelitis (HEAE). The most important distinguishing feature of acute haemorrhagic leucoencephalitis and HEAE (from ADEM and EAE respectively) is necrotising vasculitis of venules. Perivascular infiltrates consist mainly of polymorphonuclear cells. Perivascular haemorrhages are also common (*see* Table 10.1). Genetic susceptibility is possibly responsible for determining the occurrence of a particular type of encephalomyelitic variant.[22–24]

The exact molecular mechanisms that cause the death of oligodendrocytes in ADEM and its other variants are not known. Possibly, a complex interplay

Table 10.1 Pathological features of acute demyelinating disorders (modified from Scully *et al.*)[23]

Feature	ADEM	Acute multiple sclerosis	Acute haemorrhagic leucoencephalitis	Neuromyelitis optica
Perivascular infiltrates				
Lymphocytes	++	++	++	++
Macrophages or monocytes	++	++	++	++
Polymorphs	–	–	++	++
Eosinophils	–	–	–	++
Perivascular haemorrhage	–	–	++	–
Necrotising venules	–	–	++	+
Perivascular demyelination	±	±	++	++
Axonal damage	±	±	++	++

among cytokines, chemokines, and adhesion molecules is responsible for the cellular events of inflammatory encephalomyelitis. For example, tumour necrosis factor-alpha is considered an important factor in the pathogenesis of EAE.[25] It has been suggested that upregulation of Fas ligand (FasL) on autoreactive infiltrating T cells together with upregulation of Fas on resident cells in the target organ may lead to direct tissue destruction by an apoptotic pathway.[26] Active nitrogen species are overproduced in EAE and nitric oxide has been shown to mediate the death of oligodendrocytes.[27] In other suggested mechanisms, free oxygen radicals have been implicated in the death of premature oligodendrocytes.[28] Excitotoxicity could also be involved in the pathogenesis of demyelinating disorders.[29]

Clinical features

Systemic symptoms like fever, malaise, myalgias, headache, nausea, and vomiting often precede the neurological symptoms of ADEM. These systemic symptoms begin 4–21 days after the inciting event. The hallmark of clinical features of ADEM is the development of a focal or multifocal neurological disorder. The onset of the central nervous system disorder is rapid with peak dysfunction in several days. Initial clinical features include encephalopathy ranging from lethargy to coma, and focal and multifocal neurological signs like hemiparesis, cranial nerve palsies, and paraparesis. Other commonly reported findings include meningismus, ataxia, and varied movement disorders. Seizure may occur in severe cases, especially in the acute haemorrhagic form of ADEM. Optic neuritis is often bilateral and transverse myelopathy is often complete.[5,30–34]

Recovery can begin within days; on occasion complete resolution is noted within a few days, but more frequently occurs over the course of weeks or months. The mortality varies between 10% and 30%, with complete recovery in 50%. Poor prognosis is correlated with severity and abruptness of onset of the clinical syndrome. In the case series after rabies vaccine, a mortality of 18% was recorded. After a mean follow-up of 17 months, 68% of the survivors had completely recovered, and 32% had partially recovered, most with minimal deficits. In three patients in this series, a relapse of neurological deficit occurred during the recovery period. None of the patients experienced relapse once complete recovery had occurred.[6] Measles virus associated ADEM may carry a worse prognosis than vaccine-associated disease. However, with introduction of effective vaccination strategies and decline of measles, death is rare.

Young adults and children are most commonly affected, Schwarz *et al.* recently reported a follow-up study of 40 adult patients and noted that the rate of prior infection was lower.[31] Most adult patients present clinically in a fashion similar to that of children, except that there is a relatively infrequent occurrence of headache, fever and meningismus, and a higher frequency of sensory deficits. Optic neuritis is also infrequent in adult ADEM.[31]

Laboratory features

Cerebrospinal fluid

Cerebrospinal fluid may be normal but frequently it shows some changes. Typical cerebrospinal fluid changes include increased pressure, lymphocytic pleocytosis (as much as 1000/mm,[3] sometimes polymorphonuclear leucocytosis initially), and raised protein (usually <1.0 mg/l). The cerebrospinal fluid may contain increased amounts of gammaglobulin and IgG and raised levels of myelin basic protein. Glucose content is usually normal. Rarely, in cerebrospinal fluid oligoclonal band of IgG may be demonstrated. Production of intrathecal oligoclonal IgG almost ceases as the patient improves.[2,22,24]

Electroencephalography

Electroencephalographic abnormalities are common but are usually non-specific. At times, specific electroencephalographic pictures like spindle coma pattern and alternating pattern have been described. Because of low sensitivity and specificity, electrophysiological studies are not routinely used to diagnose ADEM. Hollinger *et al.* recently reported a series of 10 patients; magnetic resonance imaging (MRI) and cerebrospinal fluid findings were normal in five out of 10 patients and were only mildly abnormal in the remaining five patients. Interestingly, electroencephalography was abnormal in seven out of eight patients in whom it was performed. Abnormal electroencephalographic findings varied greatly and ranged from signs of increased sleepiness, mild generalised slowing, to severe generalised slowing with infrequent focal slowing and epileptiform discharges. Severe findings were recorded in three patients in whom electroencephalographic findings correlated fairly well with severity and the course of the clinical syndrome. In two young women, with initial suspicion of a psychiatric disease, electroencephalograms were helpful to prove the organic nature of unconsciousness.[35]

Neuroimaging

Neuroimaging is extremely valuable in establishing the diagnosis of ADEM. Computed tomography is generally normal at onset and usually becomes abnormal 5–14 days later. The typical computed tomographic appearance is that of low attenuation, multifocal lesions in the subcortical white matter. At times, constant enhancement of the lesions has been reported.[36]

Demyelinating lesions of ADEM are better visualised by MRI. These demyelinating lesions of ADEM usually exhibit no mass effect and can be seen scattered throughout the white matter of the posterior fossa and cerebral hemispheres (*see* Figures 10.1 and 10.2). Involvement of the cerebellum and brainstem is more common in children. Characteristic lesions seen on MRI appear as patchy areas of increased signal intensity on conventional T2-weighted images and on fluid attenuated inversion recovery sequence (FLAIR). Few MRI lesions may enhance after gadolinium administration. Extensive perifocal oedema may be seen. Though white matter involvement predominates grey matter can also be affected, particularly basal ganglia, thalami, and brainstem. Tumour-like lesions have also been reported in a few patients. In order to qualify as ADEM, lesions on MRI should be of the same age and no new lesion should appear on central nervous system imaging studies after the initial clinical attack. The corpus callosum is usually not involved in ADEM; infrequently its involvement has been reported, suggesting extensive lesion load. Corpus callosum involvement is more characteristic of multiple sclerosis. Thalamic involvement is exceedingly rare in multiple sclerosis but may be seen in 40% patients of ADEM, making this finding a potentially useful discriminator.[31–34,37–40] MRI changes usually appear early in the course of the disease. Honkaniemi *et al*. reported delayed MRI changes in ADEM. In their series, appearance of ADEM-associated MRI changes was associated with recovery from the disease.[41]

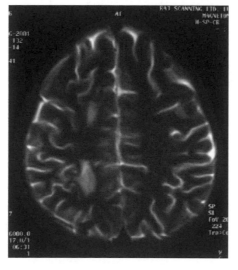

Figure 10.1 T2-weighted MRI showing multiple hyperintense lesions in the centrum semiovale of right cerebral hemisphere.

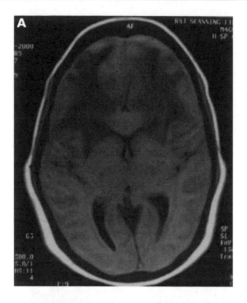

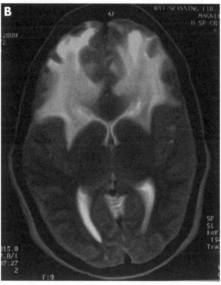

Figure 10.2 MRI of patient a week before a febrile illness. T1 (A) and T2 (B) images showing extensive bilateral demyelination of white matter of frontal lobes. This 20 year old woman presented with bilateral vision loss, cerebellar manifestations, and with extensive pyramidal signs.

Differential diagnosis

The diagnosis is considered straightforward when ADEM occurs after an exanthem or immunisation. A clear-cut latent period between systemic symptoms and neurological illness favours ADEM along with the typical pattern of diffuse and multifocal involvement of both the central nervous system and peripheral nervous system and the characteristic MRI appearance. The most important issue associated with the diagnosis of ADEM is – can this disorder be diagnosed with certainty and differentiated from the initial manifestation of multiple sclerosis?[42–44] Schwarz *et al.*, in a cohort of 40 patients who were initially diagnosed as having ADEM, noted that 35% developed clinically definite multiple sclerosis (Poser's criteria) over a mean observation period of 38 months.[31] Schwarz *et al.* look at possible discriminating clinical features but fail to identify any exclusive feature characteristic of either condition. Similarly, cerebrospinal fluid findings are not distinctive enough to allow differentiation between ADEM and multiple sclerosis in a single patient. Even MRI studies were not able to differentiate ADEM from multiple sclerosis. Approximately 50% of the patients with ADEM had MRI features that were suggestive of multiple sclerosis.[31] In general, adult patients with ADEM tend to present with a more acute, widespread central nervous system disturbance, causing loss of consciousness and multifocal signs. Fever, loss of consciousness, and meningism are infrequently observed but are highly suggestive of ADEM because these symptoms are rare in multiple sclerosis. Hynson *et al.* also noted a similar problem of differentiation between an initial attack of multiple sclerosis with ADEM, in children. These authors suggest that a viral prodrome, early onset ataxia, high lesion load on MRI, involvement of the deep cortical grey matter, and absence of oligoclonal bands are more indicative of ADEM.[34] Now it is believed that distinguishing multiple sclerosis from ADEM on single MRI examination is virtually impossible. Serial studies performed at least six months apart may prove more helpful. The findings of new lesions are highly suggestive of multiple sclerosis. In ADEM, new lesions should not appear unless a clinical relapse has occurred.[5] Gadolinium-enhanced MRI can also help to distinguish these two demyelinating disorders as a mixture of enhancing and non-enhancing lesions implies the temporal dissemination of multiple sclerosis. It is not clear whether 'relapsing ADEM' exists as a separate entity from relapsing-remitting multiple sclerosis. One should be cautious in making the diagnosis, and should refer to established criteria for the diagnosis of multiple sclerosis. The newly revised diagnostic criteria for multiple sclerosis allow the diagnosis to be made after one attack if stringent MRI criteria are met. These criteria also emphasise that in monophasic demyelinating disease such as ADEM a diagnosis of multiple sclerosis should be withheld unless new symptoms and signs or imaging abnormalities appear more than three months after clinical onset.[42,44,45]

Although ADEM is typically a disseminated process in the central nervous system, often with impaired sensorium, a few cases are dominated by spinal pathology (*see* Figure 10.3). Neuromyelitis optica (Devic's disease), sometimes caused by ADEM or systemic lupus erythematosus, may create diagnostic problems. Although stroke is the most common central nervous system feature in antiphospholipid syndrome, transverse myelitis and optic neuritis including Devic's syndrome have been described. MRI features described in patients with demyelinating disorders can also be seen in antiphospholipid syndrome. A clear distinction between an acute demyelinating disorder like ADEM and antiphospholipid syndrome can be difficult. Cuadrado *et al.* in a recent article suggested that a careful medical history, a previous history of thrombosis and/or fetal loss, an abnormal localisation of lesion on MRI, and the response to anticoagulant therapy might be helpful in the differential diagnosis of these two different diseases.[46]

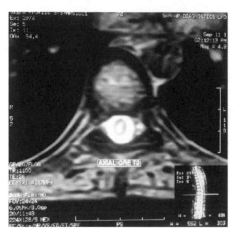

Figure 10.3 Axial T2-weighted MR image of thoracic spinal cord showing a centrally located hyper intense signal in a patient with ADEM with transverse myelopathy.

A combination of fever, seizures, altered sensorium, early parenchymal imaging abnormalities, and cerebrospinal fluid pleocytosis can cause confusion with viral encephalitis. A clear-cut latent period between systemic symptoms and neurological illness favours ADEM, because of the typical pattern of diffuse and multifocal involvement of both the central nervous system and peripheral nervous system and the usual MRI appearance.[42] Epidemic occurrence of central nervous system symptoms, absence of focal signs, and persisting systemic involvement are more likely in viral encephalitis. In an endemic region patients with ADEM may also need to be differentiated from a postmalarial neurological syndrome.[47,48] This syndrome has been defined as the acute onset of neurological or neuropsychiatric symptoms in patients recently recovered from *Plasmodium falciparum* malaria who have negative blood films at the time of onset of symptoms. There are certain similarities between ADEM and postmalarial neurological syndrome. These are latency from infection to neurological dysfunction, multifocal neurological deficits, response to steroids, good prognosis, and identical white matter MRI abnormalities. Mohsen *et al.* believe that ADEM and postmalarial neurological syndrome are indistinguishable,[48] so *P falciparum* should be added to the list of infections that are able to precipitate ADEM.

On MRI, multiple patchy areas of increased signal intensity – as demonstrated on conventional T2-weighted, proton density weighted MRI and FLAIR sequence – in the subcortical white matter have a long list of differential diagnoses (*see* Box 10.3).[5] Cerebral MRI abnormalities with other multifocal disease process that give rise to hyperintense T2-weighted lesions may have appearances and locations that are not typical of ADEM. For example, the periventricular lesions of vascular origin tend to be more peripheral than those of ADEM lesions. Multifocal hyperintensities on T2-weighted images associated with aging tend to be smaller and more randomly scattered throughout deep and subcortical white matter. These lesions are usually not visible on T1-weighted images and are confined to the patients who are more than 50 years of age. When such lesions are more extensive they tend to involve the periventricular white matter in a confluent symmetrical fashion.[35]

Box 10.3   Causes of patchy areas of increased signal intensity in T2-weighted images on MRI

- Multiple sclerosis.
- Vasculitis.
- Reversible posterior leucoencephalopathy.
- Eclampsia.
- Subcortical arteriosclerotic leucoencephalopathy.
- Neurosarcoidosis.
- Progressive multifocal leucoencephalopathy.
- HIV encephalopathy.
- Subacute sclerosing panencephalitis.
- Mitochondrial encephalopathy.
- Leucodystrophies.
- Toxic encephalopathies.
- Osmotic myelinolysis.
- Aging.

Treatment

The treatment of ADEM is targeted to suppress a presumed aberrant immune response to an infectious agent or a vaccination. Treatment with intravenous corticosteroids (methylprednisolone) or adrenocorticotrophic hormone in large doses has been shown to improve the outcome.[31,49] Approximately two thirds of the patients who are treated with corticosteroids benefit from the treatment; however, it is difficult to evaluate exact potential benefit of these therapies, as only case reports and series with small numbers of patients are available and there has been no controlled trial of their use. In some cases where corticosteroids have failed to work, use of[50] plasmapharesis or intravenous immunoglobulin[51–53] has been shown to produce dramatic improvement. Keegan *et al.* recently reviewed 59 consecutive patients with plasma exchange for acute severe attacks of central nervous system demyelination at the Mayo clinic. This series included 10 patients with ADEM and neuromyelitis optica plus 22 patients with relapsing-remitting multiple sclerosis. The remainder had miscellaneous demyelinating disorders such as acute transverse myelitis and Marburg variant of multiple sclerosis. Among 20 patients with ADEM and neuromyelitis optica 50% showed moderate or marked improvement. For the whole group of 59 patients, it was concluded that certain factors like male sex, preserved reflexes, and early initiation of treatment were associated with improvements. Successfully treated patients improved rapidly after plasma exchange and improvement was sustained.[54] In some cases cytotoxic agents have been used with success.[31]

As has been suggested previously, a persistent infection may contribute directly to the central nervous system inflammation and demyelination. It has been argued that antimicrobial therapy, if initiated soon enough, could possibly limit the infection and resulting neurotoxic immune response. Unfortunately, there are currently no effective treatments available for many of viruses implicated in ADEM, so this option remains a theoretical possibility.[5]

Prognosis

It has been observed that methylprednisolone therapy shortens the duration of neurological symptoms and immediately halts further progression. As far as long-term prognosis of ADEM is concerned, in one of the largest follow-up series of 40 adult patients (15–68 years, mean 33.5 years) with ADEM, 14 patients developed clinically definite multiple sclerosis. Out of the remaining 26 patients with a final diagnosis of ADEM, two patients died, nine had minor residual deficits, three had moderate deficits, and 12 patients had no remaining symptoms. In all patients who progressed to multiple sclerosis, the second episode occurred within the first year of initial presentation. In the longest follow-up (eight years) of 11 patients with final diagnosis of ADEM, none experienced a new clinical attack during follow-up and new white matter MRI lesions were detectable in only one patient. Recurrences in ADEM were defined as appearance of new symptoms and signs at least one month after the previous episode. The patients with the final diagnosis of ADEM were older and more often had a preceding infection, clinical signs of brainstem involvement, a higher cerebrospinal fluid albumin fraction, and infratentorial lesions.[31] In another study, Cohen *et al.* followed up 21 patients with ADEM: five patients had recurrent disease episodes, three patients had three or more recurrences. A very good response to corticosteroids was observed in each recurrence episode. Patients who relapsed tended to have more than one recurrence that usually involved (clinically and radiologically) a brain territory that was affected before. Neuropsychiatric features were the main presentation of a relapse. These authors conclude that recurrence in ADEM is more common than previously recognised; since recurrent ADEM is a corticosteroid-responsive condition, awareness about the disease and early diagnosis are mandatory.[55]

In one of the recently published series of ADEM in 31 children, 81% of patients recovered completely with various immunomodulator agents.[34] In the remaining five patients only mild neurological sequelae were recorded. None of the patients died during follow-up. In this series, four patients had relapses, and three of these had involvement of the corpus callosum on MRI (the authors considered this a feature suggestive of multiple sclerosis), even then the authors did not think that any of these patients had multiple sclerosis. In another paediatric series by Belopitova *et al.*, 25 children aged 3–18 years with an initial diagnosis of ADEM were followed up for a period of 2–8 years.[56] In 10 children there were data for clinically definite or laboratory supported definite multiple sclerosis. The remaining 15 children in this study were suspected to have multiple sclerosis. These authors think that the dynamic long-term follow-up (with the help of neuroimaging, cerebrospinal fluid, and evoked potential studies) of pathological changes is of prognostic significance for the course of the disease, which could be a definite cessation of the process in ADEM cases or transition to multiple sclerosis.

ADEM: a distinct disease or part of the multiple sclerosis spectrum?

One of the most intriguing features of ADEM is its exact relation with multiple sclerosis. Because of many similarities in clinical features, MRI findings, and pathogenesis several authors believe that ADEM is part of the multiple sclerosis spectrum.[42] The precipitants of demyelination in both conditions may be an infectious (especially viral) illness and share the major pathogenetic characteristic of an obligatory alteration of blood-brain barrier. However, the mechanisms of myelin destruction may be different. It is well known that multiple sclerosis is more prevalent in certain races because of genetic predisposition, while ADEM is seen in all races and geographical areas. In India and other developing countries ADEM is a common disease, but multiple sclerosis is infrequently seen. Here a large number of cases of ADEM occur after specific viral infections (for example, measles) or after the use of outdated vaccines and because the incidence of various specific infections that may predispose to ADEM is still high and Semple antirabies vaccine is still in use.[57] ADEM caused by Semple antirabies vaccine is often associated with involvement of the peripheral nervous system in the form of radiculoneuropathy.[30] In contrast to reports from Western countries, conversion of ADEM to multiple sclerosis has not been reported from developing countries. Modi *et al.* recently described eight black South African patients (a population with a low risk of multiple sclerosis) with a new multiphasic steroid-responsive demyelinating disorder of the central nervous system. Neuroimaging in these patients showed features consistent with those described for ADEM as well as some features that were described in multiple sclerosis. These patients had two or more distinct acute attacks of a demyelinating disorder separated in space and time generally with poor outcome and stepwise disabilities after repeated attacks. Authors were not sure about the exact diagnosis in any of the cases.[58] Therefore, it can be argued that ADEM seen in developing countries is a distinct syndrome and is not part of the multiple sclerosis spectrum.

Conclusion

ADEM is a monophasic inflammatory disease affecting the central nervous system, which usually follows an infection or vaccination. It is difficult to differentiate ADEM from a single episode of multiple sclerosis because of the largely similar clinical presentation, cerebrospinal fluid analysis, histopathological and neuroimaging appearance. Recent literature indicates that a significant proportion of adult and paediatric patients with ADEM develop clinically definite multiple sclerosis in due course. However, it is not possible to identify with certainty any clinical marker which can differentiate ADEM from the initial presentation of multiple sclerosis. Experts now believe that ADEM and multiple sclerosis are parts of the same spectrum of inflammatory demyelinating conditions. In India and other developing countries ADEM is a common neurological condition, possibly because of the high prevalence of causative infections. However, the reasons for the low occurrence of multiple sclerosis are not known.

References

1 Murthy SNK, Faden HS, Cohen ME, *et al.* Acute disseminated encephalomyelitis in children. *Pediatrics* 2002; **110**(2). www.pediatrics.org/cgi/content/full/110/2/e21.
2 Murthy JM, Yangala R, Meena AK, *et al.* Acute disseminated encephalomyelitis: clinical and MRI study from South India. *J Neurol Sci* 1999; **165**: 133–8.
3 Litvak AM, Sands IJ, Gibel H. Encephalitis complicating measles: report of 56 cases with follow-up studies in 32. *Am J Dis Child* 1943; **65**: 265–95.

4 Miller HG, Evans MJ. Prognosis in acute disseminated encephalomyelitis: with a note of neuromyelitis optica. *Q J Med* 1953; **22**: 247–79.

5 Stuve O, Zamvil SS. Pathogenesis, diagnosis and treatment of acute disseminated encephalomyelitis. *Curr Opin Neurology* 1999; **12**: 395–401.

6 Held JR, Adros HL. Neurological disease in man following administration of suckling mouse brain antirabies vaccine. *Bull World Health Organ* 1972; **46**: 321–7.

7 Label LS, Batts DH. Transverse myelitis caused by duck embryo rabies vaccine. *Arch Neurol* 1982; **39**: 426–30.

8 Swamy HS, Shankar SK, Satish Chandra P, *et al.* Neurological complications due to beta-propiolactone (BPL) inactivated antirabies vaccination. *J Neurol Sci* 1984; **63**: 111–28.

9 Hemchudha T, Griffin DE, Giffels JJ, *et al.* Myelin basic protein as an encephalitogen in encephalomyelitis and polyneuritis following rabies vaccination. *N Engl J Med* 1987; **316**: 369–74.

10 Murthy JMK. MRI in acute disseminated encephalomyelitis following Semple anti-rabies vaccine. *Neuroradiology* 1998; **40**: 420–3.

11 Chakrawarty A. Neurologic illness following post-exposure prophylaxis with purified chick embryo cell antirabies vaccine. *J Assoc Physicians India* 2001; **44**: 927–8.

12 Fenichel GM. Neurological complications of immunization. *Ann Neurol* 1982; **12**: 119–28.

13 Nalin DR. Mumps, measles and rubella vaccination and encephalitis (letter). *BMJ* 1989; **299**: 1219.

14 van Bogaert L. Post-infectious encephalomyelitis and multiple sclerosis: the significance of perivenous encephalomyelitis. *J Neuropathol Exp Neurol* 1950; **9**: 219–49.

15 Allen IV. Demyelinating diseases. In: Adams JH, Corsellis JAN, Duchen LW, eds. *Greenfield's neuropathology*. 4th edn. London: Edward Arnold, 1984: 338–84.

16 Davies JM. Molecular mimicry: can epitope mimicry induce autoimmune disease? *Immunol Cell Biol* 1997; **75**: 113–26.

17 Johnson RT. Pathogenesis of acute viral encephalitis and postinfectious encephalo-myelitis. *J Infect Dis* 1987; **155**: 359–64.

18 Zamvil SS, Steinman L. The T lymphocyte in experimental allergic encephalomyelitis. *Annu Rev Immunol* 1990; **8**: 579–621.

19 Gold R, Hartung HP, Toyka KV. Animal models for autoimmune demyelinating disorder of the nervous system. *Mol Med Today* 2000; **62**: 88–91.

20 Laouini D, Kennou MF, Khoufi S, *et al.* Antibodies to human myelin proteins and gangliosides in patients with acute neuroparalytic accident induced by brain-derived rabies vaccine. *J Neuroimmunol* 1998; **91**: 63–72.

21 't Hart BA, Brok HP, Amor S, *et al.* The major histocompatibility complex influences the ethiopathogenesis of MS-like disease in primates at multiple levels. *Hum Immunol* 2001; **62**: 1371–81.

22 Scully RE, Mark EJ, McNeely WF, *et al.* Case records of the Massachusetts General Hospital, case 37–1995. *N Engl J Med* 1995; **333**: 1485–92.

23 Scully RE, Mark EJ, McNeely WF, *et al.* Case records of the Massachusetts General Hospital, case 1–1999. *N Engl J Med* 1999; **340**: 127–35.

24 Stefansson K, Hedley-Whyte ET. Case records of the Massachusetts General Hospital, case 8–1996 – a 28 year old woman with rapid development of a major personality change and global aphasia. *N Engl J Med* 1996; **334**: 715–21.

25 Liu J, Marino MW, Wong G, *et al.* TNF is a potent anti-inflammatory cytokine in autoimmune-mediated demyelination. *Nat Med* 1998; **4**: 78–83.

26 Sabelko-Downes KA, Russell JH, Cross AH. Role of Fas–FasL interactions in the pathogenesis and regulation of autoimmune demyelinating disease. *J Neuroimmunol* 1999; **100**: 42–52.

27 Boullerne AI, Nedelkoska L, Benjamins JA. Role of calcium in nitric oxide-induced cytotoxicity: EGTA protects mouse oligodendrocytes. *J Neurosci Res* 2001; **63**: 124–35.

28 van der Goes A, Brouwer J, Hoekstra K, *et al*. Reactive oxygen species are required for the phagocytosis of myelin by macrophages. *J Neuroimmunol* 1998; **92**: 67–75.

29 Matute C, Alberdi E, Domercq M, *et al*. The link between excitotoxic oligodendroglial death and demyelinating diseases. *Trends Neurosci* 2001; **24**: 224–30.

30 Murthy JMK, Yangala R, Meena AK, *et al*. Clinical, electrophysiological and magnetic resonance imaging study of acute disseminated encephalomyelitis. *J Assoc Physicians India* 1999; **47**: 280–3.

31 Schwarz S, Mohr A, Knauth M, *et al*. Acute disseminated encephalomyelitis: a follow-up study of 40 adult patients. *Neurology* 2001; **56**: 1313–18.

32 Apak RA, Kose G, Anlar B, *et al*. Acute disseminated encephalomyelitis in childhood: report of 10 cases. *J Child Neurol* 1999; **14**: 198–201.

33 Dale RC, de Sousa C, Chong WK, *et al*. Acute disseminated encephalomyelitis, multiphasic disseminated encephalomyelitis and multiple sclerosis in children. *Brain* 2000; **123**: 2407–22.

34 Hynson JL, Kornberg AJ, Coleman LT, *et al*. Clinical and neuroradiologic features of acute disseminated encephalomyelitis in children. *Neurology* 2001; **56**: 1308–12.

35 Hollinger P, Sturzenegger M, Mathis J, *et al*. Acute disseminated encephalomyelitis in adults: a reappraisal of clinical CSF, EEG and MRI findings. *J Neurol* 2002; **249**: 320–9.

36 Lukes SA, Norman D. Computed tomography in acute disseminated encephalomyelitis. *Ann Neurol* 1983; **13**: 567–72.

37 Caldmeyer KS, Smith RR, Harris TM, *et al*. MRI in acute disseminated encephalomyelitis. *Neuroradiology* 1994; **36**: 216–20.

38 Singh S, Alexander M, Korah IP. Acute disseminated encephalomyelitis: MR imaging features. *AJR Am J Roentgenol* 1999; **173**: 1101–7.

39 O'Riordan JI, Gomez-Anson B, Moseley IF, *et al*. Long term MRI follow-up of patients with post-infectious encephalomyelitis: evidence for a monophasic disease. *J Neurol Sci* 1999; **167**: 132–6.

40 Bizzi A, Ulug AM, Crawford TO, *et al*. Quantitative proton MR spectroscopic imaging in acute disseminated encephalomyelitis. *AJNR Am J Neuroradiol* 2001; **22**: 1125–30.

41 Honkaniemi J, Dastidar P, Kahara V, *et al*. Delayed MR imaging changes in acute disseminated encephalomyelitis. *AJNR Am J Neuroradiol* 2001; **22**: 1117–24.

42 Hartung HP, Grossman RI. ADEM: distinct disease or part of MS spectrum? *Neurology* 2001; **56**: 1257–60.

43 Singh S, Prabhakar S, Korah IP, *et al*. Acute disseminated encephalomyelitis and multiple sclerosis: magnetic resonance imaging differentiation. *Australas Radiol* 2000; **44**: 404–11.

44 Barkhof F, Filippi M, Miller DH, *et al*. Comparison of MR imaging criteria at first presentation to predict conversion to clinically definite multiple sclerosis. *Brain* 1997; **120**: 2059–69.

45 Hung KL, Liao HT, Tsai ML. Post-infectious encephalomyelitis: etiologic and diagnostic trends. *J Child Neurol* 2000; **15**: 666–70.

46 Cuadrado MJ, Khamashta MA, Ballesteros A, *et al*. Can neurologic manifestations of Hughes (antiphospholipid) syndrome be distinguished from multiple sclerosis? *Medicine* 2000; **79**: 57–68.

47 Dey KB, Trikha I, Banerjee M, *et al*. Acute disseminated encephalomyelitis – another cause of postmalaria cerebeller ataxia. *J Assoc Physicians India* 2001; **49**: 756–8.

48 Mohsen AH, Mckendrick MW, Schmid ML, *et al*. Postmalaria neurological syndrome: a case of disseminated encephalomyelitis. *J Neurol Neurosurg Psychiatry* 2000; **68**: 388–90.

49 Straub J, Chofflon M, Delavelle J. Early high-dose intravenous methyl prednisolone in acute disseminated encephalomyelitis: a successful recovery. *Neurology* 1997; **49**: 1145–7.

50 Kanter DS, Horensky D, Sperling RA, *et al*. Plasmapheresis in fulminant acute disseminated encephalomyelitis. *Neurology* 1995; **45**: 824–7.

51 Pradhan S, Gupta RP, Shashank S, *et al*. Intravenous immunoglobulin therapy in acute disseminated encephalomyelitis. *J Neurol Sci* 1999; **165**: 56–61.

52 Sahlas DJ, Miller SP, Guerin M, *et al*. Treatment of acute disseminated encephalomyelitis with intravenous immunoglobulin. *Neurology* 2000; **54**: 1370–2.

53 Marchioni E, Marinou-Aktipi K, Uggetti C, *et al*. Effectiveness of intravenous immunoglobulin treatment in adult patients with steroid resistant monophasic or recurrent acute disseminated encephalomyelitis. *J Neurol* 2002; **249**: 100–4.

54 Keegan M, Pineda AA, McClelland RL, *et al*. Plasma exchange for severe attacks of CNS demyelination: predictors of response. *Neurology* 2002; **58**: 143–6.

55 Cohen O, Steiner-Birmanns B, Biran I, *et al*. Recurrence of acute disseminated encephalomyelitis at the previously affected brain site. *Arch Neurol* 2001; **38**: 797–801.

56 Belopitova L, Guergueltecheva PV, Bojinova V. Definite and suspected multiple sclerosis in children: long term follow-up and magnetic resonance imaging findings. *J Child Neurol* 2001; **16**: 317–24.

57 Chou HVV, Hien TT, Sellar R, *et al*. 'Can't you use another vaccine'? Post-rabies vaccination encephalitis [letter]. *J Neurol Neurosurg Psychiatry* 1999; **67**: 555–6.

58 Modi G, Mochan A, Modi M, *et al*. Demyelinating disorder of the central nervous system occurring in black South Africans. *J Neurol Neurosurg Psychiatry* 2001; **70**: 500–5.

Part 3

Neurodegeneration and neuroinflammation

Chapter Eleven

Management of motor neurone disease

RS Howard and RW Orrell

Motor neurone disease is a progressive neurodegenerative disorder leading to severe disability and death. It is clinically characterised by mixed upper and lower motor neurone involvement affecting bulbar, limb, and respiratory musculature. Recent guidelines have established diagnostic criteria and defined management of the condition. In a proportion of familial amyotrophic lateral sclerosis there is a mutation in the gene encoding the enzyme copper/zinc superoxide dismutase 1; this has allowed mutation screening and generated considerable laboratory-based research. The diagnosis must be given with care and consideration and close follow-up is essential. Management involves a multidisciplinary team based in the hospital and the community. Riluzole is the only drug shown to have a disease-modifying effect and has been approved by the National Institute for Clinical Excellence. The essence of care is good symptomatic management, including nutritional support with percutaneous endoscopic gastrostomy and ventilatory care with non-invasive ventilation. Palliative care should be introduced before the terminal stages after careful discussion with the patient and carers. Knowledge of this condition has grown dramatically recently with a parallel improvement in treatment and ability to deal with the most troublesome problems.

Motor neurone disease (MND) is a neurodegenerative disorder characterised by progressive involvement of the corticospinal tract and the motor neurones of the ventral cord and brainstem. Involvement of the central (upper) motor neurones leads to spasticity, weakness, and hyperreflexia, while lower motor neurone impairment will cause fasciculation, atrophy, weakness, and hyporeflexia. Amyotrophic lateral sclerosis is characterised by the involvement of upper and lower limb territories and encompasses progressive bulbar palsy. In primary lateral sclerosis there is exclusively upper motor neurone involvement, and progressive muscular atrophy involves only the lower motor neurones. Each of these conditions is a form of amyotrophic lateral sclerosis as, at necropsy, there is usually evidence of abnormalities of both upper and lower motor neurones. The condition usually spares sensation, eye movements, and sphincter function but a frontotemporal dementia may rarely coexist. The course of MND is usually rapidly progressive, impairment of mobility is common, and many patients have swallowing difficulties.

Incidence and prognosis

The annual incidence is between 1.5 and 2/100 000 and males are more commonly affected than females (1.4:1). The incidence increases with age with a mean age of onset of 63 years. Over 50% of patients die within three years and 90% within five years of the first symptom. Early respiratory or bulbar symptoms and increasing age are adverse prognostic indicators.[1–3]

Guidelines

In 1999 the Quality Standards Subcommittee of the American Academy of Neurology presented the first recommendations for the management of amyotrophic lateral sclerosis based on a prescribed review and analysis of the peer reviewed literature.[4] At the same time a UK MND advisory group, endorsed by the Association of British Neurologists, produced a series of guidelines for the management of MND.[5] Since that time there have been a number of further review articles and textbooks which have allowed further development of guidelines for best practice.[6–13] A recent study has audited the management of patients in North America after publications of the guidelines illustrating where deficiencies in provision exist.[14]

Diagnosis

The condition is characterised by the progressive development of combined upper and lower motor neurone signs in a generalised distribution without sensory involvement – however, the diagnosis is usually made at an earlier stage when the signs may be restricted. Research criteria for the diagnosis exist,[15,16] but these are rigorous and most patients are considered 'possible' or 'probable' at the time of diagnosis. Diagnostic difficulty is caused by exclusively upper or lower motor neurone monoparesis or paraparesis without sensory loss, or if there is a particularly long history, young age of onset, or the presence of significant cognitive impairment. Electrophysiology studies are required to confirm the diagnosis and these will show evidence of acute denervation and reinnervation without conduction block. Magnetic resonance imaging of the brain and spinal cord may be necessary to exclude a structural lesion and cerebrospinal fluid examination to exclude an infective or inflammatory cause. The initial clinical diagnosis is correct in more than 90% of cases.

Differential diagnosis of motor neurone disease

The most important differential diagnoses include multifocal motor neuropathy, a condition of lower motor neurone involvement due to multiple conduction block shown electrophysiologically which may be associated with the presence of GM1 ganglioside antibodies. This condition may respond to immunomodulatory treatment. Inflammatory polyneuropathies, particularly chronic inflammatory demyelinating neuropathy, may also cause progressive weakness with little or no sensory loss. Other conditions which may be confused with MND include Kennedy's syndrome (X-linked bulbospinal neuronopathy), which is associated with an older age of onset and diffuse, often severe, fasciculations as well as bulbar involvement, variable sensory ataxia, gynaecomastia, and testicular atrophy. It is known to be associated with a specific trinucleotide repeat expansion in the androgen receptor gene (Xq21–22). Adult onset spinal muscular atrophy forms a genetically heterogeneous group of disorders of progressive lower motor neurone wasting and weakness which progress at varying rates and may lead to ventilatory failure. Rarely, metabolic and inflammatory myopathy (polymyositis, inclusion body myositis, thyrotoxicosis) may present with aggressive wasting and weakness mimicking motor neurone disease. Multiple radiculopathy may also present with segmental wasting and weakness mimicking MND.

Genetics

A proved cause of MND is mutation of the gene encoding the enzyme copper/zinc superoxide dismutase 1 (SOD1). This accounts for about 2% of all cases of MND and is present in about 20% of the approximately 5% of patients with a family history. To date, over 90 different mutations have been identified. SOD1 mutation screening is available, but counselling is important before predictive testing can be undertaken.[17] Mutations in a second gene (alsin) have been described in a small number of patients with autosomal recessive inheritance.[18,19] Linkage has been described in a number of families with the gene still to be identified.

Telling the diagnosis

The communication of the diagnosis is a major and, potentially devastating, life event, which must be handled with great sensitivity.[20,21] All too often the patients complain that the diagnosis has been given in a hurried, offhand, and inappropriate manner.

   The diagnosis should be explained by a senior physician in a quiet and private room, with the patient and their chosen carer(s) with discussion and answering questions. During the consultation the patient should be allowed to dictate the pace and questioning but the neurologist must steer the discussion with sensitivity and care. A second opinion may be offered. The patient should be provided with full access to written information, which is comprehensible. During the consultation it is important to emphasise that a further follow-up appointment will be made within two weeks, ongoing follow-up can be supervised by a single named doctor, and there will be close liaison with the general practitioner (GP) and community services. The patient should be informed about the range of symptomatic and specific treatments. They should also be provided with information about the Motor Neurone Disease Association. The diagnosis and details of the information given to the patient and the management plan must be communicated to the GP without delay.

Principles of management

The management of MND involves the coordination of multidisciplinary care with a team which will include the patient's own GP and practice team, therapists, clinical nurse specialists, support and social workers, and the palliative care team. The supervising neurologist or physician should address the full continuum of care for the patient with amyotrophic lateral sclerosis from diagnosis through palliative care to the terminal phase of the disease. Each member of the team will have an individual role.[22] Physiotherapists may be involved throughout the course of the disease. In the early stages they will instruct on appropriate exercise, advice on gait, compensatory movements, and posture. In later stages passive movements may relieve musculoskeletal pain. Patients and carers will need advice on exercises, stretches, transfers, and positioning. Therapists will provide neck collars designed for patients with MND. Occupational therapists have a crucial role in the assessment and provision of aids for daily living and communication aids including environmental control systems and call systems. They will also coordinate the provision of mobility aids including wheelchairs, sticks, and walking frames. They can advise about adaptations to housing to maintain maximum independence. Social workers and other support and advice workers may counsel about financial benefits and other practical measures as well as provide assistance to patients and families in obtaining the necessary support at home.

The Motor Neurone Disease Association employs a network of regional care advisors throughout England, Wales, and Northern Ireland.[23] These individuals act as a point of contact for people with MND and their carers, and help to point to the provision of pieces of equipment such as splints and communication aids that may be needed. They also provide a telephone help line and are able to contribute to the support of relatives and carers after the death of the patient.

Disease-modifying treatment

Many putative drug treatments for MND have been reported. Such treatments have included agents which might inhibit or prevent cell damage (for example, antiglutamate, antioxidants, antiviral agents, and neurotrophic agents), to enhance neuronal repair (antigangliosides), to inhibit immune-mediated damage (immunomodulatory agents), or to enhance neuromuscular function. Apart from riluzole, none of these treatments have been shown to have an effect on the condition.

Intravenous human immunoglobulin is of benefit in patients with inflammatory neuropathic disorders including multifocal motor neuropathy. It may also result in improvement in patients with the clinical syndrome of lower motor neurone involvement in whom there is evidence of motor conduction block, and sometimes in patients where no conduction block is detected.[24]

Riluzole, which inhibits glutamate release, is the only drug which has been shown to increase survival in MND and is licensed in the UK and worldwide, with some exceptions (notably Australia and Canada).[25–31] Riluzole prolonged survival by three months after 18 months administration with little or no effect on functional deterioration in two clinical trials. Riluzole is usually well tolerated with occasional nausea and fatigue. It is taken as a tablet, as a standard dose of 50 mg twice a day. Blood count and liver function are monitored regularly and the drug is discontinued if liver function tests exceed five times the upper limit of normal. In the UK, riluzole has been recommended for use in the treatment of patients with motor neurone disease by the National Institute for Clinical

Excellence. Because of the lack of curative medication, and the progressive nature of the disease, many patients look to other possible treatments. There is no substantial evidence to support therapeutic benefit in patients with motor neurone disease. Nevertheless, based on free radical theories of MND pathogenesis, many patients take a range of antioxidant medications, including vitamin C and vitamin E. Some patients are presently also taking creatine, based on studies in a transgenic SOD1 mutant mouse model of amyotrophic lateral sclerosis. Some patients also try alternative therapies, including acupuncture, reflexology, chiropracty, and massage. The effects of these approaches are unproved, but they may contribute to the individual's personal feeling of wellbeing.

Respiratory management

Respiratory impairment is common in MND and may develop because of respiratory muscle weakness, impaired bulbar function causing aspiration or obstructive sleep apnoea, or defects in central control. Dyspnoea may be due to infection, pulmonary embolus, or airway obstruction from mucus plug or inhaled pharyngeal contents.[31] Prompt use of antibiotics should be supplemented with physiotherapy. Annual influenza vaccination should be undertaken.

Nocturnal hypoventilation may present as daytime hypersomnolence, lethargy, morning headaches, poor concentration, depression, anxiety, and irritability while obstructive sleep apnoea is characterised by snoring and restless sleep with abnormal movements.

Forced vital capacity reflects respiratory muscle strength, and serial measurements may be useful in predicting the onset of respiratory failure in MND.[32–36] Some protocols in the USA recommend initiating non-invasive ventilation when forced vital capacity is less than 50% of predicted. Other markers of impending respiratory failure include maximal inspiratory and expiratory mouth pressures and maximum sniff nasal pressure.[32] Polysomnography may detect early signs of respiratory insufficiency during sleep[37,38] and diaphragmatic electromyography and phrenic nerve conduction studies may provide useful additional information.[39] Whichever method is used, careful and detailed discussion with the patient is paramount.

It has been increasingly recognised that the provision of respiratory support can provide symptomatic relief and increase life expectancy.[39–45] However these benefits must be balanced against the difficulties of compliance in severely disabled patients, the demands on carers and relatives, the practical problems of administrating ventilatory support, the risk of iatrogenic problems,[45] increasing dependence on ventilatory support[46] causing distressing and unwanted prolongation of life, and difficulties in managing the terminal stages in these patients.[47–50] While many of these difficulties can be avoided by careful discussion with patients and their carers, many patients delay or wish to avoid decisions about embarking on ventilatory support. Elective ventilatory support is usually administered non-invasively via masks (facial or nasal), mouthpieces or nasal pillows, and initially it is usually used for improving respiratory function during sleep. Non-invasive ventilatory support has advantages as it allows speech, oral feeding, has lower costs, and leads to fewer respiratory infections,[51] but it may not be desirable in patients with severe bulbar weakness, facial abnormalities, or where aspiration has already occurred. Non-invasive ventilatory support may improve survival in

MND, reduce the work of breathing, promote good gas exchange, and improve quality of sleep. This often results in improvement of daytime symptoms such as breathlessness and excessive sleepiness. Some patients may require ventilatory support for increasing periods while awake or even continuously and may choose to undergo tracheostomy.[52–54] Tracheostomy carries a significant risk of complications and considerable difficulties in domiciliary management.[55] Pulmonary aspiration may still occur with an uncuffed tube. There remains a concern that tracheostomy may lead to prolonged survival in the face of severe disability.

Respiratory failure should be anticipated in all patients once the diagnosis of MND has been made. Optimal management of patients with MND includes protecting autonomy, giving information in advance of deterioration (particularly with regards to respiratory failure), addressing all aspects of care in a multidisciplinary environment, and discussing regularly any advance directives.[17] After careful discussion many patients will decide to use non-invasive ventilatory support if their respiratory function deteriorates and is symptomatic. The provision and supervision of respiratory support should be through a specialist centre, with experience in the management of MND.

Management of bulbar weakness

Bulbar palsy is one of the most distressing features of MND. The resulting weakness of tongue, pharynx, and facial muscles results in the loss of salivary control with slow eating, choking, drooling, dysarthria, and dysphonia.[56,57] Sialorrhoea is generally managed with anticholinergic agents including atropine or amitriptyline taken orally, hyoscine (scopolamine) transdermally, glycopyrronium bromide subcutaneously, or via gastrostomy. Side effects include confusion and exacerbation of glaucoma, particularly in the elderly.[58–60] Unilateral parotid gland irradiation and direct injection of botulinum toxin into the parotid gland have also been used.[61,62] Whereas antimuscarinic agents render secretions tenacious and viscid, β-blockers such as propranolol and metoprolol have been reported to reduce secretions without increasing tenacity.[60] Other approaches include adequate hydration and mucolytics (carbocistine or mecysteine hydrochloride).

Dysphagia

The management involves speech and language therapy assessment of swallow and advice on techniques to ease mastication and prevent aspiration.

Enteral feeding

Patients with dysphagia may have inadequate energy and fluid intake, leading to accelerated weight loss and dehydration.[63] The initial management of dysphagia in amyotrophic lateral sclerosis includes modification of food and fluid consistencies. The dietitian has an important role in ensuring maximal energy intake in as easily digested form as possible. The presence of laryngeal penetration on videofluoroscopy indicates a high risk for the development of aspiration pneumonia. As dysphagia worsens percutaneous endoscopic gastrostomy (PEG) should be considered as an alternative or supplementary route for nutrition and hydration. The immediate benefits of PEG are adequate nutritional intake, weight stabilisation, and an alternative route for medication.[64,65] People with PEG can continue to swallow liquids and solids. In amyotrophic lateral sclerosis, it is recommended that PEG should be undertaken before the forced vital capacity falls below 50% of predicted and not in the preterminal phase. Complications of the PEG procedure include transient laryngeal spasm, aspiration pneumonia, localised infection, gastric haemorrhage, failure to place PEG due to technical difficulties, and death due to respiratory arrest.[66] Gastrostomy is more successful and survival improves if it is undertaken before respiratory function deteriorates. It should be considered early, and adequate assistance be made available to the patients, their carers, and community nursing and dietetic staff. Radiological insertion of gastrostomy tube does not require sedation but is associated with a higher risk of complications.

Communication

To improve communication the speech therapist may recommend aids, ranging from pointing boards (a list of words) to computerised speech synthesisers. When a communication aid is needed it is essential that it is provided promptly.

Limb dysfunction

Musculoskeletal pain is commonly experienced and may be managed at any stage with antispasticity agents, non-steroidal anti-inflammatory agents, and stronger analgesics including opiates.[67] Skin pressure pain due to immobility may also occur. Fasciculations are common but are rarely a distressing feature. They tend to improve with disease progression but the symptoms may be eased by carbamazepine. Cramps usually affect the lower limbs, are usually nocturnal, and often uncomfortable. Quinine sulphate, diazepam, carbamazepine, and phenytoin have been used with variable results. Stiffness may be due to spasticity or muscle or joint contracture. This has been treated by increasing doses of baclofen but tizanidine is now a valuable alternative. Spasticity may compromise mobility but can aid weak legs to support the body.

Psychological factors

Depression and anxiety often follow the diagnosis of MND. Both should be treated appropriately, and not viewed as unavoidable consequences of a progressive disease. The drugs of choice for depression in this context include serotonin reuptake inhibitors, for example fluoxetine. Anxiety may be severe enough to require specific drug therapy. This may be short-term treatment with benzodiazepines but amitriptyline can also help.[68] Aggression and disinhibition may be a feature of cognitive impairment. Phenothiazines may be necessary, and psychiatric support is often helpful.

Emotional lability is usually associated with pseudobulbar palsy. It may be distressing to the patient and his carers. Emotional lability may be eased by amitriptyline or a serotonin reuptake inhibitor such as citalopram, fluoxetine, or paroxetine.[69-71]

Other symptoms

Insomnia is common in MND and may relate to physical discomfort, anxiety, or respiratory compromise. If sleep remains disturbed after relief of pain then sedatives may help. Amitriptyline is preferable to hypnotics, which are most likely to exacerbate respiratory insufficiency. Constipation is treated by dietary advice and ample fluid intake supplemented by Fybogel, lactulose, and co-danthromer.

Terminal care

Palliative care should be introduced before the terminal stages of MND.[72] Home care teams and day centres may offer respite care, with a parallel set of therapists and support staff complementing those provided elsewhere. There must be close liaison with the GP, community health care, and hospice teams. The terminal stages of the disease should be managed in close liaison with palliative care physicians.[72–75]

Terminal care often involves alleviating psychological distress and the symptoms of bulbar weakness and respiratory failure. Patients may experience a frightening sensation of choking due to episodes of laryngospasm. Benzodiazepines and agents to dry secretions may be helpful but laryngospasm usually resolves spontaneously. Oral, subcutaneous, or intravenous morphine may be indicated to relieve dyspnoea, anxiety, pain, hunger, or other distress. The effectiveness of sedatives such as diazepam, midazolam, or chlorpromazine in reducing anxiety in the terminal stages outweighs any depressive action of the drugs on respiratory function.[76–83]

The 'Breathing Space Kit', provided by the Motor Neurone Disease Association in the UK, contains medication which can be used by the carer, nurse, or GP for the emergency treatment of an acute episode of respiratory distress which often occurs in the terminal stages. These include diazepam, diamorphine, chlorpromazine, and hyoscine.

Key references from recent years

- Miller RG, Rosenberg JA, Gelinas DF, *et al.* Practice parameters. The care of the patient with amyotrophic lateral sclerosis (an evidence-based review): report of the Quality Standards Subcommittee of the American Academy of Neurology: ALS Practice Parameters Task Force. *Neurology* 1999; **52**: 1311–23.
- Exerpta Medica MND Advisory Group. *Guidelines for the management of motor neurone disease (MND)*. Endorsed by the Council of the Association of Neurologists, 1999 (www.theabn.org/downloads/mnddoc.pdp).
- Miller RG, Mitchell JD, Moore DH. Riluzole for amyotrophic lateral sclerosis/motor neurone disease (Protocol for a Cochrane review). The Cochrane Library, Issue 2, 2002. Oxford: Update Software.
- Orrell RW, Figlewicz DA. Clinical implications of the genetics of ALS and other motor neuron diseases. *Neuology* 2001; **57**: 9–17
- Bradley WG, Anderson F, Bromberg M, *et al.* Current management of ALS. *Neurology* 2001; **57**: 500–4.

Useful web sites

- www.wfnals.org World Federation of Neurology, Amyotrophic Lateral Sclerosis site
- www.mndassociation.org Motor Neurone Disease Association (England, Wales and Northern Ireland)
- www.alsmndalliance.org International Alliance of ALS/MND Associations
- www.cochrane.org The Cochrane collaboration (includes report on riluzole)
- www.theabn.org/downloads/mnddoc.pdp Guidelines for the management of motor neurone disease, endorsed by the Association of British Neurologists
- www.alsa.org ALS Association (USA).
- www.scotmnd.org.uk Scottish Motor Neurone Disease Association
- www.nice.org.uk National Institute for Clinical Excellence – includes review and recommendations for the use of riluzole

Carers

After the death of an MND sufferer the family and carers will require bereavement support.[84,85] This may be provided by the palliative care team but continuing domiciliary support may also be necessary.

Conclusion

The development of clinical guidelines for the management of MND has provided a valuable stimulus to address and improve the present provision of service for patients with MND in the UK. However, as Bradley *et al.* have illustrated in the USA,[6] there remains an overwhelming need for better access to diagnostic, rehabilitation, technical and palliative care for these patients and their carers.

Questions and answers

What is motor neurone disease?

Motor neurone disease is a neurodegenerative disease affecting upper and lower motor neurones. In many countries this is referred to as amyotrophic lateral sclerosis.

What is the cause of motor neurone disease?

The cause is largely unknown. Approximately 2% of patients have mutations in the SOD1 gene, and most of these patients show autosomal dominant inheritance. Genetic counselling may be considered in patients with a family history of motor neurone disease (around 5–10% of all patients).

What is the youngest age a patient can present with motor neurone disease?

Typically patients present in mid and late life but patients may develop the condition at any age, including the 20s and 30s. Rarely juvenile forms may occur.

Is there a curative treatment for motor neurone disease?

There is no treatment that will halt or reverse the progression of the disease. Riluzole is the only licensed medication for slowing the progression of the disease.

How may respiratory support benefit patients with motor neurone disease?

Non-invasive ventilation may provide amelioration of symptoms related to respiratory insufficiency, without causing significant extension of survival. More active and invasive respiratory support may extend survival in the face of severe disability.

What intervention has most significantly altered quality of life and survival of patients with motor neurone disease in recent years?

The active management of nutrition, including consideration of the early placement of PEG, has probably had the largest impact on the quality of life and survival by minimising cachexia, starvation, and aspiration.

What other conditions should be considered when making the diagnosis of motor neurone disease?

A wide range of neurological conditions may be confused with the initial presentation of motor neurone disease. With time the diagnosis usually becomes clear. Important treatable conditions to consider in the differential diagnoses include multifocal motor neuropathy, and other inflammatory neuropathies, which may respond to intravenous human immunoglobulin. Inflammatory myopathies, including polymyositis, may respond to steroid treatment. Also surgically treatable conditions in the brain, spinal cord, or peripheral nerves should be considered. Other rarer hereditary neuropathies, including Kennedy's disease, may have important genetic implications for the family.

References

1 Ringel SP, Murphy JR, Alderson MK, *et al*. The natural history of amyotrophic lateral sclerosis. *Neurology* 1993; **43**: 1316–22.

2 Haverkamp LJ, Appel V, Appel SH. Natural history of amyotrophic lateral sclerosis in a database population. Validation of a scoring system and a model for survival prediction. *Brain* 1995; **118**: 707–19.

3 Stambler N, Charatan M, Cedarbaum JM. Prognostic indicators of survival in ALS. ALS CNTF Treatment Study Group. *Neurology* 1998; **50**: 66–72.

4 Miller RG, Rosenberg JA, Gelinas DF, *et al*. Practice parameters. The care of the patient

with amyotrophic lateral sclerosis (an evidence-based review): report of the Quality Standards Subcommittee of the American Academy of Neurology: ALS Practice Parameters Task Force. *Neurology* 1999; **52**: 1311–23.

5 Exerpta Medica MND Advisory Group. *Guidelines for the management of motor neurone disease (MND)*. Endorsed by the Council of the Association of Neurologists, 1999 (www.theabn.org/downloads/mnddoc.pdp).

6 Bradley WG, Anderson F, Bromberg M, *et al*. Current management of ALS. *Neurology* 2001; **57**: 500–4.

7 Borasio GD. Meditation and ALS. In: Mitsumoto H, Munsat T, eds. *Amyotrophic lateral sclerosis: a comprehensive guide to management*. New York: Demos Medical Publishers, 2001: 271–6.

8 Gelinas DF, Miller RG. A treatable disease: a guide to the management of amyotrophic lateral sclerosis. In: Brown RH Jr, Meininger V, Swash M, eds. *Amyotrophic lateral sclerosis*. London: Martin Dunitz, 2000: 405–21.

9 Oliver D. Palliative care for motor neurone disease. *Practical Neurology* 2002; **2**: 68–79.

10 Miller RG, Mitchell JD, Moore DH. Riluzole for amyotrophic lateral sclerosis/motor neurone disease (Protocol for a Cochrane review). *The Cochrane Library*, Issue 2, 2002. Oxford: Update Software.

11 Hardiman O. Symptomatic treatment of respiratory and nutritional failure in amyotrophic lateral sclerosis. *J Neurol* 2000; **247**: 245–51.

12 Borasio GD, Volz R, Miller RG. Palliative care in amyotrophic lateral sclerosis. *Neurol Clin* 2001; **19**: 829–48.

13 Borasio GD, Miller RG. Clinical characteristics and management of ALS. *Semin Neurol* 2001; **21**: 155–66.

14 Bradley WG, Anderson F, Bromberg M, *et al*. Current management of ALS – comparison of the ALS CARE database and the AAN practice parameter. *Neurology* 2001; **57**: 500–4.

15 Subcommittee on Motor Neuron Diseases/Amyotrophic Lateral Sclerosis of the World Federation of Neurology Research Group on Neuromuscular Diseases, El Escorial 'Clinical Limits of Amyotrophic Lateral Sclerosis' Workshop Contributors. El Escorial World Federation of Neurology criteria for the diagnosis of amyotrophic lateral sclerosis. *J Neurol Sci* 1994; **124**(suppl): 96–107.

16 World Federation of Neurology Research Group on Motor Neuron Disease. Revised criteria for the diagnosis of Amyotrophic Lateral Sclerosis, 1998. http://wfnals.org/Articles/elescorial1998.htm.

17 Orrell RW, Figlewicz DA. Clinical implications of the genetics of ALS and other motor neuron diseases. *Neuology* 2001; **57**: 9–17.

18 Yang Y, Hentati A, Deng HX, *et al*. The gene encoding alsin, a protein with three guanine nucleotide exchange factor domains, is mutated in a form of recessive amyotrophic lateral sclerosis. *Nat Genet* 2001; **29**: 160–5.

19 Hadano S, Hand CK, Osuga H, *et al*. A gene encoding a putative GTPase regulator is mutated in familial amyotrophic lateral sclerosis. *Nat Genet* 2001; **29**: 166–73.

20 Borasio GD, Sloan R, Pongratz DE. Breaking the news in amyotrophic lateral sclerosis. *J Neurol Sci* 1998; **160**(suppl 1): S127–33.

21 Meininger V. Breaking bad news in amyotrophic lateral sclerosis. *Palliat Med* 1993; **7**: 37–40.

22 Molloy I. Rehabilitation. In: Oliver D, Borasio GD Walsh D, eds. *Palliative care in amyotrophic lateral sclerosis*. Oxford: Oxford University Press, 2000: 135–42.

23 Holmes T. MND Association of England Wales and Northern Ireland. In: Oliver D, Borasio GD, Walsh D, eds. *Palliative care in amyotrophic lateral sclerosis*. Oxford: Oxford University Press, 2000: 143–7.

24 Ellis CM, Leary S, Payan J, *et al*. Use of human intravenous immunoglobulin in lower motor neuron syndromes. *J Neurol Neurosurg Psychiatry* 1999; **67**: 15–19.

25 Bensimon G, Lacomblez L, Meininger V, *et al*. A controlled trial of riluzole in amyotrophic lateral sclerosis. *N Engl J Med* 1994; **330**: 585–91.

26 Demaerschalk BM, Strong MJ. Amyotrophic lateral sclerosis. *Current Treatment Options in Neurology* 2000; **2**: 13–22.

27 Lacomblez L, Bensimon G, Leigh PN, *et al*. Dose ranging study of riluzole in amyotrophic lateral sclerosis. *Lancet* 1996; **347**: 1425–31.

28 Meininger V, Zeisser P, Munsat T. An analysis of extended survival in patients with amyotrophic lateral sclerosis treated with riluzole. *Arch Neurol* 1998; **55**: 526–8.

29 Quality Standards Subcommittee of the American Academy of Neurology. Practice advisory on the treatment of amyotrophic lateral sclerosis with riluzole. *Neurology* 1997; **49**: 657–9.

30 Swash M. Pharmacoeconomics and motor neuron disease. *J Neurol Neurosurg Psychiatry* 2000; **68**: 401–3.

31 Howard RS, Wiles CM, Loh L. Respiratory complications and their management in motor neurone disease. *Brain* 1989; **112**: 1155–70.

32 Lyall RA, Donaldson N, Polkey MI, *et al*. Respiratory muscle strength and ventilatory failure in amyotrophic lateral sclerosis. *Brain* 2001; **124**: 2000–13.

33 Hopkins LC, Tatarian GT, Pianta TF. Management of ALS: respiratory care. *Neurology* 1996; **47**(suppl 2): 123–5.

34 Melo J, Homma A, Iturriaga E, *et al*. Pulmonary evaluation and prevalence of noninvasive ventilation in patients with amyotrophic lateral sclerosis: a multicenter survey and proposal of a pulmonary protocol. *J Neurol Sci* 1999; **169**: 114–17.

35 Brooks BR. Natural history of ALS: symptoms, strength, pulmonary function, and disability. *Neurology* 1996; **47**: S71–82.

36 Schiffman PL, Belsh JM. Pulmonary function at diagnosis of amyotrophic lateral sclerosis. Rate of deterioration. *Chest* 1993; **103**: 508–13.

37 David WS, Bundlie SR, Mahdavi Z. Polysomnographic studies in amyotrophic lateral sclerosis. *J Neurol Sci* 1997; **152**(suppl): S29–35.

38 Kimura K, Tachibana N, Kimura J, *et al*. Sleep-disordered breathing at an early stage of amyotrophic lateral sclerosis. *J Neurol Sci* 1999; **164**: 37–43.

39 Evangelista T, de Carvalho M, Pinto A, *et al*. Phrenic nerve conduction in amyotrophic lateral sclerosis. *J Neurol Sci* 1995; **129**(suppl): 35–7.

40 Aboussouan LS, Khan SU, Meeker DP, *et al*. Effect of noninvasive positive-pressure ventilation on survival in amyotrophic lateral sclerosis. *Ann Intern Med* 1997; **127**: 450–3.

41 Cazzolli PA, Oppenheimer EA. Home mechanical ventilation for amyotrophic lateral sclerosis: nasal compared to tracheostomy-intermittent positive pressure ventilation. *J Neurol Sci* 1996; **139**(suppl): 123–8.

42 Hillberg RE, Johnson DC. Non-invasive ventilation. *N Engl J Med* 1997; **337**: 1746–52.

43 Pinto AC, Evangelista T, Carvalho M, *et al*. Respiratory assistance with a non-invasive ventilator (Bipap) in MND/ALS patients: survival rates in a controlled trial. *J Neurol Sci* 1995; **129**: S19–26.

44 Kleopa AK, Sherman M, Neal B, *et al*. Bipap improves survival and rate of pulmonary function decline in patients with ALS. *J Neurol Sci* 1999; **164**: 82–8.

45 Carrey Z, Gottfried SB, Levy RD. Ventilatory muscle support in respiratory failure with nasal positive pressure ventilation. *Chest* 1990; **97**: 150–8.

46 Gelinas DF, O'Connor P, Miller RG. Quality of life for ventilator-dependent ALS patients and their caregivers. *J Neurol Sci* 1998; **160**(suppl 1): S134–6.

47 Bradley MD, Orrell RW, Clarke J, *et al*. Outcome of ventilatory support for acute respiratory failure in motor neurone disease. *J Neurol Neurosurg Psychiatry* 2002 (in press).

48 Hayashi H, Kato S, Kawada A. Amyotrophic lateral sclerosis patients living beyond respiratory failure. *J Neurol Sci* 1991; **105**: 73–8.

49 Hayashi H. Ventilatory support: Japanese experience. *J Neurol Sci* 1997; **152**(suppl 1): 97–100.

50 Hayashi H, Kato S. Total manifestations of amyotrophic lateral sclerosis. ALS in the totally locked-in state. *J Neurol Sci* 1989; **93**: 19–35.

51 Hill NS. Noninvasive ventilation positive pressure ventilation in neuromuscular disease. Enough is enough. *Chest* 1995; **105**: 337–8.

52 Moss AH, Oppenheimer EA, Casey P, *et al.* Patients with amyotrophic lateral sclerosis receiving long-term mechanical ventilation: advance care planning and outcomes. *Chest* 1996; **110**: 249–55.

53 Moss AH, Casey P, Stocking CB, *et al.* Home ventilation for amyotrophic lateral sclerosis patients: outcomes, costs, and patient, family and physician attitudes. *Neurology* 1993; **43**: 438–43.

54 Oppenheimer EA. Decision-making in the respiratory care of amyotrophic lateral sclerosis: should home mechanical ventilation be used? *Palliat Med* 1993; **5**(suppl 2): 49–64.

55 Bach JR. Amyotrophic lateral sclerosis. Communication status and survival with ventilatory support. *Am J Phys Med Rehabil* 1993; **72**: 343–9.

56 Hadjikoutis S, Eccles R, Wiles CM. Coughing and choking in motor neurone disease. *J Neurol Neurosurg Psychiatry* 2000; **68**: 601–4.

57 Leighton SEJ, Burton MJ, Lund WS, *et al.* Swallowing in motor neuron disease. *J R Soc Med* 1994; **87**: 801–5.

58 Blasco PA, Stansbury JCK. Glycopyrrolate treatment of chronic drooling. *Arch Pediatr Adolesc Med* 1996; **150**: 932–5.

59 Stern LM. Preliminary study of glycopyrrolate in the management of drooling. *J Paediatr Child Health* 1997; **33**: 52–4.

60 Newall AR, Orser R, Hunt M. The control of oral secretions in bulbar ALS/MND. *J Neurol Sci* 1996; **139**(suppl): 43–4.

61 Robinson ACR, Khoury GG, Robinson PM. Role of irradiation in the suppression of parotid secretions. *J Laryngol Otol* 1989; **103**: 594–5.

62 Giess R, Naumann M, Werner E, *et al.* Injections of botulinum toxin A into the salivary glands improve sialorrhoea in amyotrophic lateral sclerosis. *J Neurol Neurosurg Psychiatry* 2000; **69**: 121–3.

63 Kasarskis EJ, Berryman S, Vanderleest JG, *et al.* The nutritional status of patients with amyotrophic lateral sclerosis: relation to the proximity of death. *Am J Clin Nutr* 1996; **63**: 130–7.

64 Mazzini L, Corra T, Zaccala M, *et al.* Percutaneous endoscopic gastrostomy and enteral nutrition in amyotrophic lateral sclerosis. *Neurology* 1995; **242**: 695–8.

65 Mathus-Vliegen LMH, Louwerse LS, Merkus MP, *et al.* Percutaneous endoscopic gastrostomy in patients with amyotrophic lateral sclerosis and impaired pulmonary function. *Gastrointest Endosc* 1994; **40**: 463–9.

66 Light VL, Slezak FA, Porter JA, *et al.* Predictive factors for early mortality after percutaneous endoscopic gastrostomy. *Gastrointest Endosc* 1995; **42**: 330–5.

67 Newrick PG, Langton-Hewer R. Pain in motor neuron disease. *J Neurol Neurosurg Psychiatry* 1985; **48**: 838–40.

68 Caroscio JT, Cohen JA, Gudesblatt M. Amitriptyline in amyotrophic lateral sclerosis. *N Engl J Med* 1985; **313**: 1478.

69 Iannaccone S, Ferini-Strambi L. Pharmacologic treatment of emotional lability. *Clin Neuropharmacol* 1996; **19**: 532–5.

70 Schiffer RB, Cash J, Herndon RM. Treatment of emotional lability with low-dosage tricyclic antidepressants. *Psychosomatics* 1983; **24**: 1094–6.

71 Schiffer RB, Herndon RM, Rudick RA. Treatment of pathologic laughing and weeping with amitriptyline. *N Engl J Med* 1985; **312**: 1480–2.

72 Borasio GD, Voltz R. Advance directives. In: Oliver D, Borasio GD, Walsh D, eds.

Palliative care in amyotrophic lateral sclerosis. Oxford: Oxford University Press, 2000: 36–41.

73 Albert SM, Murphy PL, Del Bene ML, *et al.* Prospective study of palliative care in ALS: choice, timing and outcomes. *J Neurol Sci* 1999; **169**: 108–13.

74 Albert SM, Murphy PL, Del Bene ML, *et al.* A study of preferences and actual treatment choices in ALS. *Neurology* 1999; **53**: 278–83.

75 O'Brien T, Kelly M, Sunders C. Motor neuron disease: a hospice perspective. *BMJ* 1992; **304**: 471–3.

76 Voltz R, Borasio G. Palliative therapy in the terminal stage of neurological disease. *Neurology* 1997; **244**(suppl 4): S2–10.

77 Doyle D, O'Connell S. Breaking bad news: starting palliative care. *J R Soc Med* 1996; **89**: 590–1.

78 Oliver D, Borasio GD, Walsh D, eds. *Palliative care in amyotrophic lateral sclerosis (motor neurone disease).* Oxford: Oxford University Press, 2000.

79 Oliver D, Webb S. The involvement of specialist palliative care in the care of people with motor neuron disease. *Palliat Med* 2000; **14**: 427–8.

80 Oliver D. Opioid medication in the palliative care of motor neurone disease. *Palliat Med* 1998; **12**: 113–5.

81 Sykes N. End-of-life care in ALS. In: Oliver D, Borasio GD, Walsh D, eds. *Palliative care in amyotrophic lateral sclerosis.* Oxford: Oxford University Press, 2000: 159–68.

82 Borasio GD, Voltz R. Discontinuation of life support in patients with amyotrophic lateral sclerosis. *J Neurol* 1998; **245**: 717–22.

83 Neudert C, Oliver D, Wasner M, *et al.* The course of the terminal phase in patients with amyotrophic lateral sclerosis. *J Neurol* 2001; **248**: 612–16.

84 Goldstein LH, Adamson M, Jeffrey L, *et al.* The psychological impact of MND on patients and carers. *J Neurol Sci* 1998; **160**(suppl 1): S114–21.

85 Martin J, Turnbull J. Lasting impact, and ongoing needs, in families months to years after death from ALS. *Amyotr Lat Scler* 2000; **1**(suppl 3): 514–15.

Chapter Twelve

Motor neurone disease

K Talbot

Motor neurone disease (MND), or amyotrophic lateral sclerosis (ALS), is a neurodegenerative disorder of unknown aetiology. Progressive motor weakness and bulbar dysfunction lead to premature death, usually from respiratory failure. Confirming the diagnosis may initially be difficult until the full clinical features are manifest. For all forms of the disease there is a significant differential diagnosis to consider, including treatable conditions, and therefore specialist neurological opinion should always be sought. Clear genetic inheritance has been demonstrated in a minority of patients with familial ALS but elucidation of the biological basis of genetic subtypes is also providing important information which may lead to treatments for sporadic forms of the disease. In the absence of curative or disease-modifying therapy, management is supportive and requires a multidisciplinary approach. If, as seems likely, complex inherited and environmental factors contribute to the pathogenesis of MND, future treatment may involve a combination of molecular-based treatments or restoration of cellular integrity using stem cell grafts.

Neurologists in the 19th century recognised that muscle weakness could be due to primary disorders of muscle or secondary to loss of neuromuscular integrity, as happens when peripheral nerves are cut or when motor neurones degenerate. Furthermore, it was observed that there are forms of motor neurone degeneration which selectively affect upper motor neurones or lower motor neurones. A combination of upper and lower motor neurone dysfunction was named amyotrophic lateral sclerosis (ALS) by Charcot and Joffroy.[1] In the USA, ALS or Lou Gehrig's disease are terms used to describe all forms of the disease, whatever the combination of upper and lower motor neurone involvement. In the UK the umbrella term motor neurone disease (MND) is more common. MND is a disease of middle to late life with a mean age of onset of 58 years.[2] Although the third commonest neurodegenerative disease after Alzheimer's and Parkinson's diseases, MND is relatively rare, with an apparently uniform incidence of approximately 2/100 000 where adequate epidemiological data exists.[3,4] Despite its rarity, the disease has attracted a lot of attention, as its devastating course places it at the centre of the ethical debate about end of life decision making and physician-assisted suicide. In addition, there are a large number of diseases of diverse aetiology in which motor neurones are involved, either specifically, or as part of a more diffuse neurodegenerative process. Viral infections, toxic insults, and immune-mediated disease can all lead to motor neurone degeneration. In contrast, MND or ALS is a progressive degenerative disease of unknown aetiology. In discussing the differential diagnosis of motor neurone disorders it is useful to consider the different presentations of the condition in terms of the relative involvement of upper and lower motor neurones.

Amyotrophic lateral sclerosis ('Charcot ALS')

In its typical form with evidence of both spinal and cortical involvement, the diagnosis is usually clear. The combination of asymmetrical weakness and wasting in the limbs associated with clinical evidence of corticospinal tract damage (increased tone, brisk reflexes, extensor plantars) typically comes on insidiously over months and accounts for about 85% of all cases of MND. The disease usually begins either in one limb (foot drop or wasting of the intrinsic hand muscles) or with a combination of bulbar and corticobulbar symptoms (dysphagia, dysarthria, tongue wasting, and a brisk jaw jerk). The latter condition is particularly common in women presenting after the age of 50 and carries a poor prognosis. Despite this apparent focal onset the majority of patients have evidence of more diffuse motor involvement when first examined by a neurologist. When signs are confined to the structures below the neck (that is, there is no tongue wasting or pathologically brisk jaw jerk) then magnetic resonance imaging (MRI) must be performed to exclude spinal cord compression, which can occasionally cause a pure motor syndrome. Clinically detectable sensory involvement should raise the suspicion of an alternative diagnosis such as an inflammatory neuropathy. Diffuse fasciculation as an isolated symptom (often combined in an anxious patient with brisk reflexes) often raises the spectre of ALS but is usually due to benign fasciculations, exacerbated by caffeine, anxiety, and sympathomimetic drugs such as inhalers given for asthma. The extraocular muscles and sphincter function are spared in typical ALS. A small proportion of patients with ALS, approximately 3–5%, show clinical evidence of dementia with a predilection for abnormalities of executive function. Very rarely this can be the presenting or dominant feature and there are rare forms of inherited neurodegenerative disease in which ALS, frontotemporal dementia, or parkinsonism can exist in variable degrees within the same family.[5,6] The significance of this association is that there are likely to be common susceptibility factors shared by a number of forms of inherited and sporadic neurodegenerative diseases.

Over the last decade a number of reports of an ALS-like condition occurring in HIV positive patients have appeared. The condition is distinguished from typical ALS by a younger age of onset, progression over weeks to months, abnormal cell counts in the cerebrospinal fluid, and a response to antiretroviral drugs.[7,8] The occurrence of an ALS-like syndrome as a paraneoplastic manifestation of cancer remains controversial.[9] There are more convincing series of patients with lymphoma and ALS, but an aetiological association has not been proved.[10]

Pure lower motor neurone syndromes

A minority of patients (approximately 10%) present without upper motor neurone involvement. In the absence of typical features of ALS it is more difficult to be certain of the diagnosis until upper motor neurone signs such as brisk reflexes or extensor plantars become evident. When the tempo of the disease is the same as for ALS with progression over months then the diagnosis can usually be made firmly. Overall, MND presenting as a pure lower motor neurone syndrome (termed progressive muscular atrophy) is more slowly progressive than full blown ALS. Regional variants where involvement remains confined to the lower or upper limbs respectively are described.[11] Myasthenia gravis presenting with predominant bulbar weakness is occasionally misdiagnosed as ALS. High dose radiotherapy can lead to the appearance of a regional lower motor neurone syndrome up to 20 years after treatment.[12]

It is important to appreciate that there is a group of inherited conditions called spinal muscular atrophies in which a pure lower motor neurone pattern of weakness develops in early life and progresses very slowly.[13] While these disorders can be inherited as an X-linked, autosomal dominant or recessive trait, it is not uncommon to find apparently sporadic cases with onset in adult life. Such patients are often thought to be suffering from MND leading to an unduly pessimistic prognosis being offered. Specific genetic tests are available for X-linked bulbospinal neuronopathy (Kennedy's disease), which causes a slowly progressive lower motor neurone syndrome, sensory neuropathy, and partial androgen insensitivity leading to gynaecomastia,[14] and the recessive form of proximal spinal muscular atrophy which can occasionally come on in adult life.[15] A slowly progressive pure lower motor neurone syndrome in one limb may be due to an immune mediated condition called multifocal motor neuropathy with conduction block.[16] Typical features are profound weakness with minimal wasting, selective involvement of finger extensors, and the presence of anti-ganglioside antibodies in about 40%. It is an important condition to consider because it responds well to treatment with intravenous immunoglobulin.[17] Similarly, there is a curious form of sporadic benign focal amyotrophy which presents in males in the second or third decade and is much commoner in Japan and the Indian subcontinent than in Europe.[18,19] Wasting and weakness appears in one (usually an upper) limb over a period of months to years and then seem to plateau or to be only slowly progressive. In 40% of cases the contralateral limb is affected. The condition is of unknown aetiology. As with spinal muscular atrophy, patients are often initially suspected to have ALS.

Bilateral wasting of the limbs with either an upper or lower limb pattern can be caused by the inflammatory myopathy inclusion body myositis. While it is usually possible to distinguish this condition using electrophysiological tests, occasional patients show denervation changes.[20] Muscle biopsy can be performed to confirm the diagnosis.

Box 12.1 Potentially treatable causes of apparent MND mixed upper and lower motor neurone syndrome

- Compressive myeloradiculopathy.
- HIV infection.

Pure lower motor neurone syndrome
- Multifocal motor neuropathy with conduction block.
- Pure motor chronic inflammatory demyelinating polyneuropathy.

- Toxic neuropathies.
- Myasthenia gravis.

Pure upper motor neurone syndrome
- Cord compression.
- B12 deficiency.

Pure upper motor neurone syndromes

A small percentage of patients appear never to develop any lower motor neurone signs or at least not until very late in their illness. The term primary lateral sclerosis has been used to describe this condition which is generally considered to be aetiologically related to ALS.[21] The principal distinguishing features of primary lateral sclerosis are the symmetrical progression of a spastic tetraparesis with pseudobulbar palsy (a brisk jaw jerk, stiff slow tongue, and a characteristic spastic dysarthria in which patients are described as sounding as if they have a hot potato in their mouth), a 3:1 male to female ratio, longer survival than ALS (mean 8.5 years, range 5–15 years), relative preservation of muscle strength and prominent emotional lability, usually without cognitive impairment.[22,23] It is rare and accounts for about 1% of cases of MND. The differential diagnosis includes other causes of the syndrome of progressive spastic paraparesis such as hereditary spastic paraparesis, primary progressive multiple sclerosis, B12 deficiency and, rarely, structural lesions of the brain, including diffuse small vessel cerebrovascular disease. Electromyography may be useful if clear lower motor neurone involvement can be demonstrated but many patients with primary lateral sclerosis have normal electromyograms throughout their illness. Confusion occasionally arises between this form of MND and progressive supranuclear palsy, a degenerative condition presenting with axial rigidity, falls, loss of vertical gaze and cognitive dysfunction which usually runs a more rapidly progressive course than primary lateral sclerosis.

Investigation (see Box 12.2)

There is no specific test for ALS, which remains a clinical diagnosis. Diagnostic criteria exist, primarily for the purpose of standardising entry into clinical trials but the clinical usefulness of these schemes in individual cases where there is diagnostic uncertainty is less clear.[24] The main focus of investigation in the context of suspected MND should always be the exclusion of a treatable condition (Box 12.1) and swift resolution of diagnostic uncertainty. It is generally prudent to have a low threshold for MRI to avoid missing spinal cord compression. This is mandatory if clinical signs are restricted to the limbs. Most neurologists perform MRI of the whole neuraxis for a pure upper motor neurone syndrome. High quality diagnostic neurophysiology provides essential support to the diagnosis. It is important to appreciate that electrophysiological tests are confirmatory, not diagnostic, and must be interpreted in the context of the clinical syndrome. In typical MND motor nerve conduction velocity is normal (slow conduction suggests a neuropathy), sensory studies are normal, and electromyography reveals diffuse fibrillation and fasciculation. There is no consensus on the role of lumbar puncture, which is normal in typical ALS and should therefore be reserved for atypical cases as it introduces a delay in confirmation of the diagnosis. It is suggested that a lumbar puncture should be performed in the following clinical situations: (a) in pure upper motor neurone syndromes (spastic paraparesis) to exclude primary progressive multiple sclerosis, (b) if a paraprotein is present on serum electrophoresis or if there are other reasons to suspect an underlying paraneoplastic syndrome, and (c) in very rapidly progressive motor neurone syndromes, particularly in young patients where remote diagnostic possibilities include porphyria, poisoning, or the possibility of a treatable immunologically mediated neuropathy.

Box 12.2   Investigation of suspected MND

Mixed upper and lower motor neurone (ALS) syndrome
- Nerve conduction studies and electromyography.
- MRI of the spinal cord (brain).
- Routine blood tests, thyroid function, serum electrophoresis.
- HIV test if appropriate risk factors.

Pure lower motor neurone syndrome
- Genetic tests (if slowly progressive, suggesting spinal muscular atrophy).
- Nerve conduction studies/electromyography for conduction block.
- Routine blood tests, thyroid function, serum electrophoresis.

Pure upper motor neurone syndrome
- MRI of the spinal cord (brain) as appropriate to the level of the neurological signs.
- B12/folate.
- Central motor conduction time (using transcranial magnetic stimulation techniques, not routinely available).
- Lumbar puncture.

Making the diagnosis

As indicated in Box 12.3, MND can occasionally present to non-neurologists if the onset of symptoms is sufficiently focal to suggest local pathology. Dysphagia or dysarthria is often referred to ear, nose, and throat surgeons if malignancy is suspected. Similarly, a number of patients see orthopaedic or neurological surgeons if the first symptoms indicate the possibility of nerve root compression or cervical spondylosis. Degenerative changes are common in the age group most at risk of MND and a number of patients will undergo decompressive procedures of the cervical spine before the diagnosis of MND becomes apparent when they continue to deteriorate and develop bulbar signs. Very occasionally patients have relatively isolated weakness of respiratory muscle and may present to chest physicians with respiratory failure or obstructive sleep apnoea. Progressive decline in mobility in elderly patients with multiple comorbidities may mask MND. In this population it is suspected that the condition is under-diagnosed.

The diagnosis of MND should only be imparted to the patient by a doctor who has sufficient experience of the condition to be:

1 certain of the diagnosis
2 able to give an honest and accurate prognosis and
3 initiate appropriate supportive therapy and contact with paramedical specialists who are familiar with the management of progressive neurological disability.

In the majority of cases this will be a neurologist. Ideally the diagnosis should be made in hospital after all investigations have been performed, in an appropriately quiet setting with a close relative and a nurse present. There should be adequate time for full discussion of the implications of a diagnosis of MND. A follow-up outpatient visit should be arranged within a few weeks as many questions will not be addressed at the initial conversation.

The prognosis for patients with MND is variable and this must be emphasised at the time of diagnosis. ALS is usually relentlessly progressive and malignant in its behaviour. Approximately 50% of patients in most series are dead 2–3 years after the initial diagnosis.[2] Most patients fear that death will be by sudden asphyxiation or choking but there is evidence that the majority of people with ALS given adequate palliative care die peacefully at home or in a hospice from respiratory failure and chest infection.[25] In contrast, 20% and 5% of patients are alive at five and ten years respectively. The prognosis is generally worse if the onset of the disease is bulbar and there is early evidence of respiratory muscle compromise. A predominantly lower motor neurone picture is generally more slowly progressive, as is disease which is confined initially to the upper limbs. As mentioned above, patients with primary lateral sclerosis may survive for decades. Therefore most specialist clinics will have experience of patients who survive for many years longer than initially expected. These patients necessarily have complex needs which are often best met by a specialist neurorehabilitation team.

Box 12.3   MND presenting to non-neurological specialties

Respiratory
• Progressive respiratory failure.

Ear, nose, and throat
• Dysphagia.

Orthopaedics/neurosurgery
• Foot drop or other symptoms suggestive of compressive radiculopathy.

Elderly care
• Difficulty walking.

Pathogenesis

The aetiology of the vast majority of cases of ALS is unknown. Though the uniform incidence of MND throughout the world has been disputed,[26] with the exception of geographical isolates such as on Guam and Guadeloupe, there is remarkably little variation in published studies. This does not immediately favour either an environmental or genetic cause. An apparent increase in incidence in the disorder in the last few decades may be due to improved diagnosis, an aging population, or a genuine increase the frequency of the disease. Specific MNDs are known to be caused by dietary factors in the tropics (konzo in Africa and lathyrism in India).[27,28] Numerous theories have implicated environmental poisons such as pesticides and heavy metals, but epidemiological evidence for this as the cause of typical sporadic ALS is lacking. Rare reports of ALS after electrocution probably represent a genuine biological phenomenon,[29] but this does not seem to provide an insight into the origin of the vast majority of cases. Autoimmune factors have also been explored in some detail. While there is evidence of factors in patient serum that may damage motor neurones in culture, immunomodulation with steroids, intravenous immunoglobulin or plasma exchange has not been shown to be an effective treatment.[30] A viral aetiology is an attractive hypothesis because of the role of an enterovirus in poliomyelitis. Reports of persistent enteroviral RNA in postmortem material from ALS patients continue to occur.[31] As mentioned above, there are a small number of reports of a motor neurone syndrome in HIV positive patients. It is unclear whether this is due to direct viral tropism for motor neurones or an opportunistic infection.

The only forms of MND in which a clear cause has been established are the genetic variants listed in Box 12.4. In addition to these diseases there are numerous other inherited forms in which linkage has been established but no gene has yet been identified. Approximately 10% of cases are familial, usually with dominant inheritance. Of these cases, approximately 20% are due to mutations in the gene for superoxide dismutase type 1 (SOD-1).[32] Over 100 different mutations in the SOD-1 have been found and these can lead to changes throughout the protein. Despite the obvious assumption that disruption of SOD-1 would lead to motor neurone degeneration through a reduction in free radical scavenging, all the evidence points instead to a toxic gain of function mechanism.[33] It would appear that mutant SOD-1 protein leads to a failure in the normal protein chaperoning mechanism and subsequent degeneration of the motor neurone. Phenotypically there is no recognisable difference between SOD-1 related and sporadic ALS, raising the possibility that a greater understanding of the mechanism of cell death may shed light on the pathogenesis of sporadic disease. Other forms of genetically determined motor neurone degeneration are listed in Box 12.4.

Box 12.4   Inherited forms of MND in which a gene has been identified

ALS1
Gain of function mutations in the gene for SOD-1 leading to dominantly inherited ALS which is clinically indistinguishable from the sporadic form.[32]

ALS2
Inactivating mutations in a gene called 'alsin', a protein with rho-GEF homology and a putative role in cytoskeletal integrity. Leads to recessive primary lateral sclerosis-like picture in three families of Middle Eastern and North African origin.[34,35]

Proximal spinal muscular atrophy

Inactivating mutations in the survival motor neurone gene leading to recessive spinal muscular atrophy with onset in infancy (Werdnig-Hoffman disease) or childhood to adult life (Kugelberg-Welander syndrome).[15] Survival motor neurone has a role in ribonucleoprotein metabolism.[36]

Spinal muscular atrophy with respiratory distress

Neonatal spinal muscular atrophy with diaphragm involvement. Recessive mutations in a gene with RNA binding and helicase activity.[37]

X-linked bulbospinal neuronopathy

Kennedy's disease: bulbar spinal muscular atrophy with sensory neuropathy and androgen insensitivity. Due to gain of function mutations in the androgen receptor gene.[14]

It will be evident from this list that motor neurones are vulnerable to interference with a number of disparate metabolic pathways that do not appear to cause disease in other systems. The exact reasons for this selective vulnerability are not clear but it seems likely that the following factors contribute:

1 The extreme length of these cells imposes a high metabolic demand and necessitates specific adaptations to facilitate protein transport.
2 Pathological evidence would suggest that degenerating motor neurones in ALS show defects in protein handling. Whether this is a primary element in the pathogenesis or an epiphenomenon is unclear.
3 Motor neurones may be specifically vulnerable to defects in glutamate metabolism and to oxidative stress.[38]

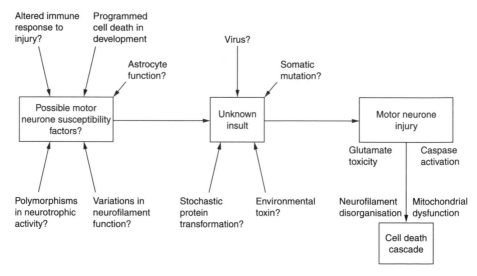

Figure 12.1 Pathogenesis of MND. Most of what we know about the biological events in the pathogenesis of ALS occur downstream of the initial motor neurone injury. The predisposing factors and the initial trigger to injury are poorly understood.

Figure 12.1 is a schematic representation of potential factors in the pathology of MND/ALS. In this model it is presumed that some as yet undefined triggering event acts on a background of susceptibility factors. Most of the molecular and cellular features of the disease for which there is good evidence belong to the series of events which occur downstream of the initiation of motor neurone death.

Management

People with MND and their carers have complex needs which can only adequately be delivered by a multidisciplinary team experienced in the management of progressive neurological disability. This should normally include a physiotherapist to advise on mobility, postural support, and prevention of contractures; a speech and language therapist to assess swallowing and provide communication aids; an occupational therapist to provide aids to maintain function (wheelchair, mobile arm supports, etc.); a dietitian to advise on maintaining weight and percutaneous endoscopic gastrostomy feeding. Liaison with patient support groups such as the Motor Neurone Disease Association (www.mnda.org) in the UK is valued by most patients and their families. For a full list of national organisations see www.alsmndalliance.org. Early contact with palliative care services and discussion of end of life decisions is an important element of care. In some areas palliative care physicians provide most of the care for MND patients once the initial diagnosis is confirmed.

Disease-modifying drug treatments

The only drug licensed for the treatment of MND is riluzole, which was designed as a specific glutamate antagonist. In two large randomised trials of patients with the ALS form of MND, the drug was shown to prolong tracheostomy-free survival by 3–6 months.[39–41] It is not known whether this effect extends to non-ALS forms of MND or if specific subgroups of patients get more prolonged survival as the follow-up period for these trials was only 18 months. As yet unpublished retrospective analyses of data from large numbers of patients taking the drug have suggested that the effect in prolonging survival may be more than the initial trials suggested but these data are confounded by the general improvements in the care of patients with ALS that has occurred over the last decade, notably greater access to specialist clinics and increased use of percutaneous endoscopic gastrostomy feeding and non-invasive ventilation. Approximately 10% of patients stop the drug because of side effects, principally gastrointestinal intolerance and asthenia. Overall, approximately 50% of patients are reported to be taking the drug, which probably reflects both patients' and physicians' perceptions of the modest effect on survival. Riluzole does not produce an improvement in symptoms. Other drugs which have been the subject of clinical trials in recent years in ALS but for which there is no evidence of benefit include high dose vitamin E, gabapentin, nerve growth factors such as brain-derived neurotrophic factor and insulin-like growth factor-1, and immunomodulatory treatments.[42] Perhaps of concern for the identification of new drugs for clinical trials is the observation that all of these agents showed benefits in animal models or cell culture systems. Despite lack of evidence many patients are taking vitamin E and creatinine. Future therapies will depend on a greater understanding of the pathogenesis but trials of stem cell therapy in animal models of MND are currently exciting much interest.

Treatment of specific symptoms

It is not widely appreciated, outside of specialist clinics, that there are a number of symptoms associated with MND which are highly amenable to treatment. The aim of these interventions is primarily palliative and aimed at maintaining quality of life rather than to prolong the duration of the illness.

Weight loss is universal in MND patients. It occurs even before calorific intake becomes limited by dysphagia and is due in part to loss of muscle mass. Careful monitoring by a dietitian and early institution of percutaneous endoscopic gastrostomy feeding is widely believed to improve quality of life and alleviate distress, though there are no randomised trials of this intervention. It is important to appreciate that it does not reduce the risk of aspiration.

Box 12.5   Principles of management of ALS/MND

- Multidisciplinary approach.
- Patient and carer support groups.
- Nutrition.
- Respiratory care.
- Palliative care.
- Drug therapy.

A number of *respiratory symptoms* occur in ALS patients including dyspnoea, orthopnoea, as well as symptoms due to carbon dioxide retention (daytime somnolence, morning headache, lack of restorative sleep, frequent nocturnal waking). Panic attacks are also very common and have a mixed aetiology but usually include some element of laryngospasm and a feeling of not being able to take a good breath. Patients often fear that they will choke to death but this is extremely rare. Panic attacks can be treated with benzodiazepines but these drugs can be hazardous in patients with incipient type II respiratory failure. The most appropriate methods for monitoring patients with ALS are still being established.[43] Vital capacity, lying and sitting, is the most practical and frequently used test in the outpatient clinic setting but is unreliable in patients with significant bulbar weakness. Many patients with ventilatory failure from ALS benefit symptomatically from non-invasive ventilation.[44] Close cooperation with colleagues in respiratory medicine is essential and appropriate patient selection is vital. Fears that this inevitably leads to pressure to proceed to tracheostomy and invasive mechanical ventilation have not proved to be justified in the UK but there is considerable international variation in the practice of long-term ventilation. The effect on carers of people with MND should be considered carefully. Inadvertent emergency ventilation by medical teams unfamiliar with the patient's diagnosis and wishes is a disaster for all concerned.

Cramps occur in most patients at some point in the disease but often wane with time and rarely need treatment. *Spasticity* can be a considerable problem leading to pain and reduction in mobility. Physiotherapy has a role, but some patients need antispasticity agents such as baclofen or tizanidine. Botulinum toxin may have an occasional role in specific situations such as jaw spasm which can lead to problems in feeding, articulation, and contribute to panic attacks.

Drooling (sialorrhoea) causes dehydration, social embarrassment, and sore lips. Transdermal hyoscine patches can be very effective without resulting in drowsiness. Botulinum toxin injections into the salivary ducts or irradiation of the salivary glands are also occasionally used successfully,[45] but the former may be hazardous and requires expertise.

Emotional lability or 'pseudobulbar affect' are slightly inaccurate terms for the commonly observed tendency of patients with corticobulbar involvement to laugh or cry inappropriately. The origin of this symptom is not precisely understood but it is not necessarily associated with an emotional experience and should not be interpreted as a sign of depression (*see* below). While it is slightly commoner in patients with cognitive involvement, it is important to appreciate that most patients with this symptom are cognitively normal. It is often a transient phenomenon that resolves over several months, but if socially embarrassing often responds well to tricyclic antidepressants.

Depression is, not unnaturally, commoner in patients with a progressive, disabling, and terminal illness. The decision to treat must be balanced by the acknowledgement that patients with a grief reaction to their illness are going through a normal psychological process with many of the features of a classical bereavement reaction. Therefore supportive counselling is as important as drug therapy.

The future

Although described in the mid-19th century, ALS-MND has proved to be one of the most puzzling neurodegenerative diseases and remains largely untreatable. Much of our knowledge of the pathogenesis of MND comes initially from analysis of postmortem material in which the disease process is advanced and many of the changes reflect the end stage of a cascade of metabolic derangements resulting in motor neurone degeneration. More recently the identification of specific genes causing MND and the creation of animal models with which to study the early events in motor neurone degeneration offer a more realistic hope of identifying the set of factors which make motor neurones peculiarly vulnerable. The underlying assumption with this approach is that the genetic forms of MND are sufficiently like sporadic ALS which is a much commoner problem. Most patients with MND have probably lost a very significant proportion of motor units by the time they are seen by a neurologist and effective treatment and arrest of the process of degeneration will require a precise profile of the molecular events that occur early in the disease process. Ultimately we need to be able to identify those individuals at risk of developing the disease in the first place. Once the disease has advanced to the point of significant functional impairment, restorative treatments will have to be developed. The current hope is that stem cells of neural or extraneural origin might be modified in vitro to differentiate into neurones that would migrate to sites of motor neurone loss and form functional connections to restore the motor pathways lost in MND. In the shorter term there is an urgent need for new therapeutic agents to emerge. Current knowledge would suggest that, whatever the initial insult triggering the disease, a number of biochemical pathways are activated downstream leading to motor neurone death, perhaps through apoptosis. By analogy with previously medically intractable disease such as haematological malignancy, it may be that combination chemotherapy with riluzole and other drugs will lead to progressive improvements in survival. It is important that quality of life, not just duration of survival, is part of the measure of effectiveness of drug regimens.

Self-assessment questions

True (T)/False (F); answers at the end of 'References'.

Q1. The following are motor neurone disorders:
(A) Primary lateral sclerosis
(B) Huntington's disease
(C) Amyotrophic lateral sclerosis
(D) Spinal muscular atrophy
(E) Lathyrism

Q2. Motor neurone disease:
(A) Shows marked variations in incidence between different regions of the world
(B) Is commoner in men
(C) Carries a worse prognosis in women
(D) Carries a worse prognosis if onset is in the lower limbs
(E) Is associated with a family history in 10% of cases

Q3. Mutations in the gene for superoxide dismutase (SOD) type 1:
(A) Cause a form of MND/ALS which is readily distinguishable clinically from sporadic disease
(B) Lead to motor neurone death through loss of free radical scavenging activity
(C) Only account for a minority of cases of dominantly inherited ALS
(D) Occur in a specific region of the SOD gene which is critical for its function in oxidative metabolism
(E) Are also associated with some forms of Parkinson's disease

Q4. The following treatments prolong life:
(A) Glial derived neurotrophic factor
(B) Riluzole
(C) Graded physiotherapy
(D) Invasive mechanical ventilation
(E) High dose vitamin E

Q5. The following are inconsistent with a diagnosis of MND:
(A) The presence of any abnormality on the MRI scan
(B) A creatine kinase level of 1500 IU
(C) Dementia
(D) Sensory changes on nerve conduction studies
(E) Involvement of eye movements

Acknowledgements

The author is funded by an MRC/GlaxoSmithKline Clinician Scientist Fellowship. The Oxford MND Care Centre is supported by a grant from the Motor Neurone Disease Association of England and Wales.

References

1 Charcot J, Joffroy A. Deux cas d'atrophie musculaire progressive avec lesions de la substance grise et des faisceaux antero-lateraux de la moelle epiniere. *Arch Physiol Neurol Pathol* 1869; **2**: 744–54.

2 Ringel SP, Murphy JR, Alderson MK, *et al.* The natural history of amyotrophic lateral sclerosis. *Neurology* 1993; **43**: 1316–22.

3 Traynor BJ, Codd MB, Corr B, *et al.* Incidence and prevalence of ALS in Ireland, 1995–1997: a population-based study. *Neurology* 1999; **52**: 504–9.

4 Piemonte and Valle d'Aosta Register for ALS. Incidence of ALS in Italy: evidence for a uniform frequency in western countries. *Neurology* 2001; **56**: 239–44.

5 Hosler BA, Siddique T, Sapp PC, *et al.* Linkage of familial amyotrophic lateral sclerosis with frontotemporal dementia to chromosome 9q21-q22. *JAMA* 2000; **284**: 1664–9.

6 Kuzuhara S, Kokubo Y, Sasaki R, *et al.* Familial amyotrophic lateral sclerosis and parkinsonism-dementia complex of the Kii Peninsula of Japan: clinical and neuropathological study and tau analysis. *Ann Neurol* 2001; **49**: 501–11.

7 Moulignier A, Moulonguet A, Pialoux G, *et al.* Reversible ALS-like disorder in HIV infection. *Neurology* 2001; **57**: 995–1001.

8 MacGowan DJ, Scelsa SN, Waldron M. An ALS-like syndrome with new HIV infection and complete response to antiretroviral therapy. *Neurology* 2001; **57**: 1094–7.

9 Forsyth PA, Dalmau J, Graus F, *et al.* Motor neuron syndromes in cancer patients. *Ann Neurol* 1997; **41**: 722–30.

10 Gordon PH, Rowland LP, Younger DS, *et al.* Lymphoproliferative disorders and motor neuron disease: an update. *Neurology* 1997; **48**: 1671–8.

11 Hu MT, Ellis CM, Al-Chalabi A, *et al.* Flail arm syndrome: a distinctive variant of amyotrophic lateral sclerosis. *J Neurol Neurosurg Psychiatry* 1998; **65**: 950–1.

12 Bowen J, Gregory R, Squier M, *et al.* The post-irradiation lower motor neuron syndrome neuronopathy or radiculopathy? *Brain* 1996; **119**(pt 5):1429–39.

13 Talbot K, Davies K. Spinal muscular atrophy. *Semin Neurol* 2001; **21**: 189–98.

14 La Spada AR, Wilson EM, Lubahn DB, *et al.* Androgen receptor gene mutations in X-linked spinal and bulbar muscular atrophy. *Nature* 1991; **352**: 77–9.

15 Lefebvre S, Burglen L, Reboullet S, *et al.* Identification and characterization of a spinal muscular atrophy-determining gene. *Cell* 1995; **80**: 155–65.

16 Pestronk A, Cornblath DR, Ilyas AA, *et al.* A treatable multifocal motor neuropathy with antibodies to GM1 ganglioside. *Ann Neurol* 1988; **24**: 73–8.

17 Chaudhry V, Corse AM, Cornblath DR, *et al.* Multifocal motor neuropathy: response to human immune globulin. *Ann Neurol* 1993; **33**: 237–42.

18 Sobue I, Saito N, Iida M, *et al.* Juvenile type of distal and segmental muscular atrophy of upper extremities. *Ann Neurol* 1978; **3**: 429–32.

19 Hirayama K, Tsubaki T, Toyokura Y, *et al.* Juvenile muscular atrophy of unilateral upper extremity. *Neurology* 1963; **13**: 373–80.

20 Dabby R, Lange DJ, Trojaborg W, *et al.* Inclusion body myositis mimicking motor neuron disease. *Arch Neurol* 2001; **58**: 1253–6.

21 Swash M, Desai J, Misra VP. What is primary lateral sclerosis? *J Neurol Sci* 1999; **170**: 5–10.

22 Le Forestier N, Maisonobe T, Piquard A, *et al.* Does primary lateral sclerosis exist? A study of 20 patients and a review of the literature. *Brain* 2001; **124**(pt 10):1989–99.

23 Pringle CE, Hudson AJ, Munoz DG, *et al.* Primary lateral sclerosis. Clinical features, neuropathology and diagnostic criteria. *Brain* 1992; 115(pt 2):495–520.

24 Traynor BJ, Codd MB, Corr B, *et al.* Clinical features of amyotrophic lateral sclerosis according to the El Escorial and Airlie House diagnostic criteria: a population-based study. *Arch Neurol* 2000; **57**: 1171–6.

25 Borasio GD, Shaw PJ, Hardiman O, *et al.* Standards of palliative care for patients with amyotrophic lateral sclerosis: results of a European survey. *Amyotroph Lateral Scler Other Motor Neuron Disord* 2001; **2**: 159–64.

26 Chancellor AM, Warlow CP. Adult onset motor neuron disease: worldwide mortality, incidence and distribution since 1950. *J Neurol Neurosurg Psychiatry* 1992; **55**: 1106–15.

27 Ludolph AC, Spencer PS. Toxic models of upper motor neuron disease. *J Neurol Sci* 1996; **139**(suppl): 53–9.

28 Howlctt WP, Brubaker GR, Mlingi N, *et al.* Konzo, an epidemic upper motor neuron disease studied in Tanzania. *Brain* 1990; 113(pt 1):223–35.

29 Jafari H, Couratier P, Camu W. Motor neuron disease after electric injury. *J Neurol Neurosurg Psychiatry* 2001; **71**: 265–7.

30 Meucci N, Nobile-Orazio E, Scarlato G. Intravenous immunoglobulin therapy in amyotrophic lateral sclerosis. *J Neurol* 1996; **243**: 117–20.

31 Berger MM, Kopp N, Vital C, *et al.* Detection and cellular localization of enterovirus RNA sequences in spinal cord of patients with ALS. *Neurology* 2000; **54**: 20–5.

32 Rosen DR, Siddique T, Patterson D, *et al.* Mutations in Cu/Zn superoxide dismutase gene are associated with familial amyotrophic lateral sclerosis. *Nature* 1993; **362**: 59–62.

33 Cleveland DW, Rothstein JD. From Charcot to Lou Gehrig: deciphering selective motor neuron death in ALS. *Nat Rev Neurosci* 2001; **2**: 806–19.

34 Hadano S, Hand CK, Osuga H, *et al.* A gene encoding a putative GTPase regulator is mutated in a familial amyotrophic lateral sclerosis 2. *Nat Genet* 2001; **29**: 166–73.

35 Yang Y, Hentati A, Deng HX, *et al.* The gene encoding alsin, a protein with three guanine-nucleotide exchange factor domains, is mutated in a form of recessive amyotrophic lateral sclerosis. *Nat Genet* 2001; **29**: 160–5.

36 Sendtner M. Molecular mechanisms in spinal muscular atrophy: models and perspectives. *Curr Opin Neurol* 2001; **14**: 629–34.

37 Grohmann K, Schuelke M, Diers A, *et al.* Mutations in the gene encoding immunoglobulin mu-binding protein 2 cause spinal muscular atrophy with respiratory distress type 1. *Nat Genet* 2001; **29**: 75–7.

38 Robberecht W. Oxidative stress in amyotrophic lateral sclerosis. *J Neurol* 2000; **247**(suppl 1): 11–16.

39 Lacomblez L, Bensimon G, Leigh PN, *et al.* A confirmatory dose-ranging study of riluzole in ALS. ALS/Riluzole Study Group-II. *Neurology* 1996; **47**(6 suppl 4): S242–50.

40 Bensimon G, Lacomblez L, Meininger V. A controlled trial of riluzole in amyotrophic lateral sclerosis. ALS/Riluzole Study Group. *N Engl J Med* 1994; **330**: 585–91.

41 Miller RG, Mitchell JD, Moore DH. Riluzole for amyotrophic lateral sclerosis (ALS)/ motor neuron disease (MND) (Cochrane Review). *Cochrane Database Systematic Reviews* 2001; **4**.

42 Turner MR, Parton MJ, Leigh PN. Clinical trials in ALS: an overview. *Semin Neurol* 2001; **21**: 167–75.

43 Lyall RA, Donaldson N, Polkey MI, *et al.* Respiratory muscle strength and ventilatory failure in amyotrophic lateral sclerosis. *Brain* 2001; **124**(pt 10):2000–13.

44 Lyall RA, Donaldson N, Fleming T, *et al.* A prospective study of quality of life in ALS patients treated with noninvasive ventilation. *Neurology* 2001; **57**: 153–6.

45 Giess R, Naumann M, Werner E, *et al.* Injections of botulinum toxin A into the salivary glands improve sialorrhoea in amyotrophic lateral sclerosis. *J Neurol Neurosurg Psychiatry* 2000; **69**: 121–3.

Answers

Q1: (A) T, (B) F, (C) T, (D) T, (E) T
Primary lateral sclerosis and amyotrophic lateral sclerosis are forms of typical MND. The spinal muscular atrophies are a group of inherited disorders of the lower motor neurone which are usually slowly progressive. Huntington's disease (chorea, personality change) does not involve motor neurones. Lathyrism is an epidemic form of upper motor neurone syndrome seen in India and due to ingestion of a toxic chickling pea.

Q2: (A) F, (B) T, (C) T, (D) F, (E) T
MND seems to have a uniform incidence in developed countries and there is an unexplained 1.6:1 male to female ratio. Females have a slightly worse prognosis, probably because a bulbar disease onset occurs in 50% of females compared with 25–30% of males. The longer the disease remains confined to a specific region such as the legs, the better the overall prognosis.

Q3: (A) F, (B) F, (C) T, (D) F, (E) F
Mutations in SOD-1 only cause ALS (20% of familial cases) and have not been associated with any other neurodegenerative disease. The SOD-1 form of ALS is clinically indistinguishable from sporadic ALS. The disease appears to result from a disorder of protein handling and SOD-1 free radical scavenging appears to be normal in most cases. The mutations are scattered throughout the gene and not confined to any functional motif of the protein.

Q4: (A) F, (B) T, (C) F, (D),T, (E) F
Riluzole is the only drug which has been shown in clinical trials to have any affect on disease duration. Invasive mechanical ventilation will prolong life by several years but the progression of paralysis (and possibly dementia) continues. For this reason few patients wish to pursue this as an option.

Q5: (A) F, (B) F, (C) F, (D) T, (E) T
MRI abnormalities (especially MRI spectroscopy) due to corticospinal tract degeneration do occur in MND. Clearly the presence of a structural lesion in the appropriate place raises an alternative explanation for the clinical presentation of MND. A creatine kinase of >1000 IU is unusual but can sometimes be seen with a lot of active denervation. Frank dementia occurs in 3% of patients. Marked sensory abnormalities on nerve conduction studies should lead to the diagnosis being questioned, as should extraocular muscle weakness which is very rare in MND.

Chapter Thirteen

Progressive supranuclear palsy (Steele-Richardson-Olszewski disease)

HR Morris, NW Wood and AJ Lees

Progressive supranuclear palsy is a neurodegenerative disease which affects the brainstem and basal ganglia. Patients present with disturbance of balance, a disorder of downward gaze and L-DOPA-unresponsive parkinsonism and usually develop progressive dysphagia and dysarthria leading to death from the complications of immobility and aspiration. Treatment remains largely supportive but, potentially, treatments based on cholinergic therapy may be useful. As in Alzheimer's disease, the neuronal degeneration is associated with the deposition of hyperphosphorylated tau protein as neurofibrillary tangles but there are important distinctions between the two diseases. Evidence from familial fronto-temporal dementia with parkinsonism linked to chromosome 17 suggests that tau protein deposition is a primary pathogenic event in some neurodegenerative diseases. The understanding of the mechanism of tau deposition in progressive supranuclear palsy is likely to be of importance in unravelling its aetiology.

Progressive supranuclear palsy (PSP) is an important but probably under-diagnosed neurodegenerative syndrome. The anatomy of PSP overlaps with that of Parkinson's disease (PD) and its microscopic pathology is similar to that of Alzheimer's disease. The distinctive clinical features of PSP, in large part due to brainstem involvement, make the diagnosis reasonably straightforward once it has been considered by the examining physician.

Historical aspects

PSP was first described as a distinct syndrome by John Steele, J Clifford Richardson, and Jerzy Olszewski in 1963 following Richardson's clinical observations on several patients with a unique syndrome in Toronto in the late 1950s.[1,2] Although experienced neurologists at that time were unable to categorise the syndrome, a number of reports from the early 20th century indicate that it is not a new disorder.[3,4] An early photograph showing the typical posture of PSP has been identified,[5] and review of the film archives of Denny-Brown have shown a number of cases which can be identified to have been early cases of PSP.[6] It is also likely that one of MacDonald Critchley's cases of 'arteriosclerotic pseudoparkinsonism', described in the 1920s, also had PSP.[7] The clinical skill of Steele and Richardson together with the expertise of Olszewski in delineating brainstem anatomy allowed this 'new' clinicopathological entity to be described and their seminal report was followed by many case reports and case series from around the world.[8] The documentation of these individual cases and case series through the 1960s, 1970s and 1980s have been followed by more recently by epidemiological studies.[9,10]

Clinical diagnosis

PSP is frequently misdiagnosed, most commonly as PD, but when PSP is considered, its distinctive features usually make it possible to make a confident diagnosis (*see* Box 13.1). Most patients present with gait disturbance and unsteadiness with a tendency to fall backwards. The gait has a characteristic reeling or staggering quality, due to the stiff posture of the trunk and neck with irregular large steps forwards, which allow a distinction to be made from the veering broad-based gait of cerebellar ataxia. Some patients present with early complaints of visual disturbance which are related to fixation instability and disruption of the control of saccadic eye movements. Unfortunately, as visual acuity itself is not affected by PSP, these symptoms may be initially thought to be psychogenic in origin until the typical disturbance of downward gaze emerges. The neuro-ophthalmological features of patients with established PSP are usually clear-cut.[11] Frontalis over-activity and a diminution of the blink rate to less than 4/minute lead to a 'surprised' facial appearance. Eye opening may be impaired either by active involuntary contraction of orbicularis oculi (blepharospasm) or by inability to voluntarily open the eyes ('apraxia of eyelid opening') (*see* Figure 13.1).[12] Fixation on a stationary object may be interrupted by visible constant velocity saccadic intrusions in which the gaze is diverted briefly away and then back to the target, described as square wave jerks.[13] In the earliest stages of the disease there may be slowness of vertical saccadic eye movements which progress to limitation of downwards vertical saccadic eye movements and then to a complete vertical gaze palsy.[11] The doll's head manoeuvre may be used to generate a normal vertical vestibular-ocular response demonstrating the integrity of the third nerve nuclei and confirming that the eye movement disorder is supranuclear. Some limitation of upgaze is a frequent accompaniment of normal ageing and may be seen in PD; limitation of downgaze is a much more specific finding suggestive of PSP. In the late stages of the disease, involvement of the horizontal eye movement system may lead to a complete supranuclear gaze palsy.[11]

Box 13.1   Diagnostic criteria for PSP[18]

Mandatory inclusion criteria
- postural instability with falls in the first year of symptoms
- slowing of vertical saccadic eye movements (clinically possible); vertical supranuclear gaze palsy (clinically probable)

Supportive criteria
- frontal/subcortical cognitive dysfunction
- axial rigidity
- pseudobulbar dysphagia and dysarthria
- blepharospasm/apraxia of eyelid opening

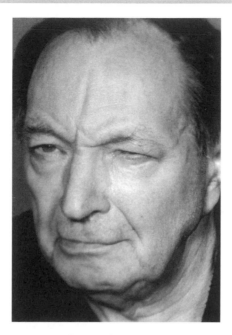

Figure 13.1 Facies of a patient with PSP showing asymmetric blepharospasm, frontalis overactivity and taut dystonic facial expression (reproduced with the patient's permission).

The extrapyramidal features of PSP are distinctive and should be separable from PD (*see* Table 13.1). Lack of spontaneous and associative movements, dysarthria and facial immobility may suggest the diagnosis of PD during conversation and history taking. However, careful observation and examination often reveals a taut spastic face, a growling dysarthria, neck held in extension with axial rigidity, and a symmetrical relatively mild distal bradykinesia, often in the presence of normal

Table 13.1 Clinical features differentiating Parkinson's disease (PD) and progressive supranuclear palsy (PSP)

	PSP	*PD*
Balance	Early postural instability	Initially well preserved gait and balance
Speech	Growling dysarthria	Hypophonic dysarthria
Facial appearance	Taut	Loose
Extrapyramidal features	Axial rigidity; relatively well preserved fine finger movements; tremor in <10%	Distal rigidity and bradykinesia; decrement in amplitude and speed of fine finger movements; tremor in 95% through disease course
Symmetry	Symmetry of symptoms and signs	Asymmetry of onset and persistent asymmetrical signs
L-DOPA	Little response to L-DOPA	Excellent response to L-DOPA

muscle tone and in the absence of rest tremor. PSP rarely responds to L-DOPA therapy and it should be considered in the differential diagnosis of L-DOPA unresponsive Parkinson's syndrome along with vascular pseudo-parkinsonism, corticobasal degeneration, and multiple system atrophy. While amnesia resulting from mesial temporal damage is not a feature of PSP, history from relatives and carers and specific bedside tests may reveal more subtle cognitive impairment. Functional imaging and clinical psychological studies show frontal hypometabolism and a deficit in frontal psychological tasks, respectively.[14] There may be a prodromal history of personality change or difficulty in carrying out day-to-day tasks which reflect frontal/subcortical disinhibition, apathy or difficulties in planning or judgement. Emotional lability and aggressive outbursts are common. Bedside testing may reveal difficulty in performing a three-stage command and markedly impaired verbal fluency in initial or category naming tests. Neuropsychological testing is often characterised by profound slowing of responses, with correct replies eventually being produced when sufficient time is allowed.[15]

The final stages of PSP are usually dominated by an increasingly severe dysarthria and dysphagia. These features are usually described as being part of a pseudo-bulbar palsy, as brisk jaw and facial jerks may be present. However, the aetiology of these bulbar features is probably multifactorial, with a contribution from damage to extrapyramidal, pyramidal and brainstem reticular structures.

Differential diagnosis

In addition to PD, a number of other conditions may be misdiagnosed as PSP, usually on the basis of a parkinsonian syndrome with gaze abnormalities (*see* Box 13.2). These conditions include corticobasal degeneration, multiple system atrophy, progressive subcortical gliosis due to prion disease, some forms of autosomal dominant cerebellar ataxia (particularly SCA-7 and SCA-2), and vascular pseudo-parkinsonism. Whipple's disease is also important to consider since, although rare, it is a treatable cause of progressive neurological disease with a gaze palsy and may be diagnosed by small bowel biopsy or cerebrospinal fluid polymerase chain reaction for *Tropheryma whippeli*. In younger patients, Niemann-Pick disease type C and occasionally other storage disorders may present in a similar way to PSP. In the elderly population, vascular pseudo-parkinsonism is common and worth considering, particularly in view of the potential to identify modifiable risk factors. Vascular pseudo-parkinsonism may be identified by a shuffling small-stepped gait with a good arm swing ('lower body parkinsonism'; 'marche à petit pas'),[16] and relative sparing of axial and upper limb function. Rarely, neurosyphilis and compressive midbrain lesions may produce a midbrain neuro-ophthalmologic disorder and these conditions should be excluded with syphilis serology and neuroimaging.[17]

Operational criteria for the research diagnosis of PSP have recently been formulated (*see* Box 13.1).[1] These criteria focus on postural instability and evidence of damage to the vertical gaze system as the two core features of the disease together with the absence of clinical or investigative features suggesting an alternative diagnosis. These criteria have been reported to have an 80% sensitivity and specificity but potentially may exclude patients with PSP who develop behavioural or personality change significantly before the occurrence of a gait disorder and those who have atypical disease without a supranuclear gaze palsy.[19,20]

Box 13.2   Causes of a vertical supranuclear gaze palsy

- progressive supranuclear palsy
- corticobasal degeneration
- fronto-temporal dementia with parkinsonism linked to chromosome 17
- prion diseases (Creutzfeld-Jakob disease, progressive subcortical gliosis)
- autosomal dominant cerebellar ataxias (particularly SCA-2 and SCA-7)
- Whipple's disease
- Niemann-Pick disease type C
- vascular pseudo-parkinsonism
- compressive midbrain syndromes (Parinaud syndrome), eg, pinealoma, glioma
- neurosyphilis

Epidemiology

A prevalence of 1.4/100 000 has been reported from New Jersey, but this is likely to be an underestimate because of the exclusion of 'atypical parkinsonism', misdiagnosed as PD.[9,21] The median life expectancy from symptom onset to death is 9 years.[9] The 1991 UK Parkinson's Disease Society brain bank study showed that 25% of clinically diagnosed PD cases had alternative pathological diagnoses; atypical PSP was the commonest misdiagnosis accounting for around 6% of the cases in this series.[21] Studies of this type suggest that PSP may be substantially under-diagnosed and that the true population prevalence of PSP may be much greater than has been reported. Case-control studies have not demonstrated any definite risk factors for the disease,[22,23] but there is increasing interest in the role of genetic susceptibility.

Pathology

PSP has a distinctive topographical and molecular pathology. The cellular hall-mark of the disease is neurofibrillary degeneration; and the distribution and intensity of damage to the brainstem and basal ganglia is used to pathologically define the syndrome.[24] The main lesions are in the substantia nigra pars compacta and reticulata, the globus pallidus, the subthalamic nucleus, and the midbrain and pontine reticular formation. This destruction of midbrain and pontine structures leads to identifiable changes of brainstem atrophy on neuroimaging with dilatation of the cerebral aqueduct, thinning of the midbrain tegmentum and dilatation of the fourth ventricle (*see* Figure 13.2).[25] A recent blinded study indicates that dilatation of the third ventricle and a midbrain diameter of less than 17 mm are useful in distinguishing PSP from other atypical parkinsonian syndromes (A Schrag, personal communication).

The renaissance of neurosurgical approaches to PD and the study of primate models of extrapyramidal dysfunction have led to reconsideration of the functional pathology of the basal ganglia. Current models are inconsistent in their explanation of the symptomatology of potentially the simplest disease, PD,[26] and the functional anatomy of PSP is even more complex and poorly

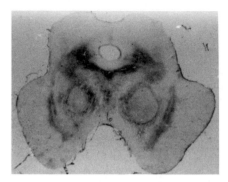

Figure 13.2 Glial stained section through the midbrain of a patient with PSP showing midbrain atrophy with dilation of the cerebral aqueduct and gliosis of the substantia nigra and peri-aqueductal region. Courtesy of Dr T Revesz, Institute of Neurology, London.

understood. PSP involves damage to both the putaminal and caudate striatal projections of the substantia nigra pars compacta (SNpc), the ventrolateral and dorsomedial areas, respectively.[27] This homogenous depletion of the SNpc is in contrast to the ventrolateral nigral selectivity of PD, which preferentially damages the putaminal nigrostriatal projection. This anatomical difference can be visualised *in vivo* with PET imaging of loss of ^{18}F-DOPA uptake by both caudate and putaminal nigrostriatal nerve terminals in PSP as opposed to preferential loss of putaminal uptake in PD[28] (*see* Figure 13.3). The treatment of PD with L-DOPA is thought to lead to a restoration of normal output from the basal ganglia with attenuation of pallidothalamic GABAergic inhibition, but in PSP the major output centres of the basal ganglia, the substantia nigra pars reticulata and the globus pallidus internus, are already severely damaged by the underlying disease process.[29] The subthalamic nucleus has been shown to be overactive in PD and lesioning or high frequency stimulation (producing suppression) of the subthalamic nucleus is proving to be a highly successful manoeuvre in ameliorating the tremor, bradykinesia and rigidity of PD.[30] The subthalamic nucleus is also damaged in patients with PSP.[31] This destruction of the major basal ganglia output areas and the subthalamic nucleus, which are intact and overactive in PD, presumably partly contributes to the clinical differences between PSP and PD (*see* Figure 13.4).

The brainstem reticular pathology in PSP includes the midbrain and pontine nuclei involved in the supranuclear control of gaze: the rostral interstitial nucleus of the medial longitudinal fasciculus, the interstitial nucleus of Cajal, the nucleus of Darkschewitsch, and the raphé nucleus interpositus.[32,33] Additionally, the cholinergic pedunculopontine nucleus is damaged, which is thought to have a role in the control of sleep and balance.[34] Contrary to the earliest reports, cortical pathology does occur in PSP and is most marked in the deepest cortical layers of the precentral gyrus, occurring to a lesser extent in prefrontal areas.[35] However, clinical and functional imaging data suggest that the major cognitive deficit in PSP is in frontal function and given the distribution of cortical neurofibrillary tangle formation, this presumably relates in part to a disturbance of reciprocal thalamocortical connections.[14,15]

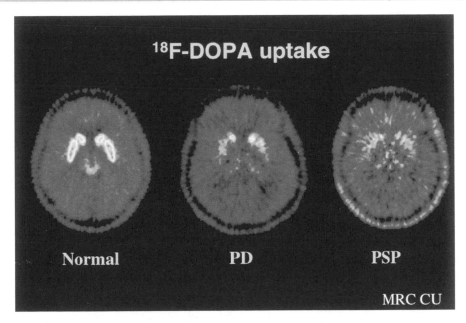

Figure 13.3 ^{18}F-DOPA uptake scan showing loss of uptake in the putamen in PD and both caudate and putamen in PSP. Courtesy of Dr P Piccini and Prof D Brooks, MRC Cyclotron Unit, Royal Postgraduate Medical School, Hammersmith Hospital, London.

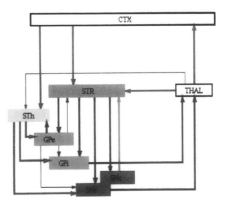

Figure 13.4 Connectivity in the basal ganglia. While in PD the substantia nigra pars compacta (SNc) is preferentially affected, in PSP the major outputs to the thalamus (THAL), the substantia nigra pars reticulata (SNr) and globus pallidus internus (GPi) are also affected in addition to the subthalamic nucleus (STh) which is overactive in PD. Other abbreviations: cerebral cortex (CTX), striatum (STR), globus pallidus externus (Gpe). Courtesy of Dr Andrew Gillies, Institute for Adaptive & Neural Computation, Division of Informatics, University of Edinburgh, Edinburgh.

Molecular pathology

PSP is one of a group of neurofibrillary tangle disorders.[36] Corticobasal degeneration, post-encephalitic parkinsonism, post-traumatic parkinsonism, some forms of frontotemporal dementia, and the parkinsonism dementia complex of Guam, all involve the deposition of hyperphosphorylated tau protein as neurofibrillary tangles.[36] The discovery of autosomal dominant mutations in the *tau* gene causing some forms of frontotemporal dementia has focused interest on the possibility that primary abnormalities in tau protein are responsible for neuronal degeneration in these conditions.[37] This suggests that therapies which alter the deposition of tau protein may be the most effective way to modify the underlying disease process. The neurofibrillary tangles deposited in PSP can be distinguished from those seen in Alzheimer's disease in a number of ways. Tau neurofibrillary tangles appear most commonly as globose tangles under the light microscope, in contrast to the flame-shaped tangles of Alzheimer's disease. Under the electron microscope, the tangles in PSP appear as straight filaments with a diameter of 15–18 nm.[38] *In vitro* work suggests that these straight filaments are preferentially formed by isoforms of the alternatively spliced *tau* gene containing four microtubule binding domains,[39] and this theory is supported by recent work confirming that *tau* protein in PSP has four repeat isoforms.[40] In Alzheimer's disease, tau is identified on immunoblotting to have three abnormal major protein bands, at 55, 64 and 68 kDa, whereas the major bands in PSP are at 64 and 68 kDa. This has also been shown to be consistent with the expression of four repeat isoforms of the *tau* gene in PSP, as opposed to expression of all six isoforms of the *tau* gene in Alzheimer's disease.[40] The link between a genetic predisposition to PSP and the differential isoform expression of the *tau* gene may be the key to explaining the pathogenesis of PSP.

Genetics

A number of families have been described with autosomal dominant PSP,[41–46] although to date neither a linked chromosomal locus nor a causative gene mutation have been identified. Analysis of sporadic PSP cases have demonstrated that one form (the A0 allele) of a variable non-protein coding site (intronic polymorphism) within the *tau* gene occurs more frequently in patients with PSP than controls.[47] This may be a predisposing factor to PSP which, similarly to the apolipoprotein E ϵ4 allele in Alzheimer's disease, increases the risk of developing PSP but is in itself neither necessary nor sufficient to cause the disease. Although this polymorphism lies before an alternatively spliced protein coding exon of the *tau* gene, it is unknown whether this polymorphism or an adjacent linked area has an effect on the alternative splicing of tau and whether this is important in the pathogenesis of the disease.

Treatment

Supportive treatment is the mainstay of management as the disease is relentlessly progressive. Explanation of the diagnosis and contact with patient support groups may be of benefit, particularly as patients may have been misdiagnosed as having PD or other disorders earlier in their illness. Physiotherapy and occupational therapy are of importance in helping with aids for balance and avoidance of falls. The early identification of problems with swallowing is important and this should prompt referral to speech therapy services for swallowing assessment and advice on appropriate measures to avoid the complications of aspiration.[48] Some patients and their families benefit from the insertion of a percutaneous gastrostomy tube but decisions on invasive interventions of this type should take into account the patient's and families' wishes in the context of the overall quality of life. Additional communication aids such as light-writers are usually not of benefit because of the concurrent eye movement disorder. Patients usually do not derive great benefit from dopaminergic medication due to widespread damage to structures in the basal ganglia.[49] Early reports suggested that amantadine may be of more benefit in improving the motor deficits in PSP, but this has not been subject to a formal randomised trial and the response is at best modest. Most interest in PSP has centred on the use of cholinergic treatments, particularly because of the suggestion that cholinergic nuclei may be responsible for the problems with balance.[50] However, although oral physostigmine and cholinergic agonists do not produce a useful symptomatic benefit in PSP,[51,52] intravenous physostigime has been shown to improve cerebral metabolism,[53] and some measures of neuropsychometric and oculomotor performance.[54] These data suggest that, if significant enhancement of central nervous system cholinergic transmission can be achieved, some symptomatic improvement might be attained. Adrenergic agents have also been used in PSP because of the adrenergic deficit resulting in part from damage to the locus coeruleus.[55] Although these agents were initially thought to improve motor performance, this has not been replicated and their use has been limited by the occurrence of cardiovascular side effects.[55,56]

Conclusions

PSP is a distinctive syndrome both clinically and pathologically and should be relatively easily diagnosed once considered by the clinician. The greater understanding of the tau gene and tau protein suggests that in the next few years there will be a much clearer understanding of the pathology and aetiology of this condition, which should lead to new potential disease-modifying agents. In the shorter term, cholinergic agents may emerge as useful symptomatic treatments for this disease. Currently, accurate diagnosis and the sympathetic provision of supportive care are the most important issues for the practising physician.

Acknowledgements

We are grateful to Dr JC Steele for helpful discussion. HRM is an MRC Clinical Training Fellow and supported by the PSP (Europe) Association. The PSP (Europe) Association provides support and advice for PSP patients and carers, and can be reached at The Old Rectory, Wappenham, Nr Towcester, Northamptonshire NN12 8SQ, UK.

References

1 Steele JC. Progressive supranuclear palsy. Historical notes. *J Neural Transm* 1994; **42**(suppl): 3–14.

2 Steele J, Richardson JC, Olszewski J. Progressive supranuclear palsy. A heterogeneous system degeneration involving brain stem, basal ganglia and cerebellum with vertical gaze and pseudobulbar palsy, nuchal dystonia and dementia. *Arch Neurol* 1964; **10**: 333–59.

3 Verhaart WJC. Degeneration of the brainstem reticular formation, other parts of the brainstem and cerebellum. An example of heterogenous systemic degeneration of the central nervous system. *J Neuropathol Exp Neurol* 1958; **17**: 382–91.

4 Chavany JA, Vanbogaert L, Godlevski S. Sur un syndrome de rigidite a predominance axiale, avec perturbation de automatismes oculopalpebraux d'origine encephalitique. *Presse Med* 1951; **59**: 958–62.

5 Goetz CG. An early photographic case of probable progressive supranuclear palsy. *Mov Disord* 1996; **1**: 617–18.

6 Robertson WM, Gilman S, Vilensky JA. The Denny-Brown collection: recognition of progressive supranuclear palsy as a unique disorder in the decade before the clinico-pathological description. *Neurology* 1997; **48**: A145.

7 Critchley M. Arteriosclerotic parkinsonism. *Brain* 1929; **52**: 22–83.

8 Brusa A, Mancardi GL, Buigiani O. Progressive supranuclear palsy 1979: an overview. *Ital J Neurol Sci* 1980; **4**: 205–22.

9 Golbe LI. The epidemiology of PSP. *J Neural Transm* 1994; **42**(suppl): 263–73.

10 Bower JH, Maraganore DM, McDonnell SK, Rocca WA. Incidence of progressive supranuclear palsy and multiple system atrophy in Olmsted County, Minnesota, 1976 to 1990. *Neurology* 1997; **49**: 1284–8.

11 Todd Troost BT, Daroff RB. The ocular motor defects in progressive supranuclear palsy. *Ann Neurol* 1977; **2**: 397–403.

12 Golbe LI, Davis PH, Lepore FE. Eyelid movement abnormalities in progressive supra-nuclear palsy. *Mov Disord* 1989; **4**: 297–302.

13 Rascol O, Sabatini U, Simonetta-Moreau M, Montastruc JL, Rascol A, Clanet M. Square wave jerks in parkinsonian syndromes. *J Neurol Neurosurg Psychiatry* 1991; **54**: 599–602.

14 Albert ML, Feldman RG, Willis AL. The 'subcortical dementia' of progressive supra-nuclear palsy. *J Neurol Neurosurg Psychiatry* 1974; **37**: 121–30.

15 Dubois B, Pillon B, Legault F, Agid Y, Lhermitte F. Slowing of cognitive processing in progressive supranuclear palsy. A comparison with Parkinson's disease. *Arch Neurol* 1988; **45**: 1194–9.

16 van Zagten M, Lodder J, Kessels F. Gait disorder and parkinsonian signs in patients with stroke related to small deep infarcts and white matter lesions. *Mov Disord* 1998; **13**: 89–95.

17 Siderowf AD, Galetta SL, Hurtig HI, Liu GT. Posey and Spiller and progressive supranuclear palsy: an incorrect attribution. *Mov Disord* 1998; **13**: 170–4.

18 Litvan I, Agid Y, Calne D, *et al.* Clinical research criteria for the diagnosis of progressive supranuclear palsy (Steele-Richardson-Olszewski syndrome): report of the NINDS-SPSP international workshop. *Neurology* 1996; **47**: 1–9.

19 Daniel SE, de Bruin VMS, Lees AJ. The clinical and pathological spectrum of Steele-Richardson-Olszewski syndrome (progressive supranuclear palsy): a reappraisal. *Brain* 1995; **118**: 759–70.

20 Davis PH, Bergeron C, McLachlan DR. Atypical presentations of progressive supra-nuclear palsy. *Ann Neurol* 1997; **17**: 337–43.

21 Hughes AJ, Daniel SE, Kilford L, Lees AJ. Accuracy of clinical diagnosis of idiopathic Parkinson's disease: a clinico-pathological study of 100 cases. *J Neurol Neurosurg Psychiatry* 1992; **55**: 181–4.

22 Davis PH, Golbe LI, Duvoisin RC, Schoenberg BS. Risk factors for progressive supra-nuclear palsy. *Neurology* 1988; **38**: 1546–52.

23 Golbe LI, Rubin RS, Cody RP, *et al.* Follow-up study of risk factors in progressive supranuclear palsy. *Neurology* 1996; **47**: 148–54.

24 Hauw J-J, Daniel SE, Dickson D, *et al.* Preliminary NINDS neuropathologic criteria for Steele-Richardson-Olszewski syndrome (progressive supranuclear palsy). *Neurology* 1994; **44**: 2015–9.

25 Aiba I, Hashizume Y, Yoshida M, Okuda S, Murakami N, Ujihira N. Relationship between brainstem MRI and pathological findings in progressive supranuclear palsy – study in autopsy cases. *J Neurol Sci* 1997; **152**: 210–17.

26 Parent A, Cicchetti F. The current model of basal ganglia organization under scrutiny. *Mov Disord* 1998; **13**: 199–202.

27 Fearnley JM, Lees AJ. Ageing and Parkinson's disease: substantia nigra regional selectivity. *Brain* 1991; **114**: 2283–301.

28 Brooks DJ, Ibanez V, Sawle GV, *et al.* Differing patterns of striatal 18F-dopa uptake in Parkinson's disease, multiple system atrophy, and progressive supranuclear palsy. *Ann Neurol* 1990; **28**: 547–55.

29 Hardman CD, McRitchie DA, Halliday GM, Cartwright HR, Morris JG. Substantia nigra pars reticulata neurons in Parkinson's disease. *Neurodegeneration* 1996; **5**: 49–55.

30 Pollak P, Benabid AL, Limousin P, *et al.* Subthalamic nucleus stimulation alleviates akinesia and rigidity in parkinsonian patients. *Adv Neurol* 1996; **69**: 591–4.

31 Hardman CD, Halliday GM, McRitchie DA, Morris JG. The subthalamic nucleus in Parkinson's disease and progressive supranuclear palsy. *J Neuropathol Exp Neurol* 1997; **56**: 132–42.

32 Juncos JL, Hirsch EC, Malessa S, Duyckaerts C, Hersh LB, Agid Y. Mesencephalic cholinergic nuclei in progressive supranuclear palsy. *Neurology* 1991; **41**: 25–30.

33 Revesz T, Sangha H, Daniel SE. The nucleus raphe interpositus in the Steele-Richardson-Olszewski syndrome (progressive supranuclear palsy). *Brain* 1996; **119**: 1137–43.

34 Mesulam MM, Geula C, Bothwell MA, Hersh LB. Human reticular formation: cholinergic neurons of the pedunculopontine and laterodorsal tegmental nuclei and some cytochemical comparisons to forebrain cholinergic neurons. *J Comp Neurol* 1989; **283**: 611–33.

35 Hauw JJ, Verny M, Delaere P, Cervera P, He Y, Duyckaerts C. Constant neurofibrillary changes in the neocortex in progressive supranuclear palsy. Basic differences with Alzheimer's disease and aging. *Neurosci Lett* 1990; **119**: 182–6.

36 Dickson DW. Neurodegenerative diseases with cytoskeletal pathology: a biochemical classification. *Ann Neurol* 1997; **42**: 541–4.

37 Hutton M, Lendon CL, Rizzu P, *et al.* Association of missense and 5'-splice-site mutations in tau with the inherited dementia FTDP-17. *Nature* 1998; **393**: 702–5.

38 Roy S, Datta CK, Hirano A, Ghatak NR, Zimmerman HM. Electron microscopic study of neurofibrillary tangles in Steele-Richardson-Olszewski syndrome. *Acta Neuropathol (Berl)* 1974; **29**: 175–9.

39 Goedert M, Jakes R, Spillantini MG, Hasegawa M, Smith MJ, Crowther RA. Assembly of microtubule-associated protein tau into Alzheimer-like filaments induced by sulphated glycosaminoglycans. *Nature* 1996; **383**: 550–3.

40 Mailliot C, Sergeant N, Bussiere T, Caillet-Boudin ML, Delacourte A, Buee L. Phosphorylation of specific sets of tau isoforms reflects different neurofibrillary degeneration processes. *FEBS Lett* 1998; **433**: 201–4.

41 Ohara S, Kondo K, Morita H, Maruyama K, Ikeda S, Yanagisawa N. Progressive supranuclear palsy-like syndrome in two siblings of a consanguineous marriage. *Neurology* 1992; **42**: 1009–14.

42 Golbe LI, Dickson DW. Familial autopsy-proven progressive supranuclear palsy. *Neurology* 1997; **45**: A255.

43 Brown J, Lantos P, Stratton M, Rocques P, Rossor M. Familial progressive supranuclear palsy. *J Neurol Neurosurg Psychiatry* 1993; **56**: 473–6.

44 Tetrud JW, Golbe LI, Forno LS, Farmer PM. Autopsy-proven progressive supranuclear palsy in two siblings. *Neurology* 1994; **46**: 931–4.

45 de Yebenes JG, Sarasa JL, Daniel SE, Lees AJ. Familial progressive supranuclear palsy Description of a pedigree and review of the literature. *Brain* 1995; **118**: 1095–103.

46 Gazely S, Maguire J. Familial progressive supranuclear palsy. *Brain Pathol* 1994; **4**: 534.

47 Conrad C, Andreadis A, Trojanowski JQ, *et al*. Genetic evidence for the involvement of tau in progressive supranuclear palsy. *Ann Neurol* 1997; **41**: 277–81.

48 Litvan I, Sastry N, Sonies BC. Characterizing swallowing abnormalities in progressive supranuclear palsy. *Neurology* 1997; **48**: 1654–62.

49 Nieforth KA, Golbe LI. Retrospective study of drug response in 87 patients with progressive supranuclear palsy. *Clin Neuropharmacol* 1993; **16**: 338–46.

50 Litvan I. Cholinergic approaches to the treatment of progressive supranuclear palsy. *J Neural Transm* 1994; **42**(suppl): 275–81.

51 Foster NL, Aldrich MS, Bluemlein L, White RF, Berent S. Failure of cholinergic agonist RS-86 to improve cognition and movement in PSP despite effects on sleep. *Neurology* 1989; **39**: 257–61.

52 Litvan I, Gomez C, Atack JR, *et al*. Physostigmine treatment of progressive supranuclear palsy. *Ann Neurol* 1989; **26**: 404–7.

53 Blin J, Mazetti P, Mazoyer B, *et al*. Does the enhancement of cholinergic neurotransmission influence brain glucose kinetics and clinical symptomatology in progressive supranuclear palsy? *Brain* 1995; **118**: 1485–95.

54 Litvan I, Blesa R, Clark K, *et al*. Pharmacological evaluation of the cholinergic system in progressive supranuclear palsy. *Ann Neurol* 1994; **36**: 55–61.

55 Ghika J, Tennis M, Hoffman E, Schoenfeld D, Growdon J. Idazoxan treatment in progressive supranuclear palsy. *Neurology* 1991; **41**: 986–91.

56 Rascol O, Sieradzan K, Peyro-Saint-Paul H, *et al*. Efaroxan, an alpha-2 antagonist, in the treatment of progressive supranuclear palsy. *Mov Disord* 1998; **13**: 673–6.

Chapter Fourteen

Pharmacological treatment of Parkinson's disease

A Münchau and KP Bhatia with SA Schneider

Parkinson's disease is a neurodegenerative disorder of unknown cause. Age is the most consistent risk factor and incidence in the general population over 75 years of age is 254:100 000.[1] With an ageing population the management of Parkinson's disease is likely to prove an increasingly important and challenging aspect of medical practice. Classically Parkinson's disease presents with resting tremor, rigidity, and akinesia often in an asymmetric fashion, but later usually bilateral. However, initial symptoms may be subtle and vague, for example discomfort or mild stiffness in the limbs, and may be misinterpreted. Moreover clinical features are variable with some patients presenting with akinesia and rigidity only and others with a tremor dominant type. About 10–20% of autopsy cases with a diagnosis of Parkinson's disease were not considered to suffer from it in life.[2] On the other hand, approximately 25% of patients with a diagnosis of Parkinson's disease in life are shown to have a different diagnosis when postmortem examination is carried out.[3,4] Diagnosis may thus be difficult particularly as there are no biological markers that unequivocally confirm the diagnosis of Parkinson's disease. The most common differential diagnoses are essential tremor, arteriosclerotic pseudoparkinsonism, drug-induced parkinsonism,[5] and the so-called Parkinson plus syndromes, namely multiple system atrophy,[6,7] progressive supranuclear palsy,[8,9] and corticobasal degeneration.[10]

Drugs used in Parkinson's disease

In the following sections a summary of drugs currently in use in the UK will be provided. The optimum use of antiparkinsonian drugs and the timing of treatment are matters of debate. This will be discussed later. Also, dose recommendations will be given later.

L-dopa

Degeneration in the basal ganglia in the brains of Parkinson's disease patients primarily affects dopaminergic neurons in the substantia nigra which results in dopamine deficiency. Exogenous L-dopa replaces endogenous deficient neurotransmitter. L-dopa is taken up by remaining dopaminergic neurons where it undergoes decarboxylation in the presynaptic terminal to form dopamine.

Usually L-dopa is combined with benserazide or carbidopa. They do not cross the blood-brain barrier but inhibit the conversion of L-dopa to dopamine peripherally by blocking the enzyme aromatic acid decarboxylase that catalyses this reaction. Dopaminergic adverse effects are thus reduced, central delivery is amplified, and dosage of L-dopa can be reduced.[11] By giving long acting controlled release preparations fluctuations in plasma concentration of L-dopa can be reduced.[12-14]

L-dopa remains the single most effective drug for the treatment of Parkinson's disease.[11,15] For the first five to ten years after starting L-dopa treatment all symptoms usually improve, although higher doses may be needed to treat tremor. The drug is tolerated well and side effects, particularly psychiatric symptoms, orthostatic hypotension, and nausea, are limited. After several years of a favourable response to L-dopa (the 'L-dopa honeymoon') patients often develop disabling motor complications including fluctuations between the 'on' and 'off' state and dyskinesias.[16] This is mainly related to an increasing loss of dopaminergic nerve terminals. L-dopa can no longer be stored in these terminals and patients' symptoms begin to fluctuate according to the plasma concentration of circulating L-dopa.

In addition to the development of treatment-related complications there is theoretical concern that L-dopa is neurotoxic as it has the potential to form free radicals and other toxic metabolites as breakdown products when metabolised.[17,18] These free radicals might injure surviving dopaminergic neurons and thus speed the progression of Parkinson's disease.[19] However, in vivo toxicity of L-dopa to neurons in the substantia nigra has not been demonstrated[20,21] and the emphasis on the toxic potential of L-dopa has been criticised.[22]

Nevertheless, it appears prudent to delay treatment with L-dopa, provided adequate improvement of parkinsonian symptoms is achieved with other drugs.

Alternatives to L-dopa are dopamine agonists, amantadine, anticholinergic drugs, and selegeline.

Dopamine agonists

Drugs belonging to this class act directly on dopamine receptors, mimicking the endogenous neurotransmitter. They can be classified into ergot derivates (bromocriptine, pergolide, lisuride, and cabergoline) and the nonergolines (apomorphine, pramipexole, and ropinirole).

There are several theoretical advantages of dopamine agonists over L-dopa. Firstly, they usually have a long duration of action that more closely mimics the physiological tonic release of dopamine from normal nigral neurons and may help to prevent or reduce motor fluctuations.[23] However, half-life varies between agonists as well as between individual patients.[24,25] Secondly, they can have a L-dopa sparing effect. Thirdly, due to sparing of L-dopa and stimulation of presynaptic autoreceptors resulting in a decrease of dopamine turnover including potentially toxic metabolisms, they may also be neuroprotective. Moreover, dopamine agonists are not metabolised by oxidative pathways and do not produce free radical metabolites.[26] They may also have direct antioxidative effects.[27]

In clinical practice dopamine agonists have been shown to be efficacious in Parkinson's disease.[28] They are commonly used as adjunctive therapy to L-dopa after motor complications have developed[29,30] but may also be considered as monotherapy before starting L-dopa, particularly in younger patients.[31] On dopamine agonist monotherapy patients often do not show motor fluctuations until L-dopa is added to the regimen.[32] They usually take longer than L-dopa to reach effective doses and require supplementary L-dopa for relief of symptoms after a varying period of time.[15]

A common side effect of dopamine agonists is nausea due to stimulation of the area postrema in the medulla, a region that is outside the blood-brain barrier. The peripherally acting dopamine antagonist domperidone can alleviate this symptom without worsening parkinsonian symptoms.[30,33] Psychiatric side effects such as hallucinations are similar to those caused by L-dopa.[34]

Most long-term studies assessing dopamine agonist monotherapy in previously untreated Parkinson patients have investigated bromocriptine. About one third of these patient have shown a good response to this drug and some may not require L-dopa for 2–5 years.[15] A recent study found support for the usefulness of bromocriptine monotherapy at an early stage of Parkinson's disease with adjunctive L-dopa when necessary.[35]

Pergolide, which stimulates both D1 and D2 receptors, unlike bromocriptine, which only stimulates D2 receptors, has been demonstrated to be beneficial in Parkinson's disease.[36,37] In a comparative review of pergolide and bromocriptine as adjunctive to L-dopa, pergolide was shown to be more effective than bromocriptine.[29]

Newer dopamine agonists including pramipexole,[38] ropinirole,[39] and cabergoline[40] were demonstrated to have some benefit in previously untreated patients but it is not yet known whether they have better long-term efficacy with fewer complications than bromocriptine or pergolide.

An electrophysiological study has shown that pramipexole binds selectively and with high affinity to dopamine D2 and D3 receptors and has a greater efficacy for stimulating dopamine receptors than ergoline dopamine agonist.[41] It appears to be safe, well tolerated, and effective as an add-on therapy in advanced Parkinson's disease with treatment complications such as motor fluctuations.[38]

Ropinirole is a specific D2 and D3 receptor non-ergoline dopamine agonist, that is probably equally effective as L-dopa in mild, early Parkinson's disease.[42] A report of an ongoing study suggests that monotherapy with ropinirole might be more effective than monotherapy with bromocriptine.[43] As an adjunct to L-dopa in patients with motor fluctuations it has been shown to improve parkinsonism and to decrease time spent in the 'off' state[44,45] and permits a reduction in L-dopa dose.[44]

Cabergoline, a long acting predominantly D2 receptor agonist, is effective as adjunct therapy in advanced Parkinson's disease and also as monotherapy in de novo patients.[40,46] In a trial comparing L-dopa with cabergoline monotherapy for up to one year cabergoline was slightly less effective than L-dopa.[40]

Apomorphine

The use of apomorphine in Parkinson's disease was first reported by Schwab *et al.*,[47] who noticed improvement in tremor and rigidity. It was later shown that oral apomorphine reduced 'on'/'off' effects but treatment was limited by nausea, vomiting, postural hypotension, and sedation.[48] However, given subcutaneously by repeated injections or by continuous infusion under domperidone cover it is a well tolerated treatment that effectively reduces daily 'off' periods.[49–51] Due to rapid subcutaneous absorption response to a bolus occurs after 10–15 minutes and the effect lasts for 20–60 minutes. Infusion pumps are generally well tolerated but widespread application is limited by the complexity of the technique. Alternatively, rectal, intranasal, or sublingual preparations have proved effective.[52–54] Side effects are postural hypotension, cognitive impairment, and disabling dyskinesias during 'on' phases. When infusion pumps are used, particular attention to the subcutaneous infusion site is needed, as allergic reactions, aseptic necrosis, or infection may occur.

Monoamine oxidase B inhibitors

Selegeline is an example of this class of drug. It selectively and irreversibly inhibits intracellular and extracellular monoamine oxidase B (MAO B) and therefore reduces or delays the breakdown of dopamine to dihydroxyphenylacetic acid (DOPAC) and hydrogen peroxide. The latter has been implicated in oxidative damage in dopaminergic neurons in the substantia nigra. It also inhibits reuptake of dopamine from the synaptic cleft. Adding selegeline to L-dopa may allow a reduction of the L-dopa dose of 10–15%, occasionally up to 30%.[31] Mild L-dopa response fluctuations can often be reduced by adding selegeline. Monotherapy in de novo patients delays the need for additional treatment by approximately a year.[55,56] Possible neuroprotective effects will be discussed later (*see* 'neuroprotection'). Side effects of L-dopa, including dyskinesias and psychiatric problems, are potentially enhanced by selegeline. Orthostatic hypotension may also occur.[57]

Amantadine

This antiviral agent has been used in Parkinson's disease for almost 30 years[58] and several possible mechanisms of action have been advocated. It may increase dopamine synthesis, it may be a dopamine and noradrenaline presynaptic reuptake blocker, and it also has a mild anticholinergic action.[31,59,60] Amantadine influences predominantly akinesia and rigor but has also a mild effect on rest tremor. Two thirds of parkinsonian patients show an improvement on amantadine monotherapy.[61] The beneficial effects of amantadine may be short lived. Recently an NMDA antagonism (NMDA is one of the receptors that binds the excitatory neurotransmitter glutamate) was proposed for amantadine.[62] This might have implications for the treatment of dyskinesias as functional over-activity of glutaminergic projections to the basal ganglia has been shown to be of importance in the development of dyskinesias.[23] A recent study has indeed confirmed that amantadine can reduce L-dopa induced dyskinesias in patients with Parkinson's disease without altering the antiparkinsonian effects of L-dopa.[63]

Cautious use of amantadine is recommended in renal failure as it is excreted in the urine. Side effects include hallucinations, insomnia, nightmares, livedo reticularis, and ankle oedema.

Anticholinergics

Current drugs available in the UK are biperiden, procyclidine, orphenadrine, benzhexol, and benztropine. Anticholinergic drugs improve tremor and stiffness to a greater degree than akinesia and are overall mildly effective.[64] Due to a peripheral parasympathomimetic action, side effects such as glaucoma, dryness of the mouth, blurred vision, urinary retention, and constipation can occur. Anticholinergics have a relatively high potential for causing or worsening confusional states and impairing concentration.[65] They should therefore be used very cautiously in the elderly.

Catechol o-methyl transferase inhibitors

L-dopa is converted to dopamine by a reaction catalysed by the enzyme aromatic acid decarboxylase which is inhibited by carbidopa and benserazide. Significant peripheral metabolism of L-dopa is also mediated by catechol-omethyltransferase (COMT) which catalyses the O-methylation of L-dopa to 3-Omethyldopa. As aromatic acid decarboxylase is inhibited by conventional L-dopa preparations the peripheral metabolism is shunted towards the reactions catalysed by COMT. The addition of a COMT inhibitor as adjunctive therapy to L-dopa plus either carbidopa or benserazide reduces peripheral metabolism of L-dopa, prolongs the plasma half-life of L-dopa and increases the amount available in the brain.[66] Peak concentration of L-dopa is not altered by adding COMT inhibitors.[67] In the brain COMT activity catalyses the metabolism of L-dopa to 3-OMD and of DOPAC to homovanillic acid.

COMT inhibition translates into less fluctuation of L-dopa plasma concentrations so that levels remain within the therapeutic range and benefit from each dose of L-dopa will be prolonged.

Tolcapone inhibits COMT both peripherally and centrally[68] whereas entacapone acts only peripherally.[69,70] It could be demonstrated that tolcapone reduces 'off' time by an average of 40% and increases 'on' time by about 25% in fluctuating Parkinson patients.[71] Doses of L-dopa could significantly be reduced. In a double blind, multicentre, randomised trial tolcapone reduced the wearing-off time and reduced the requirements for L-dopa in patients with fluctuating disease.[72]

Oral entacapone generally improves the duration of daily 'on' time by 30 to 60 minutes, especially in patients who have a low proportion of 'on' time.[73–76] Patients' daily 'off' time was found to be reduced by approximately 1.3 hours.[74] The mean daily L-dopa dosage could be reduced by 12% in two multicentre, double blind randomised placebo controlled studies.[74,76]

Side effects of COMT inhibitors include potentiation of dyskinesias, nausea, orange discoloration of the urine, and sleep disturbances. Chronic tolcapone use can result in diarrhoea that can be severe. Elevations of liver enzymes have been associated with tolcapone. Because of two cases of fatal toxic hepatitis, tolcapone was recently withdrawn from the market in Europe. Entacapone is currently the only available COMT inhibitor in the UK. No association between the drug and liver toxicity has been shown[77] and elevations of liver enzymes have not been reported. The dosage should be reduced in patients with hepatic impairment in whom the bioavailablility of entacapone is increased. Overall, entacapone appears to be a safe drug. It did not cause significant changes in biochemical or haematological parameters in clinical studies of up to six months' duration or in the report of a 12 month tolerability study.[74,76,78]

No significant change of autonomic function and no significant haemodynamic effects have been observed in patients with Parkinson's disease.[77]

Treatment strategies

In neurodegenerative disorders like Parkinson's disease any therapeutic intervention that halts or reverses the progression of the disease would be desirable. We shall therefore first consider possible neuroprotective agents and then discuss symptomatic treatment.

Neuroprotection

Until now no drug has been convincingly shown to halt the degenerative process in Parkinson's disease. As the disease progresses an increasing number of dopaminergic neurons in the substantia nigra die. The reduction of the population of these cells in turn stimulates dopaminergic turnover of the remaining neurons with an increase of hydrogen peroxide that is a by-product of dopamine metabolism (MAO-B pathway). Hydroxide peroxide gives rise to the formation to toxic hydroxyl radicals that can cause further cell damage by membrane disruption.[79]

Box 14.1 Drugs used in Parkinson's disease

- The aim of medical treatment is the restoration of abnormal neurotransmitter function in the basal ganglia.
- L-dopa combined with a peripheral decarboxylase inhibitor remains the single most effective drug to improve parkinsonian symptoms but chronic use is associated with motor fluctuations and dyskinesias. L-dopa can be given as a standard formulation or as a slow release preparation.
- Dopamine agonists offer several advantages over L-dopa and can be tried before introducing L-dopa therapy but they are not as effective as L-dopa and sooner or later supplementary L-dopa is required. They are useful as an adjunct to L-dopa in later stages of the disease.
- Selegeline can delay the introduction of L-dopa. Its neuroprotective properties remain controversial.
- Amantadine can give symptomatic relief and may improve dyskinesias in later stages of the disease.
- Anticholinergics may improve tremor but are otherwise only mildly effective. They should be avoided in the elderly.
- COMT inhibitors increase 'on' time, reduce time spent in the 'off' state and may allow a reduction of the daily L-dopa dose.

Selegeline inhibits MAO-B and it was therefore postulated that administration of this drug will protect remaining neurons in the substantia nigra.[80] Moreover in animal experiments selegeline, by inhibiting MAO-B, blocked the conversion of MPTP to MPP+, an exogenous neurotoxin that damages neurons in the substantia nigra,[81] and prevented MPTP induced parkinsonism in primates. On the basis of these experiments it was hypothesised that MAO-B inhibition might also retard the progression of Parkinson's disease in humans, although this is different from MPTP induced parkinsonism in animals.

Several studies have been undertaken to prove this hypothesis. In the DATA-TOP study[82] selegeline very significantly delayed the need for L-dopa by about nine months. However, after three years of follow-up, no difference with respect to clinical symptoms was found between the group treated with placebo and L-dopa and the group treated with selegeline and L-dopa. Furthermore methods of the original DATATOP study have been criticised.[83] An open label, long-term, prospective randomised UK study comparing treatment with either L-dopa alone or in combination with selegeline failed to demonstrate a clinical benefit of the combined treatment.[84]

Compelling evidence to support selegeline as a neuroprotective agent is there-fore lacking. Moreover in the UK study[84] mortality was significantly higher with combination treatment which led to doubts on the chronic use of selegeline in Parkinson's disease. An extension of this study also showed excess mortality in patients treated with combined L-dopa and selegeline.[85] Other groups[56] and a recent meta-analysis[86] could not confirm this and the issue thus remains a matter of debate.

As outlined above dopamine agonists may have a neuroprotective effect by sparing L-dopa, decreasing dopamine metabolism, and possibly also by a direct antioxidative affect. It has also been suggested that amantadine may have a neuroprotective effect by inhibition of NMDA glutamate receptors.[87] One study has shown an improved survival of Parkinson's disease patients treated with amantadine[88] but this requires confirmation.

Apart from preventing oxidative stress and inhibiting excitatory neurotoxicity, future neuroprotective strategies may also focus on antiapoptotic agents as apoptosis (programmed cell death) appears to play a part in the pathogenesis of Parkinson's disease.[89] The administration of brain derived neurotrophic factors, antioxidants, or iron chelates to overcome neurodegeneration in the substantia nigra[90] is still experimental.

Symptomatic treatment

The optimal management of Parkinson's disease is still controversial and mainly based on empirical experience as properly designed clinical trials are scarce.[30] First it has to be decided when treatment is started. This obviously depends on the patient's needs. Although delaying treatment for as long as possible appears prudent since treatment will foster motor complications this is often not feasible, particularly in young patients whose employment may be threatened by the symptoms of Parkinson's disease. On the other hand, delaying treatment in elderly patients may compromise physical independence.

Once treatment has been started the choice of drug becomes the main issue. Ever since the introduction of bromocriptine the controversy emerged whether drug treatment of Parkinson's disease should be started with a dopamine agonist or with L-dopa and this controversy continues.[91,92] Treatment of early disease generally differs from later stages when various complications occur. It is also influenced by the patients' age. Younger patients usually develop motor compli-cations earlier than older patients and these symptoms can be severe.[93,94] This has to be taken into account when commencing symptomatic treatment. On the other hand dementia is less common in younger patients who may better be able to tolerate individual but potentially complicated drug regimens that would be inadequate for older patients. We will therefore outline recommendations for young patients (under the age of 50 years) and older patients (above the age of 70 years). For the group of patients between 50 and 70 years a more flexible approach is recommended.

Early treatment in young patients (age <50 years)

In view of problematic motor complications, L-dopa treatment is best delayed for as long as possible. As selegeline delays the introduction of L-dopa it may be considered as an early treatment. Selegeline can be administered once a day (10 mg).

Amantadine and anticholinergics can be tried, although they usually give only modest benefit that may not be enough for a young patient who is still employed and depends on a reliable medication to improve motor function. The recommended dose for amantadine is 100 mg daily increased after one week to 100 mg twice daily. The dose of anticholinergics has to be increased very gradually over several weeks to avoid side effects (particularly dry mouth, dizziness, blurred vision, and mental confusion). For instance, benzhexol should be started with 0.5 mg at night and increased by 0.5 mg every five days up to 6 mg daily in two or three divided doses.

Dopamine agonists are possibly the first line treatment as they are most likely to give enough benefit without provoking dyskinesias and often allow delaying L-dopa for at least a year.[31] Even after a delayed introduction of L-dopa dyskinesias are still less common than if L-dopa had been started earlier.[95] The same might be true for early combination therapy of L-dopa and a dopamine agonist[96,97] but this remains controversial.[98] Dopamine agonists should be introduced with domperidone cover (20 mg three times a day) and should gradually be increased. For most dopamine agonists starter packs are available with detailed but simple instructions on how to increase the dose. Dopamine agonists are generally given three times a day, apart from cabergoline that can be taken once a day. Dose equivalents among the different available dopamine agonists is difficult to know with certainty but has been estimated as follows: 30 mg of bromocriptine, 15 mg of ropinirole, 4.5 mg of pramipexole, and 3.0 mg of pergolide.[99] Recommended daily doses for bromocriptine are 10–40 mg, for ropinirole 3–9 mg, for pergolide 3 mg, for cabergoline 2–6 mg, for lisuride 5 mg, and for pramipexole 4.5 mg.

Eventually symptoms will not be sufficiently controlled and L-dopa has to be added. When introducing L-dopa one can opt for standard formulations (starting with 50–100 mg three times a day) or sustained release preparations (100 mg three times a day). The latter may be more suitable early in the course of the disease as receptor stimulation in the basal ganglia will be continuous and hence more physiological compared with standard formulations that produce rapid excessive plasma peaks followed by troughs and result in the brain being alternately flooded and starved.

Early treatment in old patients (age >70 years)

In elderly patients L-dopa remains the treatment of choice even in early stages as it is the drug with the best therapeutic window particularly with regard to psychiatric side effects. In view of their high potential of causing confusion anticholinergics should best be avoided but dopamine agonist and amantadine can be tried. Again, selegeline may be considered but the advantage of delaying L-dopa for several months is less meaningful in this age group.

Box 14.2 Treatment strategies: early stages

- None of the currently available drugs has a proved neuroprotective effect. Potential neuroprotective agents are under study.
- Treatment should be tailored to the individual patient's needs. The choice of drugs is mainly influenced by age.
- Young patients are more prone to develop motor complications. L-dopa therapy should therefore be delayed for as long as other drugs, particularly dopamine agonist, adequately relieve symptoms.
- In elderly patients L-dopa has the best therapeutic index and is the first line treatment.

Management of later stages

After the first five years about half the patients develop motor fluctuations or dyskinesias[100,101] that may be difficult to treat. Commonly the first fluctuations to occur are early morning akinesia and end-of-dose deterioration, also referred to as wearing off. These are predictable periods of immobility or greater severity of other parkinsonian symptoms when the effect of L-dopa wears off. They usually develop gradually over a period of several minutes up to an hour and are related to the timing of antiparkinsonian medication.

To overcome wearing off, more frequent doses of standard L-dopa are sometimes helpful, for example, five or six instead of three daily doses. Alternatively, changing from a standard L-dopa preparation to a slow release formulation can be tried. The bioavailability of these drugs is usually 70% of that of standard L-dopa. Although they last longer, initial absorption is slower and peak dose concentrations are lower so that patients often need a kick start dose of standard L-dopa first thing in the morning to compensate for that. They may also need occasional top-up doses of L-dopa during the day. Occasionally only very small doses are required. In these situations patients may benefit from dispersible L-dopa to titrate their individual doses.

COMT inhibitors can help to reduce wearing-off phenomena, increase the 'on' time and allow an overall reduction of the daily dose of L-dopa. [71–76,78,102] All published studies that have assessed the efficacy of COMT inhibitors in patients with Parkinson's disease have been conducted in patients with an end-of-dose deterioration.[78,102] It needs to be clarified whether COMT inhibitors also have a role in the treatment of drug naive de novo Parkinson's disease patients. Entacapone, currently the only available COMT inhibitor, is taken with each dose of L-dopa (three up to 10 doses per day). A dose of 200 mg (with each L-dopa dose) is associated with the optimal pharmacokinetic effect on L-dopa.[103] Another option for the treatment of the wearing off is to partially substitute L-dopa with a long lasting agonist drug.[29,30]

Box 14.3   Management of later stages

- Later stages of the disease are complicated mainly by motor fluctuations, dyskinesias, and psychiatric problems.
- Wearing-off phenomena can be overcome by more frequent doses of standard L-dopa, switching from standard L-dopa to slow release preparation, COMT inhibitors, or long lasting dopamine agonists.
- Abrupt fluctuations can be caused by delayed gastric emptying or delayed absorption of L-dopa and may be improved by adding cisapride or changing the diet.
- Dyskinesias sometimes improve by partial replacement of L-dopa by a dopamine agonist or adding amantadine.
- 'Off' period dystonia may respond to lithium therapy and can be relieved by botulinum toxin injections into dystonic muscles.
- When psychiatric complications occur, drugs with the least therapeutic benefit and highest potential to cause alterations of the mental state should be stopped first before reducing the dose of L-dopa.
- Symptomatic treatment of psychosis and delusions without worsening parkinsonian symptoms is possible with clozapine.

Fluctuations may be abrupt and patients may switch from the 'on' to the 'off' in a rather unpredictable way within seconds. Also, dose failure might occur. Both indicates a threshold effect of L-dopa which is explained by the fact that in later stages of the disease when exogenous L-dopa can no longer be stored in dopaminergic neurons the effect of L-dopa will solely depend on the plasma level. Small changes in plasma levels may then have dramatic effects.

A delayed 'on' or dose failures may be related to delayed gastric emptying[104] and hence inadequate plasma concentrations of L-dopa. This may improve in response to agents that promote gastric motility like cisapride.[105] Amino acids from proteins in the food may interfere with the absorption of L-dopa[105,106] and confining protein intake may help reducing fluctuations.

The duration of 'off' periods may effectively be reduced by subcutaneous administration of apomorphine either as a single rescue dose (2–5 mg, in rare cases up to 10 mg) or as continuous infusion (3–6 mg apomorphine/hour).[49–51]

Questions

Answers can be found at the end of 'References'.

1   What are the main differential diagnoses of idiopathic Parkinson's disease?
2   Why do motor complications occur?
3   What are the theoretical advantages of the use of dopamine agonists?
4   Which drug has proved neuroprotective properties?
5   Which drug that relieves parkinsonian symptoms has recently been shown to improve dyskinesias?
6   What are the benefits of COMT inhibitors?
7   Why should L-dopa therapy be delayed, particularly in young patients?

8   Which drug can effectively and reliably reduce refractory 'off' periods?
9   What is the most effective drug for symptomatic treatment of psychosis and delusions?

Dyskinesias are difficult to manage. Tackling peak dose dyskinesias or 'square wave' dyskinesias (that persist throughout the 'on' period) is sometimes possible by reducing the dose of L-dopa or partial replacement of L-dopa by a dopamine agonist. Diphasic dyskinesias that occur at the beginning or the end of a dose can be very severe and are often refractory to medical treatment. They are more common in young onset Parkinson's disease.[30] Adding an agonist sometimes helps. Overlapping L-dopa doses can be useful. Amantadine has recently been shown to be effective in reducing L-dopa induced dyskinesias without altering the antiparkinsonian effects of L-dopa.[63]

'Off' period dystonia commonly occurs in the morning and can sometimes be avoided by taking a dispersible L-dopa preparation on waking or can be overcome by apomorphine injections. Lithium is also sometimes helpful[107] and patients often benefit from botulinum toxin injections into dystonic muscles.[108]

During 'off' periods patients may experience dysphoria[109] including panic attacks, depression, and occasionally delusions or hallucinations. These symptoms resolve when patients turn 'on' again and are best managed by reducing the time the patients spend in an 'off' state. When sustained depression develops, which is the case in about one third of patients, treatment with antidepressants is warranted. Selective serotonin reuptake inhibitors have the potential to worsen parkinsonism[110] and can adversely interact with selegeline.[111]

In case of an organic confusional state or psychosis antiparkinsonian drugs should in principle be discontinued following the rule 'last in, first out'. If that rule is not applicable as the patient has not changed his medication recently the following order is suggested: anticholinergics, selegeline, amantadine, dopamine agonist. L-dopa has the best therapeutic index and should therefore be stopped last. If antipsychotic treatment is necessary clozapine is probably the drug of choice.[112,113] It appears to be specific for the subclass of dopamine receptors mediating psychosis and does not worsen parkinsonian symptoms.[112,113] Full blood count has to be monitored regularly as agranulocytosis may occur under clozapine treatment. Alternatively, olanzapine, the newest atypical neuroleptic drug, has become an option to treat psychosis in Parkinson patients.[114] It has not been associated with agranulocytosis but may worsen parkinsonian symptoms.[115] Ondansetron, an antagonist of the 5-hydroxytryptamine$_3$ receptor, has also been shown to be effective for visual hallucinations and delusions without worsening parkinsonian symptoms.[116]

Acknowledgement

Dr Alexander Münchau was supported by the Ernst Jung-Stiftung für Wissenschaft und Forschung in Hamburg, Germany and by the Eugene Brehm Bequest, UK.

References

1   Rajput AH, Offort K, Beard CM, *et al*. Epidemiologic survey of dementia in parkinsonism and control population. *Adv Neurol* 1984; **40**: 229–34.

2 Hughes AJ, Daniel SE, Lees, AJ. The clinical features of Parkinson's disease in 100 histologically proven cases. *Adv Neurol* 1993; **60**: 595–9.

3 Rajput AH, Rozdilski B, Rajput A. Accuracy of clinical diagnosis in parkinsonism – a prospective study. *Can J Neurol Sci* 1991; **18**: 275–8.

4 Hughes AJ, Daniel SE, Kilford L, *et al*. Accuracy of clinical diagnosis of idiopathic Parkinson's disease: a clinicopathological study of 100 cases. *J Neurol Neurosurg Psychiatry* 1992; **55**: 181–4.

5 Marti-Masso JF, Poza JJ, Lopez de Munain A. Drugs inducing or aggravating parkinsonism: a review. *Therapie* 1996; **51**: 568–77.

6 Shy GM, Drager GA. A neurological syndrome associated with orthostatic hypotension. *Arch Neurol* 1960; **2**: 511–27.

7 Wenning GK, Ben Shlomo Y, Magalhaes M, *et al*. Clinical features and natural history of multiple system atrophy. *Brain* 1994; **117**: 835–45.

8 Lees AJ. The Steele-Richardson-Olsewski syndrome (progressive supranuclear palsy). In: Marsden CD, Fahn S, eds. *Neurology 7, Movement disorders 2*. Butterworth International Medical Reviews. London: Butterworth, 1987: 272–87.

9 Steele JC, Richardson JC, Olszewski J. Progressive supranuclear palsy. A heterogeneous degeneration involving the brainstem, basal ganglia and cerebellum with vertical gaze and pseudobulbar palsy, nuchal dystonia and dementia. *Arch Neurol* 1964; **10**: 333–59.

10 Litvan I. Progressive supranuclear palsy and corticobasal degeneration. *Baillieres Clin Neurol* 1997; **6**: 167–85.

11 Silva MA, Mattern C, Hacker R, *et al*. Increased neostriatal dopamine activity after intraperitoneal or intranasal administration of L-dopa: on the role of benserazide pretreatment. *Synapse* 1997; **27**: 294–302.

12 Koller WC, Pahwa R. Treating motor fluctuations with controlled-release levodopa preparations. *Neurology* 1994; **44**(suppl 6):S23–8.

13 MacMahon DG, Sachdev D, Boddie HG, *et al*. A comparison of the effects of controlled-release levodopa in late Parkinson's disease. *J Neurol Neurosurg Psychiatry* 1990; **53**: 220–3.

14 Pahwa R, Lyons K, McGuire D, *et al*. Comparison of standard carbidopa-levodopa and sustained-release carbidopalevodopa in Parkinson's disease: pharmacokinetic and quality-of-life measures. *Mov Disord* 1997; **12**: 677–81.

15 Lang AE, Lozano AM. Medical progress: Parkinson's disease. *N Engl J Med* 1998; **339**: 1130–43.

16 Lesser RD, Fahn S, Snider SR, *et al*. Analysis of the clinical problems in parkinsonism and the complications of long-term levodopa therapy. *Neurology* 1979; **29**: 1253–60.

17 Basma AN, Morris EJ, Nicklas WJ, *et al*. L-dopa cytotoxicity to PC12 cells in culture is via its autooxidation. *J Neurochem* 1995; **64**: 825–32.

18 Graham DG. Oxidative pathways for catecholamines in the genesis of neuromelanin and cytotoxic quinones. *Mol Pharmacol* 1978; **14**: 633–43.

19 Fahn S. Is levodopa toxic? *Neurology* 1996; **47**(suppl 3):S184–95.

20 Quinn N, Parkes D, Janota I, *et al*. Preservation of the substantia nigra and locus coeruleus in a patient receiving levodopa (2 kg) plus decarboxylase inhibitor over a four year period. *Mov Disord* 1986; **1**: 65–8.

21 Rajput AH, Fenton ME, Birdi S, *et al*. Is levodopa toxic to human substantia nigra? *Mov Disord* 1997; **5**: 634–8.

22 Agid Y. Levodopa: is toxicity a myth? *Neurology* 1998; **50**: 858–63.

23 Chase TN, Engber TM, Mouradian MM. Contribution of dopaminergic and glutamatergic mechanisms to the pathogenesis of motor response complications in Parkinson's disease. *Adv Neurol* 1996; **69**: 497–501.

24 Goetz CG, Tanner CM, Glantz RH, *et al*. Chronic agonist therapy for Parkinson's disease: a 5-year study of bromocriptine and pergolide. *Neurology* 1985; **35**: 749–51.

25 Mizuno Y, Kondo T, Narabayashi H. Pergolide in the treatment of Parkinson's disease. *Neurology* 1995:**45**(suppl 3): S13–21.

26 Mena MA, Pardo B, Casarejas JJ, *et al*. Neurotoxicity of levodopa on catecholamine-rich neurons. *Mov Disord* 1992; **7**: 23–31.

27 Yoshikawa T, Minamiyama Y, Naito Y, *et al*. Antioxidant properties of bromocriptine, a dopamine agonist. *J Neurochem* 1994; **62**: 1034–8.

28 Uitti RJ, Ahlskog JE. Comparative review of dopamine receptor agonists in Parkinson's disease. *CNS Drugs* 1996; **5**: 369–88.

29 Nohria V, Partiot A. A review of the efficacy of the dopamine agonists pergolide and bromocriptine in the treatment of Parkinson's disease. *Eur J Neurol* 1997; **4**: 537–43.

30 Quinn N. Drug treatment of Parkinson's disease. *BMJ* 1995; **310**: 575–9.

31 Oertel WH, Quinn NP. Parkinsonism. In: Brandt T, Caplan LR, Dichgans J, *et al*., eds. *Neurological disorders. Course and treatment*. San Diego: Academic Press, 1996: 715–72.

32 Hely MA, Morris JG, Reid WG, *et al*. The Sydney Multicentre Study of Parkinson's disease: a randomized, prospective five year study comparing low dose bromocriptine with low dose levodopa-carbidopa. *J Neurol Neurosurg Psychiatry* 1994; **57**: 903–10.

33 Soykan I, Sarosiek I, Shifflet J, *et al*.Effect of oral domperidone therapy on gastrointestinal symptoms and gastric emptying in patients with Parkinson's disease. *Mov Disord* 1997; **12**: 952–7.

34 Factor SA, Molho ES, Podskalny GD, *et al*. Parkinson's disease: drug-induced psychiatric states. *Adv Neurol* 1995; **65**: 115–38.

35 Ogawa N, Kanazawa I, Kowa H, *et al*. Nationwide multicenter prospective study on the long-term effects of bromocriptine for Parkinson's disease. Final report of a ten-year follow-up. *Eur Neurol* 1997; **38**: 37–49.

36 Pezzoli G, Canesi M, Pesenti A, *et al*. Pergolide mesylate in Parkinson's disease treatment. *J Neurol Transm* 1995; **45**(suppl): 203–12.

37 Schwartz J, Scheidtmann K, Trenkwalder C. Improvement of motor fluctuations in patients with Parkinson's disease following treatment with high doses of pergolide and cessation of levodopa. *Eur Neurol* 1997; **37**: 236–8.

38 Guttman M. Double-blind comparison of pramipexole and bromocriptine treatment with placebo in advanced Parkinson's disease. International Pramipexole-Bromocriptine Study Group. *Neurology* 1997; **49**: 1060–5.

39 Adler CH, Sethi DK, Hauser RA, *et al*. Ropinirole for the treatment of early Parkinson's disease. *Neurology* 1997; **49**: 393–9.

40 Rinne UK, Bracco F, Chouza C, *et al*. Cabergoline in the treatment of early Parkinson's disease: results of the first year treatment in a double-blind comparison of cabergoline and levodopa. The PKDS0009 Collaborative Study Group. *Neurology* 1997; **48**: 363–8.

41 Piercey MF, Hoffmann WE, Smith MW, *et al*. Inhibition of dopamine neuron firing by pramipexole, a dopamine D3 receptor-preferring agonist: comparison to other dopamine receptor agonists. *Eur J Pharmacol* 1996; **312**: 35–44.

42 Rascol O, Brooks DJ, Brunt ER, *et al*. Ropinirole in the treatment of early Parkinson's disease: a 6-month interim report of a 5-year levodopa-controlled study. *Mov Disord* 1998; **13**: 39–45.

43 Korczyn AD, Brooks DJ, Brunt ER, *et al*. Ropinirole vs bromocriptine in the treatment of early Parkinson's disease: a 6-months interim report of a 3-year study. *Mov Disord* 1998; **13**: 46–51.

44 Lieberman A, Olanow CW, Sethi K, *et al*. A multicenter trial of ropinirole as adjunct for Parkinson's disease. *Neurology* 1998; **51**: 1057–62.

45 Rascol O, Lees AJ, Senard JM, *et al*. Ropinirole in the treatment of levodopa-induced motor fluctuations in patients with Parkinson's disease. *Clin Neuropharmacol* 1996; **19**: 234–45.

46 Del Dotto P, Colzi A, Musatti E, *et al.* Clinical and pharmacokinetic evaluation of L-dopa and cabergoline cotreatment in Parkinson's disease. *Clin Neuropharmacol* 1997; **20**: 455–65.

47 Schwab RS, Amador LV, Lettvin LY. Apomorphine in Parkinson's disease. *Trans Am Neurol Assoc* 1951; **76**: 251–3.

48 Cotzias GC, Papavasiliou PS, Fehling C, *et al.* Similarities between neurologic effect of L-dopa and of apomorphine. *N Engl J Med* 1970; **282**: 31–3.

49 Ostergaard l, Werdelin L, Lindvall O, *et al.* Pen injected apomorphine against off phenomena in late Parkinson's disease: a double blind, placebo controlled study. *J Neurol Neurosurg Psychiatry* 1995; **58**: 681–7.

50 Stibe CMH, Lees AJ, Kempster PA, *et al.* Subcutaneous apomorphine in parkinsonian on-off-oscillations. *Lancet* 1988; **i**: 403–6.

51 Frankel JP, Lees AJ, Kempster PA, *et al.* Subcutaneous apomorphine in the treatment of Parkinson's disease. *J Neurol Neurosurg Psychiatry* 1990; **53**: 96–101.

52 Kapoor R, Turjanski N, Frankel J, *et al.* Intranasal apomorphine: a new treatment in Parkinson's disease (letter). *J Neurol Neurosurg Psychiatry* 1990; **53**: 1015.

53 Hughes AJ, Bishop S, Lees AJ, *et al.* Rectal apomorphine in Parkinson's disease (letter). *Lancet* 1991; **337**: 118.

54 Lees AJ, Montastruc JL, Turjanski N, *et al.* Sublingual apomorphine and Parkinson's disease (letter). *J Neurol Neurosurg Psychiatry* 1989; **52**: 1440.

55 Parkinson Study Group. Effect of deprenyl on the progression of disability in early Parkinson's disease. *N Engl J Med* 1989; **321**: 1364–71.

56 Parkinson Study Group. Mortality in DATATOP: a multicenter trial in early Parkinson's disease. *Ann Neurol* 1998; **43**: 318–25.

57 Churchyard A, Mathias CJ, Boonkonchuen P, *et al.* Autonomic effects of selegeline: possible cardio-vascular toxicity in Parkinson's disease. *J Neurol Neurosurg Psychiatry* 1997; **63**: 228–34.

58 Schwab RS, England AC, Poskanzer DC, *et al.* Amantadine in the treatment of Parkinson's disease. *JAMA* 1969; **208**: 1168–70.

59 Bailey EV, Stone PW. The mechanism of action of amantadine in parkinsonism: a review. *Arch Int Pharmacodynam Ther* 1975; **216**: 246–60.

60 Kulisevsky J, Tolosa E. Amantadine in Parkinson's disease. In: Koller WC, Paulson G, eds. *Therapy of Parkinson's disease*. New York: Marcel Dekker, 1990: 143–60.

61 Kornhuber J, Streifler M. Amantadine. In: Riederer P, Laux G, Pöldinger W, eds. *Neuro-psychopharmaka*. Vol 5. New York: Springer, 1992: 59–76.

62 Kornhuber J, Bormann J, Hubers M, *et al.* Effects of the 1-amino-adamantanes at the MK-801-binding site of the NMDA-receptor-gated ion channel: a human post-mortem brain study. *Eur J Pharmacol* 1991; **206**: 297–300.

63 Verhagen Metman L, Del Dotto P, van den Munckhof P, *et al.* Amantadine as treatment for dyskinesias and motor fluctuations in Parkinson's disease. *Neurology* 1998; **50**: 1323–6.

64 Duvoisin RC. Cholinergic-anticholinergic antagonisms in parkinsonism. *Arch Neurol* 1967; **17**: 124–36.

65 Pondal M, Del Ser T, Berjemo F. Anticholinergic therapy and dementia in patients with Parkinson's disease. *J Neurol* 1996; **243**: 543–6.

66 Kaakkola S, Gordin A, Männisto PT. General properties and clinical possibilities of new selective inhibitors of catechol-o-methyltransferase. *Gen Pharmacol* 1994; **25**: 813–24.

67 Keräenen T, Gordin A, Harjola V-P, *et al.* The effect of catechol-O-methyltransferase inhibition by entacapone on the pharmacokinetics and metabolism of levodopa in healthy volunteers. *Clin Neuropharmacol* 1993; **16**: 145–56.

68 Roberts JW, Cora-Locatelli G, Bravi D, *et al.* Catechol-O-methyl transferase inhibitor tolcapone prolongs levodopa/carbidopa action in parkinsonian patients. *Neurology* 1993; **43**: 2685–8.

69 Nutt JG, Woodward WR, Beckner RM, *et al*. Effect of peripheral catechol-O-methyl transferase inhibition on the pharmacokinetics and pharmacodynamics of levodopa in parkinsonian patients. *Neurology* 1994; **44**: 913–19.

70 Kurth MC, Adler CH. COMT inhibition: a new treatment strategy for Parkinson's disease. *Neurology* 1998; **50**(suppl 5): S3–14.

71 Kurth MC, Adler CH, Saint Hilaire M-H, *et al*. Tolcapone improves motor function and reduces levodopa requirement in patients with Parkinson's disease experiencing motor fluctuations: a multicenter, double-blind, randomized, placebo-controlled trial. *Neurology* 1997; **48**: 81–7.

72 Baas H, Beiske AG, Ghika J, *et al*. COMT inhibition with tolcapone reduces 'wearing-off' phenomenon and levodopa requirements in fluctuating parkinsonian patients. *J Neurol Neurosurg Psychiatry* 1997; **63**: 421–8.

73 Kieburtz K, Rinne UK. The COMP inhibitor entacapone increases 'on' time in levodopa-treated PD patients with motor fluctuations: report of two randomized, placebo-controlled trials (abstract). *Mov Disord* 1996; **11**: 595–6.

74 Rinne UK, Larsen JP, Siden A, *et al*., and the Nomecomt Study Group. Entacapone enhances the response to levodopa in parkinsonian patients with motor fluctuations. *Neurology* 1998; **51**: 1309–14.

75 Ruottinen HM, Rinne UK. Entacapone prolongs levodopa response in a one month double blind study in parkinsonian patients with levodopa related fluctuations. *J Neurol Neurosurg Psychiatry* 1996; **60**: 36–40.

76 Parkinson Study Group. Entacapone improves motor fluctuations in levodopa-treated Parkinson's disease patients. *Ann Neurol* 1997; **42**: 747–55.

77 Lyytinen J, Kaakkola S, Teräväinen H, *et al*. Comparison between the effects of L-dopa + entacapone and L-dopa + placebo on exercise capacity, haemodynamics and autonomic function in patients with Parkinson's disease (abstract). *Mov Disord* 1997; **12**(suppl 1): 103.

78 Holm KJ, Spencer CM. Entacapone. A review of its use in Parkinson's disease. *Drugs* 1999; **58**: 159–77.

79 Chiueh CC, Wu RM, Mohanakumar KP, *et al*. In vivo generation of hydroxyl radicals and MPTP-induced dopaminergic toxicity in the basal ganglia. *Ann NY Acad Sci* 1994; **738**: 25–36.

80 Marsden CD. Parkinson's disease. *Lancet* 1990; **335**: 948–52.

81 Heikkila RF, Manzino L, Cabbat FS, *et al*. Protection against the dopaminergic neurotoxicity of 1-methyl-1,2,5,6-tetrahydropyridine by monoamine oxidase inhibitors. *Nature* 1984; **311**: 467–9.

82 The Parkinson Study Group. Effects of tocopherol and deprenyl on the progression of disability in early Parkinson's disease. *N Engl J Med* 1993; **328**: 176–83.

83 Landau WM. Clinical neuromythology IX. Pyramid sale in the bucket shop: DATATOP bottoms out. *Neurology* 1990; **40**: 1337–9.

84 Lees AJ, Parkinson Disease Research Group of the United Kingdom. Comparison of therapeutic effects and mortality data of levodopa and levodopa combined with selegeline in patients with early, mild Parkinson's disease. *BMJ* 1995; **311**: 1602–7.

85 Ben-Shlomo Y, Churchyard A, Head J, *et al*. Investigation by Parkinson's disease research group of United Kingdom into excess mortality seen with combined levodopa and selegeline treatment in patients with early, mild Parkinson's disease: further results of randomised trial and confidential inquiry. *BMJ* 1998; **316**: 1191–6.

86 Olanow CW, Myllylä VV, Sotaniemi KA, *et al*. Effects of selegeline on mortality in patients with Parkinson's disease. A meta-analysis. *Neurology* 1998; **51**: 825–30.

87 Kornhuber J, Weller M. Psychogenicity and N-methyl-D-aspartate receptor antagonism: implications for neuroprotective pharmacotherapy. *Biol Psychiatry* 1997; **41**: 135–44.

88 Uitti RJ, Rajput AH, Ahlskog JE, *et al*. Amantadine treatment is an independent predictor of improved survival in Parkinson's disease. *Neurology* 1996; **46**: 1551–6.

89 Ziv I, Melamed E. Role of apoptosis in the pathogenesis of Parkinson's disease: a novel therapeutic opportunity? *Mov Disord* 1998; **13**: 865–70.

90 Ebadi M, Srinivasan SK, Baxi MD. Oxidative stress and antioxidant therapy in Parkinson's disease. *Prog Neurobiol* 1996; **48**: 1–19.

91 Weiner W. The initial treatment of Parkinson's disease should begin with levodopa. *Mov Disord* 1999; **14**: 716–24.

92 Montastruc JL, Rascol O, Senard J-M. Treatment of Parksinson's disease should begin with a dopamine agonist. *Mov Disord* 1999; **14**: 725–30.

93 Quinn N, Critchley P, Marsden CD. Young onset Parkinson's disease. *Mov Disord* 1987; **2**: 73–91.

94 Schrag A, Ben-Shlomo Y, Brown R, *et al*. Young-onset Parkinson's disease revisited-clinical features, natural history, and mortality. *Mov Disord* 1998; **13**: 885–94.

95 Montastruc JL, Rascol O, Senard JM, *et al*. A randomized controlled study comparing bromocriptine to which levodopa was later added, with levodopa alone in previously untreated patients with Parkinson's disease: a five year follow up. *J Neurol Neurosurg Psychiatry* 1994:**57**: 1034–8.

96 Rinne UK. Early combination of bromocriptine and levodopa in the treatment of Parkinson's disease: a 5-year-follow-up. *Neurology* 1987; **57**: 1034–8.

97 Rinne UK. Lisuride, a dopamine agonist in the treatment of early Parkinson's disease. *Neurology* 1989; **39**: 336–9.

98 Weiner WJ, Factor SA, Sanchez-Ramos JR, *et al*. Early combination therapy (bromocriptine and levodopa) does not prevent motor fluctuations in Parkinson's disease. *Neurology* 1993; **43**: 21–7.

99 Hobson DE, Pourcher E, Martin WR. Ropinirole and pramipexole, the new agonists. *Can J Neurol Sci* 1999; **26**(suppl 2): S27–33.

100 Marsden CD, Parkes JD. 'On-off'effects in patients with Parkinson's disease on chronic levodopa therapy. *Lancet* 1976; **i**: 292–6.

101 Riley DE, Lang AE. The spectrum of levodopa-related fluctuations in Parkinson's disease. *Neurology* 1993; **43**: 1459–64.

102 Ruottinen HM, Rinne UK. COMT inhibition in the treatment of Parkinson's disease. *J Neurol* 1998; **245**(suppl 3): P25–34.

103 Ruottinen HM, Rinne UK. A double-blind pharmacokinetic and clinical dose-response study of entacapone as an adjuvant to levodopa therapy in advanced Parkinson's disease. *Clin Neuropharmacol* 1996; **19**: 283–96.

104 Djaldetti R, Baron J, Ziv I, *et al*. Gastric emptying in Parkinson's disease: patients with and without response fluctuations. *Neurology* 1996; **46**: 1051–4.

105 Nutt JG, Woodward WR, Hammerstad JP, *et al*. The 'on-off' phenomenon in Parkinson's disease: relation to levodopa absorption and transport. *N Engl J Med* 1984; **310**: 483–8.

106 Pincus JH, Barry K. Protein redistribution diet restores motor function in patients with dopa-resistant 'off' periods. *Neurology* 1987; **38**: 481–3.

107 Quinn N, Marsden CD. Lithium for painful dystonia in Parkinson's disease (letter). *Lancet* 1986; **i**: 1377.

108 Pacchetti C, Albani G, Martignoni G, *et al*. 'Off' painful dystonia in Parkinson's disease treated with botulinum toxin. *Mov Disord* 1995; **10**: 333–6.

109 Nissenbaum H, Quinn NP, Brown RG, *et al*. Mood swings associated with the 'on-off' phenomenon in Parkinson's disease. *Psychol Med* 1987; **17**: 899–904.

110 Miyawaki E, Meah Y, Koller WC. Serotonine, dopamine, and motor effects in Parkinson's disease. *Clin Neuropharmacol* 1997; **20**: 300–10.

111 Richard IH, Kurlan R, Tanner C, *et al*. Serotonin syndrome and the combined use of deprenyl and an anti-depressant in Parkinson's disease. *Neurology* 1997; **48**: 1070–7.

112 Factor SA, Friedman JH. The emerging role of clozapine in the treatment of movement disorders. *Mov Disord* 1997; **12**: 483–96.

113 Friedman JH, Lannon MC. Clozapine in the treatment of psychosis in Parkinson's disease. *Neurology* 1989; **39**: 1219–20.

114 Wolters EC, Jansen EN, Tuynman-Qua, *et al*. Olanzapine in the treatment of dopaminomimetic psychosis in patients with Parkison's disease. *Neurology* 1996; **47**: 1085–7.

115 Friedman JH, Goldstein S, Jacques C. Substituting clozapine for olanzapine in psychiatrically stable Parkinson's disease patients: results of an open label pilot study. *Clin Neuropharmacol* 1998; **21**: 285–8.

116 Zoldan J, Friedberg G, Weizman A, *et al*. Ondansetron, a 5-HT$_3$ antagonist for visual hallucinations and paranoid delusional disorders associated with chronic L-DOPA therapy in advanced Parkinson's disease. *Adv Neurol* 1996; **69**: 541–4.

Answers

1 Essential tremor, drug-induced parkinsonism, multiple system atrophy, progressive supranuclear palsy, and corticobasal degeneration.

2 This is probably due to non-physiological pulsatile stimulation of dopamine receptors in the basal ganglia. In early stages exogenous L-dopa is taken up by remaining neurons in the substantia nigra and L-dopa release is more or less continuous. This changes in later stages when an increasing number of dopaminergic neurons die. Consequently L-dopa can no longer be stored and L-dopa levels fluctuate according to plasma levels. Dyskinesias do not occur when L-dopa is administered continuously by intravenous infusion supporting this concept.

3 Dopamine agonists have a longer mode of action and therefore resemble physiological continuous dopamine receptor stimulation. They have a L-dopa sparing effect and may have neuroprotective properties.

4 None of the currently available drugs.

5 Amantadine.

6 COMT inhibitors reduce 'off' periods, prolong the 'on' time and allow a reduction of the L-dopa dose. They do not, however, have a L-dopa sparing effect.

7 There is theoretical concern that L-dopa may be neurotoxic. Moreover, and more importantly, L-dopa invariably induces motor complications after chronic use.

8 Apomorphine that can be given as single subcutaneous injections or as a continuous infusion via a pump.

9 Clozapine. Full blood count must be monitored regularly when using this drug as it may cause agranulocytosis.

Chapter Fifteen

Young onset dementia

EL Sampson, JD Warren and MN Rossor

Young onset dementia is a challenging clinical problem with potentially devastating medical and social consequences. The differential diagnosis is wide, and includes a number of rare sporadic and hereditary diseases. However, accurate diagnosis is often possible, and all patients should be thoroughly investigated to identify treatable processes. This review presents an approach to the diagnosis, investigation, and management of patients with young onset dementia, with particular reference to common and treatable causes.

Dementia in younger people (young onset dementia, YOD) is increasingly recognised as an important clinical and social problem, with frequently devastating consequences for both the sufferer and those who care for them.[1] Prevalence rates of YOD have been estimated between 67 to 81 per 100 000 in the 45 to 65 year old age group;[2,3] thus there are currently approximately 10 000 patients with YOD in the United Kingdom alone. YOD poses a diagnostic challenge and may present with a wide variety of subtle behavioural, cognitive, psychiatric, or neurological symptoms. While the degenerative dementias characteristically affect older patients, they are also an important cause of YOD: indeed, Alzheimer's disease is the commonest single cause of YOD with an estimated 3000 cases in the United Kingdom, followed by vascular dementia and the frontotemporal lobar degenerations (*see* Table 15.1). The young onset forms of these diseases are frequently familial.[4] Some degenerative dementias such as variant Creutzfeldt-Jakob disease typically occur in the young patient. In contrast, Lewy body dementia, which accounts for 20% of cases in patients over 65 years of age, accounts for only a small proportion of YOD.

The differential diagnosis of YOD is wide (*see* Tables 15.2 and 15.3). Dementia is very rare before the age of 40: in young adults and adolescents, genetic and metabolic disorders predominate and many present as a 'dementia-plus' syndrome, where cognitive impairment occurs in the setting of more widespread neurological disturbance. The additional features of pyramidal, extrapyramidal, cerebellar, or peripheral nerve involvement are key diagnostic clues in this group (*see* Table 15.3) and help to direct investigations. Most inherited disorders of metabolism are autosomal recessive: in these diseases, the absence or partial inactivity of the affected enzyme leads to accumulation of abnormal material in lysosomes or peroxisomes.[5] Mitochondrial diseases have variable inheritance, as components of the respiratory chain are encoded both by nuclear DNA and maternally inherited mitochondrial DNA.[6] Many of the dementia-plus syndromes and metabolic disorders have 'subcortical' cognitive impairment that may be misinterpreted as a pseudodementia. Changes in personality and mood, apathy and cognitive slowing are common, whereas memory may be relatively spared. In addition, drugs and toxic exposures should always be considered in younger adults: in approximately 10% of cases, YOD is a consequence of chronic alcohol abuse.[2]

This review will focus on common and treatable causes of YOD and outline general principles of investigation and management.

Primary neurodegenerations

Alzheimer's disease

Presenile Alzheimer's disease may manifest as early as the fourth decade, and it is frequently familial. Inheritance in familial Alzheimer's disease is autosomal dominant with essentially complete penetrance. It is genetically heterogeneous (see Table 15.3): the majority of cases are due to mutations in the presenilin (PS)1 gene on chromosome 14;[7] rarely, pathogenetic mutations occur in the β-amyloid precursor protein gene on chromosome 21 (initially targeted because of the strikingly increased incidence of young onset Alzheimer's disease in Down's syndrome)[8] or in the PS-2 gene on chromosome 1.[9] The identification of these mutations has greatly advanced our understanding of the molecular pathology of Alzheimer's disease. Amyloid precursor protein is a trans-membrane protein that undergoes alternative proteolysis, either by α-secretase to generate a non-amyloidogenic product, or by the sequential action of β- and γ-secretase to generate Aβ peptides including highly amyloidogenic Aβ1–42 (the most abundant species in neuritic plaques). According to the 'amyloid hypothesis', Alzheimer's disease results from a pathogenetic cascade driven by the accumulation of abnormally aggregated β-amyloid that leads to secondary neuronal injury and accumulation of tau in neurofibrillary tangles.[10] A central role for amyloid, though contentious,[11] is consistent both with the location of the pathogenetic amyloid precursor protein mutations, which are all clustered near protease cleavage sites within the β-amyloid domain, and with evidence implicating the PS genes in γ-secretase cleavage of amyloid precursor protein, leading to over-production of Aβ1–42.

The neuropathological hallmarks of Alzheimer's disease are neuritic (senile) plaques and neurofibrillary tangles. Neuritic plaques are extracellular and composed of dystrophic axons and dendrites clustered round a central core, predominantly consisting of β-amyloid (Aβ). Neurofibrillary tangles are intracellular and composed of abnormally phosphorylated microtubule associated tau protein. Involvement of basal forebrain nuclei leads to a widespread deficit in cholinergic transmission in cortical projection areas.

The clinical phenotype is similar in young onset and older onset Alzheimer's disease, and in familial and sporadic cases. Typically, early involvement of medial temporal lobe structures (hippocampus and entorhinal cortex) leads initially to forgetfulness for daily events (episodic memory loss). The patient may become lost in a familiar area (topographical memory impairment). Parietal dysfunction manifests as dyspraxia and visuospatial defects including visual disorientation:

Table 15.1 Epidemiology of young onset dementia (onset 30–64 years) (after Harvey *et al.*)[2]

Young onset dementia	Prevalence/100 000	Proportion of total (%)
Alzheimer's disease	21.7	30
Vascular dementia	10.9	15
Frontotemporal lobar degenerations	9.3	13
Alcohol-related dementia	8.3	12
Dementia with Lewy bodies	6	4
Huntington's disease	4.7	
Dementia in multiple sclerosis	4.1	
Dementia in Down's syndrome	1.6	
Corticobasal degeneration	1.0	
Prion disease	1.0	25
Dementia in Parkinson's disease	1.0	
Dementia due to carbon monoxide poisoning	0.5	
Other causes	4.1	

typically, parietal signs appear after memory loss, however in a subgroup of patients with posterior cortical atrophy they are the presenting features. In contrast to the frontotemporal lobar degenerations, language and social functioning are generally preserved until late in the course. Delusions, hallucinations, and aggression commonly occur later in the illness and often precipitate admission to institutional care. In familial Alzheimer's disease, myoclonus tends to be more florid and naming may be spared until later in the course.[12] Age at onset and age at death vary widely within the same kindred.[13] Specific mutations may give rise to characteristic clinical features such as early behavioural change,[14] a speech production deficit,[15] or spastic paraparesis with white matter changes.[16]

In familial cases, genotyping may enable Alzheimer's disease to be diagnosed at an early stage. As is true of the neurodegenerative dementias generally, definitive diagnosis in sporadic cases must still await histopathological examination. However volumetric magnetic resonance imaging (MRI) techniques can identify and quantify patterns of regional atrophy,[17] in particular medial temporal lobe structures (*see* Figure 15.1(A)), that reflect neuronal destruction. Studies of 'at risk' members of familial Alzheimer's disease pedigrees indicate that increased rates of tissue loss and neuropsychological deficits (in particular, verbal recognition memory and performance IQ) precede symptoms by several years.[18]

Frontotemporal lobar degenerations

The frontotemporal lobar degenerations (FTLD) are a group of disorders characterised by focal degeneration of frontal and temporal lobes. The recent development of consensus diagnostic criteria for FTLD[19] has led to an increase in the number of cases diagnosed, and the recognition that FTLD and Alzheimer's disease have similar prevalence in YOD populations.[3] However, FTLD remains a source of considerable nosological confusion, largely on account of its histo-pathological and genetic heterogeneity.

The usual age at onset is 45–60 (range 20–75 years); males may be more frequently affected.[3] Family history is positive in up to 50% of patients[4] and a number of genetic causes have been identified (*see* Table 15.3). The largest single group has mutations in the tau gene on chromosome 17: FTDP-17 (frontotem-poral dementia with parkinsonism linked to chromosome 17).[20] The clinical phenotype is often highly variable within a kindred.

A wide variety of histopathological findings have been described in FTLD. Mild spongiform change with neuronal loss and non-specific gliosis may occur without inclusion bodies (dementia lacking distinctive histopathology).[21] Many cases are associated with tau inclusions; microtubular instability secondary to tau dysfunc-tion may contribute to the pathogenesis of such 'tauopathies'.[20] The number of microtubule binding domains in the tau isoform provides a partial basis for classifying the tauopathies; thus, inclusions with three-repeat tau isoform are associated with classical Pick's disease with Pick bodies, while inclusions with four-repeat tau are associated with corticobasal type inclusions. Ubiquitin positive, tau negative inclusions similar to those in motor neurone disease may occur without motor neurone involvement.[22] New histopathological patterns continue to be defined.[23] There is no consistent relationship between histopathol-ogy and the clinical phenotype, which is largely determined by the distribution rather than the type of pathology.

In frontotemporal dementia, the clinical presentation is variable and often subtle, and may be dominated by behavioural disturbances, personality change, loss of empathy or motivation.[24] Loss of planning and judgment may force early retirement. Families and carers may attribute behavioural changes to marital difficulties or 'mid-life crisis' and misdiagnoses as treatment resistant depression or Alzheimer's disease are frequent. As the disease advances, behavioural rigidity, disinhibition, loss of social skills, fatuousness, emotional lability and impulsivity often develop, accompanied by executive dysfunction, decreased verbal fluency, impaired abstraction, difficulty shifting set and motor and verbal perseveration and stereotypies. Hyperorality and development of a sweet tooth are characteristic. Disproportionate frontal atrophy may be evident on MRI (*see* Figure 15.1(C)); however, this is often subtle.

Semantic dementia resembles a progressive fluent aphasia, with increasingly empty and circumlocutory (but grammatically correct) speech due to loss of semantic knowledge about the meanings of words and objects.[25] Anatomically, it is characterised by focal, predominantly left anterior temporal lobe atrophy (*see* Figure 15.1(B)): this asymmetry and the existence of an anteroposterior gradient of atrophy can distinguish semantic dementia from Alzheimer's disease on MRI.[26] For unknown reasons, selective right anterior temporal atrophy is observed much more rarely; it presents as a progressive difficulty interpreting facial expressions and emotions, facial impassivity, loss of empathy, and behavioural symptoms.[27] Primary progressive non-fluent aphasia manifests as an insidious deterioration in speech production with phonemic and syntactic errors and word-finding diffi-culties, frequently accompanied by orofacial apraxia. It is associated with circumscribed left perisylvian atrophy.[28] In these focal syndromes, other cognitive functions are typically well preserved at presentation; generalised intellectual decline tends to occur only at the later stages of the illness. FTLD may be

Table 15.2 Causes of young onset dementia: sporadic and acquired (bold, treatable condition; *, often absent)

Disease	Clues to diagnosis	
	Clinical features	Investigations
Primary neurodegenerations		
Alzheimer's disease	History of becoming lost, biparietal signs	EEG: absent α rhythm MRI: early hippocampal atrophy
Frontotemporal lobar degenerations:		
Frontotemporal dementia	Early behavioural change, frontal features	EEG: preserved α rhythm
Semantic dementia[25]	Early circumscribed semantic impairment	MRI: selective anterior left temporal atrophy
Primary progressive non-fluent aphasia[28]	Progressive speech production impairment	MRI: circumscribed left perisylvian atrophy
Frontal dementia (motor neurone disease)[29]	Orofacial apraxia, bulbar features, fasciculations (especially deltoid), amyotrophy	EMG: changes of denervation*
Dementia with Lewy bodies[30]	Visual hallucinations, extrapyramidal syndrome, fluctuation	
Multiple system atrophy[71]	Dysautonomia, cerebellar, extrapyramidal features	MRI: midbrain atrophy, 'hot cross bun sign'* (increased signal in cerebellum, middle cerebellar peduncles, pons)
Corticobasal degeneration[72]	Early asymmetric apraxia and rigidity, dystonia, cortical sensory deficit, alien limb	
Parkinson's disease[73]	Established typical parkinsonian syndrome predating cognitive decline	
Progressive supranuclear palsy (Steele-Richardson-Olszewski)[72]	Early falls, vertical supranuclear gaze palsy, axial rigidity, no tremor	MRI: midbrain atrophy/hyperintensity*
Neurofilament inclusion body disease[23]	Rapidly progressive frontotemporal or corticobasal syndrome, early falls, mutism	
Vascular		
Strategic infarct[42]	Discrete thalamic, basal ganglia, or capsular infarct	Computed tomography/MRI: discrete infarction
Multiple cortical infarcts	Stepwise cognitive decline; predisposing factors	
Small vessel disease	Predisposing factors, brisk facial reflexes, frontal gait disorder	Computed tomography/MRI: lacunar state (generally involving basal ganglia and brainstem)

Table 15.2 (*continued*)

Disease	Clues to diagnosis	
	Clinical features	*Investigations*
Prion		
Classical Creutzfeldt-Jakob disease[34]	Rapid, florid myoclonus, cortical blindness	EEG: triphasic periodic complexes
		MRI: basal ganglia high signal
Iatrogenic Creutzfeldt-Jakob disease[36]	History of dural or corneal grafts, exposure to donor human growth hormone; features as in sporadic Creutzfeldt-Jakob disease	CSF: positive 14-3-3 protein
New variant Creutzfeldt-Jakob disease[38]	Rapid, early psychiatric symptoms, dysaesthesiae	MRI: pulvinar sign
Inflammatory		
Multiple sclerosis[52]	History of acute demyelinating episodes*, frontal-subcortical features, absent abdominal reflexes	VERs/BAERs/SSEPs: delayed
		MRI: demyelinating changes in brain (corpus callosum involved) and/or spinal cord
		CSF: unmatched oligoclonal bands
Vasculitis associated with systemic disorders	Rapid course, headache, fluctuation, seizures, systemic features	EEG: slowing of rhythms
		MRI: ischaemic lesions
		CSF: >3 cells, oligoclonal bands
Primary angiitis of central nervous system*[47]	Rapid course, headache, seizures, fluctuation	EEG: slowing of rhythms
		MRI: ischaemic lesions
		CSF: >3 cells, oligoclonal bands
Neurosarcoidosis[74]	Systemic features, uveitis, hypothalamic dysfunction, cranial nerve signs, or polyradiculopathy	CXR: various patterns
		MRI: white matter lesions ± meningeal enhancement
		CSF: chronic lymphocytic meningitis
Behçet's disease[75]	Racial predilection (especially Turkish/Japanese), oral and genital ulcers, uveitis, skin lesions; posterior circulation strokes	MRI: brainstem, basal ganglia lesions
		CSF: chronic lymphocytic meningitis
Neoplastic/paraneoplastic		
Tumours (especially frontal/ callosal, midbrain)[76]	Signs of raised intracranial pressure*, focal neurological signs, frontal disconnection syndromes	Computed tomography/MRI: mass lesion(s)
Limbic encephalitis[56]	Often smoker, constitutional upset, weight loss, rapid course, prominent behavioural changes, hallucinations, seizures	MRI: abnormal temporal lobe signal
		CSF: oligoclonal bands
		Serum: positive antineuronal/ antivoltage gated potassium channel antibodies

Table 15.2 (*continued*)

| Disease | Clues to diagnosis | |
	Clinical features	Investigations
Infections		
Tuberculosis/fungal/ 'atypical' meningitis[77]	Risk factors* (including racial origin in tuberculosis, immunosuppression); systemic features, chronic meningitis ± cranial nerve signs	CXR: frequently abnormal Computed tomography/MRI: may have mass lesions (tuberculoma) CSF: lymphocytic meningitis
HIV (AIDS-dementia complex)[53]	Risk factors; systemic features, AIDS related illnesses, advanced immunosuppression, gait disorder, seizures	MRI: confluent white matter changes Serum: positive HIV serology, low CD4 count
Whipple's disease[78]	Arthralgia, gut symptoms, facial movement disorder (oculomasticatory myorrhythmia)	CSF: positive Whipple's polymerase chain reaction
Lyme disease[79]	Suspicion of tick bite/travel to endemic area, skin lesion, arthritis, radiculopathies/ mononeuropathies	CSF: lymphocytic meningitis Serum: positive Lyme serology*
Neurosyphilis[62]	Risk factors (now rare); chronic meningitis, multiple strokes, Argyll Robertson pupils (light-near dissociation), tremor, seizures, dorsal column signs (tabes dorsalis)	CSF: mononuclear pleocytosis, oligoclonal bands Serum: positive syphilis serology
Subacute sclerosing panencephalitis[80]	Usually child or adolescent; history of measles, rapid course, florid myoclonus and seizures	EEG: periodic burst suppression CSF: oligoclonal bands (measles specific antibody)
Progressive multifocal leukoencephalopathy[81]	Immunosuppression/ haematological malignancies, posterior cortical syndrome	MRI: confluent posterior white matter changes CSF: positive JC virus polymerase chain reaction
Metabolic[62]		
Endocrinopathies	Clinical and/or biochemical features of specific diagnosis	
Nutritional deficiency	History of food faddism, features of malabsorption	
Uraemia	Usually obvious from clinical setting	
Hepatic encephalopathy	Usually obvious from clinical setting	
Epilepsy[61]	Discrete episodes, fluctuating course, topographical amnesia	EEG: epileptiform discharges (especially temporal lobe origin) MRI: abnormal mesial temporal signal

Table 15.2 (*continued*)

Disease	Clues to diagnosis	
	Clinical features	*Investigations*
Alcohol[50]	Usually obvious from clinical setting; may be associated nutritional deficiency	
Toxic (including carbon monoxide poisoning,[82] lead,[83] prescribed drugs including lithium,[84] interferon α[85]	Suspicion of overt or covert exposure (for example, occupational/environmental, recreational drug use)	Specific screens if available
Post-irradiation[86]	History of cranial irradiation (may be delayed), corticospinal signs, ataxia, seizures	MRI: confluent white matter changes
Other		
Obstructive sleep apnoea[87]	Obesity, morning headaches, daytime somnolence, excessive snoring	Sleep study: findings consistent with obstructive sleep apnoea
Chronic subdural haematoma[62]	History of head trauma*, frontal-subcortical signs	Computed tomography: subdural haematoma (may be isodense depending on chronicity; may be bilateral)
Hydrocephalus (any cause)[62]	History of meningitis, subarachnoid haemorrhage or neurosurgical procedure; gait apraxia, urinary incontinence	Computed tomography/MRI: findings of hydrocephalus (disproportionate ventricular enlargement) and/or causative lesion
Dementia pugilistica[88]	History of repeated head trauma; parkinsonism	

BAERs, brainstem auditory evoked potentials; CSF, cerebrospinal fluid; CXR, chest radiograph; EEG, electroencephalography; EMG, electromyography; MRI, magnetic resonance imaging; SSEPs, somatosensory evoked potentials; VERs, visual evoked potentials.

associated with motor neurone disease; the age of onset is similar to that of classical motor neurone disease, and frontal dementia (often associated with expressive language difficulties) commonly precedes the development of amyotrophy. Dysarthria and dysphagia caused by progressive bulbar palsy may develop rapidly, and progression is more rapid than in FTLD alone.[29]

Lewy body dementia

Lewy body dementia appears to be relatively uncommon in younger populations; the clinical presentation is similar to that in older patients, with fluctuating cognitive impairment, vivid visual hallucinations, parkinsonian symptoms, frontal-subcortical features, and autonomic instability.[30] The tempo of evolution is usually similar to Alzheimer's disease; occasional patients show a rapid clinical course. Lewy bodies are neuronal inclusions, composed of abnormally phosphorylated neurofilament proteins aggregated with ubiquitin and α-synuclein, that are deposited widely in brainstem nuclei, paralimbic, and neocortical areas.

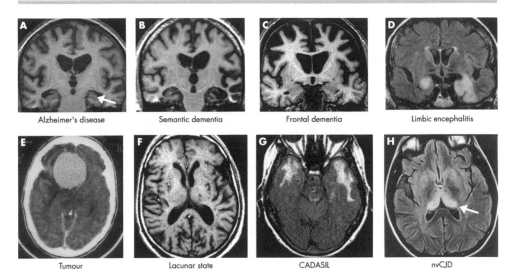

Figure 15.1 Coronal (above) and axial (below) views of brain imaging findings in selected young onset dementias (images reproduced by kind permission of Dr Hadi Manji and Dr Nick Fox, Institute of Neurology). All images are presented in radiological convention (the left hemisphere is on the right). (A) Magnetic resonance imaging (MRI), T1 sequence of Alzheimer's disease: disproportionate bilateral atrophy of hippocampi (white arrow). (B) MRI, T1 sequence, semantic dementia variant of frontotemporal lobar degeneration: disproportionate, asymmetric atrophy of anterior left temporal lobe. (C) MRI, T1 sequence, frontal variant of frontotemporal lobar degeneration: diffuse bilateral frontal atrophy relatively sparing temporal lobes. (D) MRI, fluid attenuated inversion recovery (FLAIR) sequence, paraneoplastic limbic encephalitis: focal bilateral alteration in mesial temporal lobe signal. (E) Computed tomogram, large frontal meningioma. (F) MRI, T1 sequence, small vessel disease: multiple lacunes in cerebral white matter and basal ganglia. (G) MRI, FLAIR sequence, cerebral autosomal dominant arteriopathy with subcortical infarcts and leukoencephalopathy (CADASIL): bilateral abnormal high signal in anterior temporal lobes. (H) MRI, FLAIR sequence, new variant Creutzfeldt-Jakob disease (nvCJD): bilateral abnormal high signal focally affecting posterior thalami ('pulvinar sign'; white arrow).

Neuritic plaques similar to those in Alzheimer's disease are frequent. Involvement of cholinergic projection pathways produces a profound cholinergic deficit.

Huntington's disease

Huntington's disease is caused by the expansion of a CAG trinucleotide repeat sequence on the short arm of chromosome 4.[31] It is inherited in autosomal dominant fashion, penetrance is complete, and new mutations are very rare; most apparently sporadic cases reflect an incomplete family history or non-paternity. The prevalence in Europe is approximately 0.5–8/100 000.[32] The gene encodes a protein, huntingtin, of unknown function. Pathologically, there is neuronal loss and gliosis mainly affecting the frontal lobes and the caudate nucleus; polyglutamine nuclear inclusions are present. Onset is generally in middle life, with relentless progression of cognitive and behavioural decline in most cases. Neuropsychiatric symptoms of depression, apathy, aggression, disinhibition, and social disintegration are common and may predate chorea and other extrapyramidal signs;[33] a subcortical dementia with gaze apraxia typically develops. Bilateral atrophy of the head of the caudate nucleus may be seen on brain imaging. Diagnostic and predictive genetic testing is now widely available.

Prion dementias

The prion diseases are transmissible neurodegenerations characterised pathologically by diffuse brain spongiosis and deposition of an abnormal fibrillar prion glycoprotein, PrP, which is encoded by the PRNP gene on chromosome 20.[34] Different PrP conformations and glycosylation patterns give rise to various strains, which show species specificity. The paradigm for these disorders is scrapie, a disease of sheep and goats, for which analogues exist in a number of other species. Human prion diseases occur in sporadic (approximately 90% of cases), acquired (generally iatrogenic), and inherited forms. Creutzfeldt-Jakob disease (CJD) is the most common, with an approximate incidence of one case per million worldwide. Kuru, described in the Fore linguistic group of New Guinea highlanders, was transmitted by ritual cannibalism; the disease has largely disappeared since this practice was abolished in the 1950s, although occasional new cases may occur, suggesting a very long presymptomatic phase. The inherited prion diseases comprise familial CJD, fatal familial insomnia, Gerstmann-Sträussler-Scheinker syndrome, and atypical Alzheimer-like illnesses. All have autosomal dominant inheritance.

Prion diseases are examples of 'conformational dementias',[35] arising from the aggregation of a conformational isomer (PrP^{Sc}) of the native prion protein, PrP^C. Sporadic disease results from rare spontaneous post-translational conversions of PrP^{Sc} to PrP^C, whereas the inherited prion diseases arise from mutations in the PRNP gene. Due to its relative insolubility, resistance to digestion by intracellular proteases and propensity to self-aggregate, the PrP^{Sc} isomer accumulates in neurones as β-sheet amyloid fibrils (quite distinct from the amyloid deposited in Alzheimer's disease, which is composed of $A\beta$ peptide). The mechanisms by which accumulation leads to cell death remain unclear. There are approximately 270 well documented cases worldwide in which CJD has been transmitted to humans by neurosurgical procedures, dural and corneal grafts, and pooled donor pituitary extract before the advent of recombinant human growth hormone;[36] presumably such iatrogenic cases result from 'seeding' of the conformational conversion by introduced PrP^{Sc}. Susceptibility to acquired and sporadic CJD is determined by a common polymorphism (valine or methionine) at codon 129 of the PRNP gene, heterozygotes being relatively protected against development of disease.

Intense interest in the human prion diseases has been generated by growing concern that so-called new variant Creutzfeldt-Jakob disease (nvCJD), first identified in the United Kingdom in 1996,[37] was transmitted by ingestion of beef products contaminated with central nervous tissue from cattle with bovine spongiform encephalopathy (BSE), then epidemic in Britain. A number of lines of evidence, including molecular strain typing and transmission studies in animals, indicate that BSE and nvCJD are caused by the same prion strain.[38] To date, a small but steadily increasing number of cases have appeared in the United Kingdom; the full public health implications are yet to be realised. New variant CJD is histopathologically distinct from the sporadic disease, with characteristic 'florid plaques'. All patients so far have been homozygous for methionine at codon 129 of the PRNP gene (compared with approximately 40% of controls and 80% of patients with sporadic CJD), and no mutation has been identified.

Clinically, classical (sporadic) CJD is a rapidly progressive dementia of middle life, generally proceeding relentlessly to death within six months, although some patients have a more prolonged course. Prodromal insomnia, depression, and general malaise are common. Myoclonus generally becomes prominent, and may be accompanied by seizures, extrapyramidal signs, cerebellar ataxia, and cortical blindness. In nvCJD, psychiatric disturbances and limb dysaesthesiae are often early features, and the spectrum of cognitive and neurological deficits is similar to sporadic disease, however patients as a group have been younger and the course tends to be more indolent, with a median survival of 14 months. Familial CJD is clinically indistinguishable from sporadic CJD; the other inherited prion diseases have characteristic clinical features (early prominent cerebellar ataxia in Gerstmann-Sträussler-Scheinker syndrome and progressive insomnia with dysautonomia in fatal familial insomnia), although genotype:phenotype correlation is problematic.

The differential diagnosis is limited but includes a number of potentially treatable causes of rapidly progressive dementia (*see* Table 15.4). In advanced sporadic (though not new variant) CJD, the electroencephalogram frequently shows characteristic triphasic periodic (1–2 Hz) complexes superimposed on a slow, disorganised background cerebral rhythm. Routine examination of cerebrospinal fluid is generally unremarkable; markers of rapid neuronal destruction such as the 14-3-3 protein are frequently raised in sporadic CJD, though not in nvCJD. A number of brain MRI abnormalities have been described:[39] in sporadic CJD, high signal changes in putamen and caudate head and cortical hyperintensity on FLAIR sequences, and in nvCJD, increased signal in the pulvinar (*see* Figure 15.1(H)). In nvCJD, prion protein immunostaining is positive in lymphoid tissue, and the diagnosis can be made reliably on tonsillar biopsy.[40] Lymphoid staining is negative in sporadic CJD, and a brain biopsy is required to exclude a potentially treatable, inflammatory disorder if there are atypical features. After discussion with the patient's relatives, genetic typing of prion proteins in peripheral white blood cells for epidemiological and research purposes should be undertaken in sporadic and nvCJD, and mutation analysis with formal genetic counselling in familial cases.

Vascular dementia

Vascular dementia is a common cause of YOD.[2] Patients developing young onset vascular dementia may lack conventional vascular risk factors, and unusual haematological, metabolic, and genetic causes (*see* Tables 15.2 and 15.3) should always be considered. Diagnosis is based on the clinical picture, brain imaging findings, and the identification of predisposing factors; however, no standard diagnostic criteria, even for neuropathology, are yet available.[41] Three broad clinicopathological syndromes have been described. Strategic infarcts especially involving the thalamus, basal ganglia, or internal capsule may produce a frontal-subcortical disconnection.[42] Multiple cortical infarcts lead to stepwise erosion of cognitive function with a mixture of cortical and subcortical impairments. Small vessel disease produces a clinical syndrome of subcortical frontal executive dysfunction, gait 'apraxia', pseudobulbar palsy and urinary incontinence, associated with brain imaging findings (*see* Figure 15.1(F)) of lacunes in deep grey

Table 15.3 Causes of young onset dementia: inherited (bold, treatable condition; *, various combinations possible; †, neurological manifestations usually treatment resistant)

Disease	Chromosome and inheritance pattern	Protein	Cardinal features*				Other
			Ataxia	Pyramidal signs	Extrapyramidal syndrome	Peripheral neuropathy	
Neurodegenerations							
Alzheimer's disease[7]	21	APP (rare)	–	–	–	–	Biparietal signs, myoclonus
	14	Presenilin 1					EEG: loss of α rhythm
	1	Presenilin 2 (Volga Germans)					MRI: early hippocampal atrophy
FTDP-17[20]	17	Tau	–	–	+	–	May have amytotrophy
	AD						EEG: preserved α rhythm
Familial frontotemporal dementia	17[89] or NK	NK	–	–	–	–	EEG: preserved α rhythm
	AD						
	9[90]	NK	–	–	–	–	Association with inclusion body myopathy and Paget's disease
	AD						
Familial non-specific dementia[91]	3	NK	–	+	+	–	Danish kindred
	AD						FTLD, neurological signs late
Dementia (motor neurone disease)[92]	9	NK	–	+	–	–	Orofacial apraxia, bulbar features, fasciculations (especially deltoid), amyotrophy
	AD						

Disorder	Chromosome / inheritance	Gene/protein					Clinical features
Huntington's disease[33]	4 CAG triplet repeat AD	Huntingtin	+	−	+	−	Various movement disorders possible, gaze apraxia MRI: atrophy of caudate head
Dentato-rubro-pallido-luysian atrophy[93]	12 AD	Atrophin 1 CAG triplet repeat disorder	+	−	+	−	Seizures More common in Japanese
Neuroacanthocytosis[94]	9 or X-linked	Chorein (chromosome 9) XK protein (X-linked)	+	−	+	+	Orofacial movement disorder, seizures Acanthocytes on wet smears Raised serum creatine kinase
Familial encephalopathy with neuroserpin inclusion bodies[95]	3 AD	Neuroserpin	−	−	−	−	Frontal-subcortical dementia Collins bodies (intraneuronal inclusions)
Neuroferritinopathy[96]	19	Ferritin light polypeptide	−	−	+	−	Palatal tremor AD MRI: iron in basal ganglia
Hallervorden-Spatz (PKAN)[97]	20 AR	Pantothenate kinase (PANK2)	+	+	+	+	Seizures MRI: 'eye of the tiger' (iron in globus pallidus)
Spinocerebellar ataxias[98]	Various CAG triplet repeats AD	Various	+	+	+	+	Often abnormal saccades; predominant executive dysfunction, usually mild

Table 15.3 *(continued)*

Disease	Chromosome and inheritance pattern	Protein	Cardinal features*				
			Ataxia	Pyramidal signs	Extrapyramidal syndrome	Peripheral neuropathy	Other
Metabolic							
Wilson's disease[55]	13	Human copper-transporting	+	-	+	-	Psychiatric disturbances, corneal Kayser-Fleischer rings
	AR	ATPase ATP7B					Cirrhosis, haemolytic anaemia
							MRI: 'face of the giant panda' sign
							Decreased serum copper and caeruloplasmin, increased urinary copper excretion
Cerebrotendinous xanthomatosis[99]	2	Mitochondrial sterol 27-hydroxylase	-	-	-	-	Tendon xanthomas, cataracts
	AR						Characteristic MRI features
							Raised levels of cholestanol (bile acid intermediate) in serum, nervous tissue, tendons
Ornithine transcarbamylase deficiency[100]	X-linked	Ornithine transcarbamylase (urea cycle enzyme)	+	+	-	-	Episodes of unexplained vomiting and stupor, hyperammonaemia
Prion							
Creutzfeldt-Jakob disease[34]	20 (PRNP)	Prion protein	+	+	+	-	Florid myoclonus, cortical blindness
	AD						Periodic triphasic complexes on EEG

	Mutation codon 178 (codon 129 val)				MRI: basal ganglia high signal
Gerstmann-Sträussler-Scheinker	Mutation codon 102	+	+	−	May have gaze palsy, deafness, pseudobulbar palsy, cortical blindness
Fatal familial insomnia	Mutation codon 178 (codon 129 methionine)	+	+	−	Disordered sleep, oneiric behaviour, dysautonomia, myoclonus
Vascular/arteriopathies					
Cerebral autosomal dominant arteriopathy with subcortical infarcts and leukoencephalopathy (CADASIL)[43]	19 Notch3	In context of vascular events	−		Psychiatric disturbances, migraine, strokes
	AD				Lack of conventional risk factors
					MRI: anterior temporal and external capsule high signal
					Osmophilic perivascular material on electron microscopy of skin, muscle, peripheral nerve, brain
Fabry's disease[101]	X-linked Alpha-galactosidase A	In context of vascular events	+		Small vessel disease
					Renal disease, skin changes (angiokeratoma corporis diffusum), extremity pain

Table 15.3 (continued)

Disease	Chromosome and inheritance pattern	Protein	Cardinal features*				Other
			Ataxia	Pyramidal signs	Extrapyramidal syndrome	Peripheral neuropathy	
Vascular/arteriopathies (continued)							
Cerebral amyloid angiopathies:[46]							
British (Worster-Drought)[45]	13 point mutation AD	BRI	+	+	–	–	MRI: prominent white matter disease (no haemorrhages)
Danish	13 duplication AD		+		–	–	Cataracts, deafness
Dutch (HCHWA-D)	21	APP	–	–	–	–	Recurrent lobar cerebral haemorrhages
Icelandic (HCHWA-I)	20	Cystatin C	–	–	–	–	
Meningovascular	18	Transthyretin	+	+	–	–	
Lysosomal storage disorders							
Adult GM2 gangliosidosis[102]	15/5 AR	Hexosaminidase A	+	+	+	+	Amyotrophy Particularly common in Ashkenazi Jews
Globoid cell leukodystrophy (Krabbe's)[103]	14 AR	Galactocere-brosidase	+	+	–	+	Visual loss Characteristic MRI features

Disease	Chromosome	Inheritance	Defective protein/enzyme				Clinical features
Niemann-Pick type C[104]	18	AR	NPC1 protein	+	+	−	Psychosis, vertical supranuclear gaze palsy, seizures Organomegaly Sea-blue histiocytes on bone marrow biopsy Abnormal cholesterol esterification in cultured fibroblasts
Metachromic leukodystrophy[105]	22	AR	Arylsulphatase A	+	+	+	May have early behavioural changes; wide range of age at onset MRI: white matter changes Urinary metachromatic deposits
Gaucher's type 3[106]	1	AR	Glucocerebrosidase	+	+	−	Horizontal supranuclear gaze palsy, progressive myoclonic epilepsy† Bone pain, hepatospenomegaly, anaemia, thrombocytopenia Increased plasma non-prostatic acid phosphatase Gaucher's cells in bone marrow
Ceroid lipofuscinosis (Kufs')[107]	NK various		NK	+	−	−	Psychiatric features, progressive myoclonic epilepsy, facial dyskinesias
Sialidosis (mucolipidosis I)[108]	6	AR	Sialidase (alpha-N-acetyl neuraminidase)	+	−	−	Progressive myoclonic epilepsy, retinal cherry red spot
Adult Pelizaeus-Merzbacher[109]	X-linked		Proteolipid	+	+	−	MRI: cerebral demyelination

Table 15.3 (continued)

Disease	Chromosome and inheritance pattern	Protein	Cardinal features*				Other
			Ataxia	Pyramidal signs	Extrapyramidal syndrome	Peripheral neuropathy	
Peroxisomal storage disorders							
Adrenoleuko-dystrophy[110]	X-linked	Adrenoleuko-dystrophy protein	+	+	−	+	Adrenal insufficiency; MRI: diffuse cerebral white matter change; Increased plasma very long chain fatty acid esters
Other storage disorders							
Lafora body disease[111]	6 AR	Laforin	+	−	−	−	Progressive myoclonic epilepsy; Lafora bodies on axillary skin biopsy
Adult polyglucosan body disease[112]	Various AR	Various (including glycogen branching enzyme)	+	+	+	+	Urinary incontinence; Polyglucosan bodies on axillary skin biopsy

	Gene/protein	Chromosome/DNA	Inheritance				Clinical features
Mitochondrial disorders[6]	Respiratory chain components	mtDNA or nuclear DNA	Various (often maternal)	+	+	+	Various phenotypes (mixtures common); brain infarcts, cerebral white matter disease, seizures, myopathy, CPEO, sensorineural hearing loss, fundal abnormalities. Diabetes mellitus, lactic acidosis, short stature. *May have ragged red fibres on muscle biopsy*
Novel mechanisms							
Polycystic lipomembranous osteodysplasia with sclerosing leukoencephalopathy: Nasu-Hakola[113]	DAP12	19 or NK	AR	−	−	−	Frontal dementia and bone cysts, postural dyspraxia. MRI: atrophy, periventricular high signal

AD, autosomal dominant; APP, amyloid precursor protein; AR, autosomal recessive; CPEO, chronic progressive external ophthalmoplegia; EEG, electroencephalography; FTDP-17, frontotemporal dementia parkinsonism linked to chromosome 17; MRI, magnetic resonance imaging; mtDNA, mitochondrial DNA; NK, not known.

Table 15.4 Differential diagnosis of rapidly progressive dementia

Reversible processes
  Non-convulsive status epilepticus
  Cerebral vasculitis/other inflammatory conditions
  Non-inflammatory cerebrovascular disease
  Drug toxicities (especially lithium)
  Tuberculosis/fungal meningitis
  Parenchymal Whipple's disease
  Chronic subdural haematoma/cerebral tumour
  Paraneoplastic limbic encephalitis (may improve with treatment of tumour)
  Antivoltage gated potassium channel antibody syndrome[59]
  ?Hashimoto's encephalopathy

Irreversible processes
  Rapidly progressive neurodegenerative variants:
  Dementia with Lewy bodies, multiple system atrophy, Alzheimer's disease
  Dementia (motor neurone disease) syndromes
  Neurofilament inclusion body disease[23]
  Prion diseases:
    Sporadic, familial, and new variant Creutzfeldt-Jakob disease
    Progressive multifocal leukoencephalopathy
    Subacute sclerosing panencephalitis (sequela of measles)

matter nuclei and leukoaraiosis (diffuse white matter ischaemic changes) and histopathological features of deep periventricular ischaemic demyelination ('Binswanger's disease'); this form of vascular dementia presents insidiously, often without a history of stroke.

A number of genetic arteriopathies are recognised. CADASIL (cerebral autosomal dominant arteriopathy with subcortical infarcts and leukoencephalopathy)[43] is an uncommon cause of young onset subcortical strokes and dementia (mean age of onset 45 years) associated with migraine and psychiatric symptoms, which may be the presenting feature. The clinical picture is highly variable within families. MRI reveals diffuse white matter lesions of the cerebral hemispheres, notably the anterior temporal lobes and external capsules (*see* Figure 15.1(G)). CADASIL is caused by mutations of the Notch3 gene on chromosome 19. Light microscopy of skin biopsies may reveal non-specific periodic acid Schiff staining of vessel walls and electron microscopy frequently demonstrates characteristic granular osmophilic material of uncertain origin in proximity to vascular smooth muscle cells in skin, muscle, peripheral nerve, and brain. Genetic testing may be diagnostic; immunostaining of skin biopsies using Notch3 monoclonal antibody is a promising alternative diagnostic test.[44] Various hereditary cerebral amyloid angiopathies have been identified (*see* Table 15.3): these include the familial British and Danish dementias associated with mutations in the BRI gene on chromosome 13 which produce complex neurological syndromes.[45,46]

Cerebral vasculitis

Vasculitis rarely affects the central nervous system in isolation but must always be considered as it is a potentially treatable cause of YOD.[47,48] The differential diagnosis is wide (*see* Table 15.4) and includes primary vasculitides such as Wegener's granulomatosis, temporal arteritis, polyarteritis nodosa, and Churg-Strauss syndrome; systemic diseases that may produce vasculitis such as systemic lupus, sarcoidosis, Behçet's disease and cryoglobulinaemia; infectious agents such as herpes zoster; and other rare conditions such as intravascular lymphoma. Special mention should be made of primary angiitis of the central nervous system, which is almost exclusively confined to brain and less commonly spinal cord; the aetiology remains unknown, however pathologically there is patchy inflammation (which may be granulomatous, necrotising or lymphocytic) preferentially affecting small leptomeningeal and parenchymal vessels. Clinical presentations are highly variable, ranging from an acute encephalopathy and multiple sclerosis-like illnesses to an indolent subcortical dementia. Headache is common but not universal; symptoms may fluctuate, and seizures may occur. Findings on investigation that suggest cerebral vasculitis include raised inflammatory markers and/or autoantibodies, vascular lesions on brain imaging, an encephalopathic electro-encephalogram, cerebrospinal fluid pleocytosis with unmatched oligoclonal bands, and beading of vessels on cerebral angiography; however, none in isolation can substitute for histopathology, and unconfirmed suspicion of cerebral vasculitis remains one of the few indications for biopsy of brain and meninges before committing the patient to immunosuppressive therapy.

Other causes

Alcohol-related dementia

Progressive intellectual deterioration is part of the spectrum of neurological and psychiatric sequelae of chronic alcohol abuse and represents a substantial social burden (*see* Table 15.1);[2] improvement may occur if abstinence is achieved.[49] Executive function and autobiographical memory appear especially vulnerable and confabulation may occur. However, the concept of alcohol-related dementia has raised considerable nosological difficulties: many patients have clinical features of Wernicke-Korsakoff syndrome (thiamine deficiency), other nutritional deficiencies, or hepatic encephalopathy.[50] Brain imaging often shows generalised cerebral atrophy with frontal predominance; however, appearances are non-specific. Neuropathological findings have been variable and heterogeneous, consistent with a multifactorial aetiology.[50]

Multiple sclerosis

Cognitive impairment may be the presenting feature of multiple sclerosis and it is common late in the course;[51,52] most cases have predominantly frontal executive dysfunction, resulting from frontosubcortical disconnection with extensive cerebral white matter disease. Intellectual deterioration generally progresses slowly, however cognitive impairment is more severe in chronic progressive than in relapsing-remitting disease. Cognitive impairment correlates with total lesion load and degree of atrophy of the corpus callosum on MRI,[52] and probably reflects axonal loss rather than demyelination *per se*.

AIDS dementia complex

AIDS dementia complex should not be overlooked as a cause of YOD. It generally presents as a subcortical dementia associated with gait ataxia and seizures. Brain MRI reveals diffuse cerebral atrophy with white matter hyperintensities. It is probably the direct result of central nervous HIV infection, and it is a diagnosis of exclusion in patients with known AIDS who develop cerebral symptoms. It is associated with a relatively low CD4 count[53] and is seen less frequently since the advent of highly active antiretroviral therapy.[54]

Wilson's disease

Wilson's disease is a treatable cause of YOD. It is an autosomal recessive disorder of copper transport with a prevalence of approximately 1/50 000.[55] Accumulated tissue copper causes progressive toxicity to the nervous system, liver, blood, and other organs. Abnormalities in behaviour and personality, depression, and cognitive deterioration are common. Neurological manifestations include tremor, dystonia, chorea, ataxia, dysarthria, a characteristic grimacing facial expression, and the pathognomonic corneal Kayser-Fleischer ring (which may require slit lamp examination for detection). The diagnosis is confirmed by low serum caeruloplasmin and total copper levels and increased 24 hour urinary copper excretion. Treatment is based on copper chelation. Copper studies should be part of the routine work-up of any patient presenting with psychiatric illness, dementia, or a movement disorder before the fifth decade.

Paraneoplastic limbic encephalitis

The rare entity of paraneoplastic limbic encephalitis arises from an autoimmune response to tumour antigens and usually precedes diagnosis of the underlying malignancy. It is characterised by mood and personality changes, hallucinations, seizures, and dementia,[56] often coupled with symptoms and signs referable to other areas of the nervous system (ataxia, sensory neuronopathy). Mesial temporal involvement is typical, however extralimbic areas (including hypothalamus and brainstem) are also frequently affected; histopathological features include inflammatory infiltrates and neuronal loss. Clues may include an inflammatory cerebrospinal fluid (with oligoclonal bands in the cerebrospinal fluid but absent in serum, indicating local immunoglobulin synthesis, in a high proportion), and focal temporal lobe abnormalities on MRI (*see* Figure 15.1(D)) and electroencephalography. Approximately 60% of cases have positive anti-neuronal antibodies (predominantly anti-Hu), and this finding mandates an exhaustive search for malignancy, usually including thoracoabdominal computed tomography or whole body positron emission tomography if available. The most common associated cancers are lung, testis, and breast. Therapeutic options are limited but some patients improve after treatment of the underlying malignancy.

'Steroid-responsive' and autoimmune encephalopathies

A small proportion of patients with YOD improve with immunosuppressive therapy. The 'steroid-responsive encephalopathies' are likely to represent a heterogeneous group of disorders which produce tissue damage via autoimmune mechanisms. This group is currently the focus of considerable interest and nosological controversy. Some patients may have an underlying cerebral vasculitis. Circulating autoantibodies can sometimes be identified (notably thyroid autoantibodies in 'Hashimoto's encephalopathy'), however their pathogenetic role remains undefined.[57] Similar reservations apply to dementia in association with antigliadin antibodies and coeliac disease.[58] The recent identification of autoantibodies directed against voltage gated potassium channels in patients with reversible dementia[59] raises the possibility that ion channel dysfunction plays a part in some cases.

An approach to diagnosis in young onset dementia

Clinical assessment

All young patients presenting with suspected dementia need specialist referral. As in any patient with dementia, a corroborating history should always be obtained, exploring different cognitive domains (not simply memory) and impact on work and daily life. It is particularly important to establish the mode of onset and tempo of evolution. A psychiatric history is mandatory because behavioural symptoms are frequently the presenting feature. Issues of safety need to be considered,[60] for example, whether the patient is still driving, or whether they have they developed aggressive or sexually disinhibited behaviours. The past medical and family history must be detailed; relatives who develop 'mental instability' or personality change in younger life or unaccountably 'disappear' may indicate a previously undiagnosed familial dementia. The physical examination must be thorough: although the neurological examination is often normal in the early stages of many degenerative dementias, the presence of additional pyramidal, extrapyramidal, and cerebellar signs will direct the diagnosis towards one of the 'dementia-plus' syndromes (*see* Tables 15.2 and 15.3). The general examination may provide specific clues such as hepatosplenomegaly and evidence of treatable comorbidity such as hypertension. Where available, neuropsychometry is very valuable in delineating the cognitive syndrome in detail and in identifying involvement of cognitive domains that may not have been evident clinically, indicating a more widespread impairment.

It is sometimes difficult to distinguish between organic and functional cognitive symptoms. This applies to diseases in which behavioural and emotional disturbances are integral to the disease process (such as FTLD) or where neurological symptoms may appear bizarre (as in some biparietal presentations of Alzheimer's disease), as well as disorders in which prominent mood symptoms may be a manifestation of retained insight. The opposite error is also frequent, for example misdiagnosing Alzheimer's disease in a depressed patient whose presenting complaint is poor memory, or FTLD in schizophrenia with prominent negative symptoms. The mode of onset of the symptoms and previous psychiatric history are of particular importance. Certain symptoms and signs should always arouse suspicion of an organic process (for example, isolated visual hallucinations, incontinence, ataxia, micrographia, or frontal phenomena such as utilisation behaviour, perseveration, or echolalia). Clues to a psychiatric disorder include a relatively abrupt onset, the presence of an identifiable emotional precipitant, and lack of progression. There may be inconsistencies on formal testing and perform-ance inferior to that expected from the history (for example, the patient who, having found his way to clinic unaccompanied, is quite unable to recall test material or gives 'Don't know' responses): in contrast, many FTLD patients perform well on formal testing despite social disintegration. However, in practice, the distinction between organic and psychiatric disease may be difficult and the possibility of an elaborated, underlying organic impairment should always be considered. Clinical reassessment over time is the key to resolving this dilemma.

Investigations

The first priority of investigation is the identification of a treatable process (*see* Table 15.5). In addition, accurate diagnosis has implications for prognosis and possibly genetic counselling of other family members. The standard dementia screen used in older patients needs to be supplemented by additional investigations (*see* Table 15.5). This applies particularly to dementia in young adults and adolescents: accurate diagnosis is worthwhile in this group, as some of these disorders are treatable or have substantial genetic implications, however specialised techniques such as white cell or fibroblast enzyme assays, tissue histochemistry, and electron microscopy and molecular genetic studies are often required (*see* Table 15.5).

Certain investigations, such as HIV serology and diagnostic genetic testing, require the consent of the patient and family after detailed discussion, and predictive genetic testing of family members requires formal genetic counselling in collaboration with a clinical genetics service. All patients with suspected YOD should have electroencephalography: this may assist diagnosis in the neuro-degenerations (it is usually normal in FTLD) and is particularly important in detecting unrecognised complex partial seizures that may produce an epileptic pseudodementia.[61] The brain imaging modality of choice in YOD is MRI, which provides more accurate visualisation of regional atrophy (*see* Figure 15.1) and signal change than computed tomography. Computed tomography can however exclude hydrocephalus or large mass lesions (*see* Figure 15.1(E)). Cerebrospinal fluid examination is recommended for all younger patients and in cases where there is an unusual presentation or rapid course.[62] Tissue biopsies can be of value in a number of diagnoses such as skin in CADASIL and Lafora body disease, and muscle in mitochodrial cytopathies and Kufs' disease. Tonsillar biopsy can provide a definitive diagnosis in nvCJD.[40] Rarely cerebral biopsy (usually non-dominant frontal and including cortex, white matter, and meninges) is required if vasculitis is suspected. Quarantining of instruments is necessary if CJD is in the differential diagnosis.

Principles of management

The management of the patient with YOD is complex and a multidisciplinary approach is essential. However, many areas in the United Kingdom lack specific services for YOD. Many patients with YOD lack insight and judgement and associated behavioural disturbances often place a heavy burden on carers. Patients with cognitive impairment who wish to drive are legally obliged to inform their car insurance company and the Driver and Vehicle Licensing Agency, which will then make a decision as to whether the patient should hold

Table 15.5 Investigation of the young patient with suspected dementia
(* , specific counselling required; † *see* Table 15.3)

Investigation		Rationale
Routine		
Neuropsycho-metry		Delineation of cognitive syndrome, identification of 'subclinical' areas of impairment
Haematology	Full blood count	Screen for anaemia, polycythaemia, eosinophilia
Inflammatory markers	Erythrocyte sedimentation rate/C-reactive protein	Screen for inflammatory process
Biochemistry	Urea and electrolytes, renal function, liver function, thyroid function, B12 and folate, lipids	Screen for treatable causes of dementia and vascular risk factors
Treponemal serology		Exclude tertiary syphilis
Immunology	ANCA, thyroid antimicrosomal, antigastric parietal, antiphospholipd, antineuronal, VGKC, serum electrophoresis	Screen for vasculitides, atrophic gastritis, Hashimoto's encephalopathy, paraneoplastic syndromes
Imaging	Chest radiography	Screen for pulmonary neoplasm, tuberculosis, some systemic disorders (for example, sarcoid)
	Brain computed tomography	Generalised atrophy, large space occupying lesions
	Brain MRI	Visualisation of regional atrophy and signal change
Neurophysiology	Electroencephalography	May help distinguish Alzheimer's from frontotemporal dementia (loss of α rhythm); diagnosis of CJD, epilepsy, acute encephalopathies
Cardiac	Electroencephalography, echocardiography	May reveal cardiac arrythmia or sources of emboli
For specific indication		
Copper studies	Slit lamp examination, serum caeruloplasmin, serum copper, 24 hour urine copper excretion	Wilson's disease where clinical suspicion or patient <age 40
Thrombophilia screens		Unexplained cerebrovascular disease
White cell enzymes†		Metabolic disorder/patient <age 40
Plasma long chain fatty acids		Metabolic disorder/patient <age 40
Heavy metal screens		Chronic intoxication
Drug screens		Chronic illicit drug use
HIV serology		Risk factors*

Table 15.5 (*continued*)

Investigation		Rationale
For specific indication (*continued*)		
Genetic testing†		For mutation analysis where specific genetic disorder suspected*
Imaging	Computed tomography of chest/ abdomen, whole body PET	To identify neoplasm in suspected paraneoplastic syndrome
	Brain SPECT/PET	Occasionally if normal structural imaging (usually suspected frontal dementias)
	Gallium scan	Some inflammatory disorders (for example, sarcoidosis)
	Gadolinium brain MRI	Meningeal enhancement after contrast
Neurophysiology	EEG telemetry	Frequent covert seizures
	EMG	Motor neurone disease/amyotrophy
	Sphincter EMG	Multiple system atrophy
	VERs/BAERs/SSEPs	Demyelination; characteristics of myoclonus
Sleep study		Obstructive sleep apnoea
Cerebrospinal fluid examination	Glucose, cell count, protein, electrophoresis for oligoclonal bands	Any rapidly progressing or unusual dementia and/or patient >age 55
	Human herpes virus serology	Infection (especially if complex partial seizures)
	Whipple's polymerase chain reaction	Infection (especially if oculofacial movement disorder)
	Measles antibodies	Subacute sclerosing panencephalitis
	JC virus polymerase chain reaction	PML
	Neuronal marker proteins	14-3-3 in setting of rapid neuronal destruction (for example, CJD); S100, tau in research settings
Tissue biopsy	Skin	CADASIL; some storage diseases (for example, Kufs'; must have axillary skin for apocrine sweat glands)
	Muscle	Vasculitis; mitochondrial disease
	Small bowel	Whipple's disease; coeliac disease
	Bone marrow	Niemann-Pick type C; lymphoma/other haematological malignancies
	Tonsil	New variant CJD
	Brain (cortex, white matter + meninges)	Cerebral vasculitis

ANCA, antineutrophil cytoplasmic antibodies; BAERs, brainstem auditory evoked potentials; EEG, electroencephalography; EMG, electromyography; PET, positron emission tomography; PML, progressive multifocal leukoencephalopathy; SPECT, single photon emission tomography; SSEPs, somatosensory evoked potentials; VERs, visual evoked potentials; VGKC, voltage gated potassium channel antibodies.

Table 15.6 Voluntary societies offering advice and support to patients and carers

Society	Web address
Alzheimer's Society	www.alzheimers.org.uk
Pick's Disease (FTLD) Support Group	www.pdsg.org.uk
Huntington's Society	www.hda.org.uk
Gaucher's Association	www.gaucher.org.uk

a driver's licence. Early diagnosis of YOD and a comprehensive social needs assessment allow patients and carers to plan for the future and make pre-emptive decisions such as living wills or enduring power of attorney while they still have legal capacity. Volunteer support groups for YOD patients and their carers are an important resource (*see* Table 15.6).

Non-pharmacological management

All behavioural problems need thorough assessment and an 'Antecedent, Behaviour, and Consequences' (ABC) chart can be useful in documenting and then formulating management. Techniques include distraction by engaging the patient in activities (jigsaws and word puzzles may be particularly effective in FTLD), or environmental modifications such as restricting access to food. Occupational and speech therapists may be able to suggest alternative ways in which patients can communicate. In the later stages, physical dependency may increase greatly such that patients need intensive nursing from district nurses or residential nursing care; in this phase a palliative care approach may be appropriate. The question of brain donation should be visited sensitively with the family wherever practical.

Multiple choice questions

Answers appear at the end of 'References'.

Q1. Regarding the epidemiology of young onset dementia:
A. Lewy body dementia is the commonest cause
B. Alzheimer's disease is rare
C. Approximately 10% is alcohol-related
D. Prion disease is rare

Q2. Characteristics of early onset Alzheimer's disease include:
A. Early disinhibition and personality change
B. 75% of patients have a family history of dementia
C. Supranuclear gaze palsy
D. Parietal signs

Q3. Patients with frontotemporal lobar degeneration present with:
A. Lack of insight
B. Hepatosplenomegaly
C. Disinhibition
D. Cerebellar ataxia

Q4. Which of the following investigations are mandatory in YOD?
A. EEG
B. Genetic testing
C. Cerebral biopsy
D. Tonsillar biopsy

Q5. Cholinesterase inhibitors may be of symptomatic benefit in:
A. Frontotemporal lobar degeneration
B. Vascular dementia
C. Alzheimer's disease
D. Huntington's disease

Pharmacological management

Depression frequently occurs in YOD; mood symptoms should be inquired about specifically, and there should be a low threshold for treatment with antidepressants. Selective serotonin reuptake inhibitors are the class of choice as tricyclic compounds have anticholinergic effects and may worsen cognition. If the patient is severely agitated, there are psychotic symptoms, there is danger to the patient or others or all other behavioural measures have failed, the use of sedative or neuroleptic medication may be appropriate, however many patients (notably those with Lewy body dementia and FTLD)[63] are exquisitely sensitive to neuroleptics and can develop life-threatening extrapyramidal syndromes. If absolutely necessary, atypical neuroleptics such as risperidone or olanzapine are preferable; these agents should be used for the shortest time possible, under close supervision, and at low dosage (for example, risperidone 0.5 mg twice a day).

Few specific therapies are available for most forms of YOD. Close attention to vascular risk factors can modify the course of vascular dementia and may also have a role in preventing progression of Alzheimer's disease. The prevalence of Alzheimer's disease is lower in patients receiving statins,[64] suggesting that these lipid lowering drugs may be protective against Alzheimer's disease, although the mechanism is unclear. Based on observations that raised plasma homocysteine is associated with an increased risk of developing Alzheimer's disease, it has been suggested that folate may have a protective effect; however this remains unproven.[65]

The acetylcholinesterase inhibitors donepezil, rivastigmine, and galantamine (*see* Table 15.7) can be effective as symptomatic therapies to partly redress the cholinergic deficit in Alzheimer's disease and may delay entry to residential care, however they have not been shown to influence the underlying disease process. Overall probably fewer than 50% of patients will experience an improvement in cognitive function, however the drugs may also have benefits for activities of daily living, mood, and general wellbeing which are difficult to quantify. The drugs should be prescribed according to the current United Kingdom National Institute for Clinical Excellence[66] guidelines (for patients with Mini-Mental State Examination Score 12–26/30 and arrangements for recommended follow-up and monitoring). Acetylcholinesterase inhibitors may also be helpful in Lewy body

Table 15.7 Acetylcholinesterase inhibitors currently licensed in United Kingdom

| Drug | Dosage schedule | | Side effects |
	Start	Maintenance	
Donepezil (Aricept)	5 mg at night	10 mg at night	Usually minor; may include gastrointestinal upset, sedation, agitation, sleep disturbance, headache, muscle cramps, urinary incontinence, atrioventricular block
Rivastigmine (Exelon)	1.5 mg twice a day	Up to 6 mg twice a day	
Galantamine (Reminyl)	8 mg/day	Up to 12 mg twice a day	

dementia[67] and vascular dementia,[68] although they are not currently licensed for use in these diseases. They may worsen behavioural disturbance in FTLD.[69] The N-methyl-D-aspartate receptor antagonist Memantine (Ebixa) may reduce glutamate-mediated neuronal excitotoxicity and has produced modest symptomatic benefit in severe Alzheimer's disease;[70] it is now licensed for this indication in the United Kingdom.

Acknowledgements

The authors thank Dr Nick Fox for helpful discussion and Dr Hadi Manji for permission to reproduce brain images.

References

1 Health Advisory Service. *Heading for better care: commissioning and providing mental health services for people who have acquired brain injury, early onset dementia or Huntington's disease.* London: HMSO, 1997.

2 Harvey RJ, Rossor MN, Skelton-Robinson M, *et al. Young onset dementia: epidemiology, clinical symptoms, family burden, support and outcome.* London: Dementia Research Group, 1998.

3 Ratnavalli E, Brayne C, Dawson K, *et al.* The prevalence of frontotemporal dementia. *Neurology* 2002; **58**: 1615–21.

4 Schott JM, Fox NC, Rossor MN. Genetics of the dementias. *J Neurol Neurosurg Psychiatry* 2002; **73**: 141–7.

5 Wenger DA, Coppola S, Liu SL. Insights into the diagnosis and treatment of lysosomal storage diseases. *Arch Neurol* 2003; **60**: 322–8.

6 Schapira AH. Primary and secondary defects of the mitochondrial respiratory chain. *J Inherit Metab Dis* 2002; **25**: 207–14.

7 Janssen JC, Beck JA, Campbell TA, *et al.* Early onset familial Alzheimer's disease: mutation frequency in 31 families. *Neurology* 2003; **60**: 235–9.

8 Holland AJ, Oliver C. Down's syndrome and the links with Alzheimer's disease. *J Neurol Neurosurg Psychiatry* 1995; **59**: 111–14.

9 Mann DM, Iwatsubo T, Nochlin D, *et al.* Amyloid (Abeta) deposition in chromosome 1-linked Alzheimer's disease: the Volga German families. *Ann Neurol* 1997; **41**: 52–7.

10 Hardy J, Selkoe DJ. The amyloid hypothesis of Alzheimer's disease: progress and problems on the road to therapeutics. *Science* 2002; **297**: 353–6.

11 Lovestone S, McLoughlin DM. Protein aggregates and dementia: is there a common toxicity? *J Neurol Neurosurg Psychiatry* 2002; **72**: 152–61.

12 Rossor MN, Janssen JC, Fox NC, *et al.* Lessons in familial Alzheimer's disease. In: Tanka C, McGeer PL, Ihara Y, eds. *Neuroscientific basis of dementia*. Basel: Birkhauser Verlag, 2001: 259–65.

13 Lippa CF, Swearer JM, Kane KJ, *et al.* Familial Alzheimer's disease: site of mutation influences clinical phenotype. *Ann Neurol* 2000; **48**: 376–9.

14 Queralt R, Ezquerra M, Lleo A, *et al.* A novel mutation (V89L) in the presenilin 1 gene in a family with early onset Alzheimer's disease and marked behavioural disturbances. *J Neurol Neurosurg Psychiatry* 2002; **72**: 266–9.

15 Kennedy AM, Newman SK, Frackowiak RSJ, *et al.* Chromosome 14 linked familial Alzheimer's disease: a clinico-pathological study of a single pedigree. *Brain* 1995; **118**: 185–205.

16 O'Riordan S, McMonagle P, Janssen JC, *et al.* Presenilin-1 mutation (E280G), spastic paraparesis, and cranial MRI white-matter abnormalities. *Neurology* 2002; **59**: 1108–10.

17 Fox NC, Scahill RI, Crum WR, *et al.* Correlation between rates of brain atrophy and cognitive decline in AD. *Neurology* 1999; **52**: 1687–9.

18 Fox NC, Warrington EK, Seiffer AL, *et al.* Presymptomatic cognitive deficits in individuals at risk of familial Alzheimer's disease: a longitudinal prospective study. *Brain* 1998; **121**: 1631–9.

19 Neary D, Snowden JS, Gustafson L, *et al.* Frontotemporal lobar degeneration: a consensus on clinical diagnostic criteria. *Neurology* 1998; **51**: 1546–54.

20 Rosso SM, Van Swieten JC. New developments in frontotemporal dementia and parkinsonism linked to chromosome 17. *Curr Opin Neurol* 2002; **15**: 423–8.

21 Knopman DS, Mastri AR, Frey WH, *et al.* Dementia lacking distinctive histologic features: a common non-Alzheimer degenerative dementia. *Neurology* 1990; **40**: 251–6.

22 Rossor MN, Revesz T, Lantos PL, *et al.* Semantic dementia with ubiquitin-positive tau-negative inclusion bodies. *Brain* 2000; **123**: 267–76.

23 Josephs KA, Holton JL, Rossor MN, *et al.* Neurofilament inclusion body disease: a new proteinopathy. *Brain* 2003; **126**: 2291–303.

24 Miller BL, Darby A, Benson DF, *et al.* Aggressive, socially disruptive and antisocial behaviour associated with fronto-temporal dementia. *Br J Psychiatry* 1997; **170**: 150–4.

25 Garrard P, Hodges JR. Semantic dementia: clinical, radiological and pathological perspectives. *J Neurol* 2000; **247**: 409–22.

26 Chan D, Fox NC, Scahill RI, *et al.* Patterns of temporal lobe atrophy in semantic dementia and Alzheimer's disease. *Ann Neurol* 2001; **49**: 433–42.

27 Rosen HJ, Perry RJ, Murphy J, *et al.* Emotion comprehension in the temporal variant of frontotemporal dementia. *Brain* 2002; **125**: 2286–95.

28 Turner RS, Kenyon LC, Trojanowski JQ, *et al.* Clinical, neuroimaging and pathologic features of progressive non-fluent aphasia. *Ann Neurol* 1996; **39**: 166–73.

29 Bak TH, O'Donovan DG, Xuereb JH, *et al.* Selective impairment of verb processing associated with pathological changes in Brodmann areas 44 and 45 in the motor neurone disease-dementia-aphasia syndrome. *Brain* 2001; **124**: 103–20.

30 McKeith IG. Dementia with Lewy bodies. *Br J Psychiatry* 2002; **180**: 144–7.

31 Gusella JF, MacDonald ME, Ambrose CM, *et al.* Molecular genetics of Huntington's disease. *Arch Neurol* 1993; **50**: 1157–63.

32 Harper PS. The epidemiology of Huntington's disease. *Hum Genet* 1992; **89**: 365–76.

33 Paulsen JS, Ready RE, Hamilton JM, *et al.* Neuropsychiatric aspects of Huntington's disease. *J Neurol Neurosurg Psychiatry* 2001; **71**: 310–14.

34 Collinge J. Prion diseases of humans and animals: their causes and molecular basis. *Annu Rev Neurosci* 2001; **24**: 519–50.

35 Carrell RW, Lomas DA. Conformational disease. *Lancet* 1997; **350**: 134–8.

36 Brown P, Preece M, Brandel JP, *et al*. Iatrogenic Creutzfeldt-Jakob disease at the millennium. *Neurology* 2000; **55**: 1075–81.

37 Will RG, Ironside JW, Zeidler M, *et al*. A new variant of Creutzfeldt-Jakob disease in the UK. *Lancet* 1996; **347**: 921–25.

38 Collinge J, Brandner S, Kennedy A, *et al*. A 38-year-old man with a 9 month history of neurological and cognitive impairment. *Lancet Neurology* 2003; **2**: 189–94.

39 Collie DA, Sellar RJ, Zeidler M, *et al*. MRI of Creutzfeldt-Jakob disease: imaging features and recommended MRI protocol. *Clin Radiol* 2001; **56**: 726–39.

40 Hill AF, Butterworth RJ, Joiner S, *et al*. Investigation of variant Creutzfeldt-Jakob disease and other human prion diseases with tonsil biopsy samples. *Lancet* 1999; **353**: 183–9.

41 Chui H. Vascular dementia, a new beginning: shifting focus from clinical phenotype to ischemic brain injury. *Neurol Clin* 2000; **18**: 951–78.

42 Schott JM, Crutch SJ, Fox NC, *et al*. Development of selective verbal memory impairment secondary to a left thalamic infarct: a longitudinal case study. *J Neurol Neurosurg Psychiatry* 2003; **74**: 255–7.

43 Markus HS, Martin RJ, Simpson MA, *et al*. Diagnostic strategies in CADASIL. *Neurology* 2002; **59**: 1134–8.

44 Joutel A, Favrole P, Labauge P, *et al*. Skin biopsy immunostaining with a Notch3 monoclonal antibody for CADASIL diagnosis. *Lancet* 2001; **358**: 2049–51.

45 Mead S, James-Galton M, Revesz T, *et al*. Familial British dementia with amyloid angiopathy. Early clinical, neuropsychological and imaging findings. *Brain* 2000; **123**: 975–91.

46 Revesz T, Holton JL, Lashley T, *et al*. Sporadic and familial cerebral amyloid angiopathies. *Brain Pathol* 2002; **12**: 343–57.

47 Scolding NJ, Jayne DRW, Zajicek JP, *et al*. Cerebral vasculitis – recognition, diagnosis and management. *Q J Med* 1997; **90**: 61–73.

48 Joseph FG, Scolding NJ. Cerebral vasculitis: a practical approach. *Practical Neurology* 2002; **2**: 80–93.

49 Tuck RR, Brew BJ, Britton AM, *et al*. Alcohol and brain damage. *Br J Addict* 1984; **79**: 251–9.

50 Victor M. Alcoholic dementia. *Can J Neurol Sci* 1994; **21**: 88–99.

51 DeSousa EA, Albert RH, Kalman B. Cognitive impairments in multiple sclerosis: a review. *Am J Alzheimers Dis Other Demen* 2002; **17**: 23–9.

52 Bobholz JA, Rao SM. Cognitive dysfunction in multiple sclerosis: a review of recent developments (review). *Current Opin Neurol* 2003; **16**: 283–8.

53 Wesselingh SL, Thompson KA. Immunopathogenesis of HIV-associated dementia. *Curr Opin Neurol* 2001; **14**: 375–9.

54 Sacktor NC, Skolasky RL, Lyles RH, *et al*. Improvement in HIV-associated motor slowing after antiretroviral therapy including protease inhibitors. *J Neurovirol* 2000; **6**: 84–8.

55 Pfeil SA, Lynn DJ. Wilson's disease: copper unfettered (review). *J Clin Gastroenterol* 1999; **29**: 22–31.

56 Gultekin SH, Rosenfeld MR, Voltz R, *et al*. Paraneoplastic limbic encephalitis: neurological symptoms, immunological findings and tumour association in 50 patients. *Brain* 2000; **123**: 1481–94.

57 Chong JY, Rowland LP, Utiger RD. Hashimoto encephalopathy: syndrome or myth? *Arch Neurol* 2003; **60**: 164–71.

58 Collin P, Pirttila T, Nurmikko T, *et al*. Celiac disease, brain atrophy and dementia. *Neurology* 1991; **41**: 372–5.

59 Schott JM, Harkness K, Barnes J, *et al.* Amnesia, cerebral atrophy and autoimmunity: a treatable dementia associated with voltage-gated potassium channel antibodies. *Lancet* 2003; **361**: 1266.

60 Talerico KA, Evans LK. Responding to safety issues in frontotemporal dementias. *Neurology* 2001; **56**(suppl 4): S52–5.

61 Hoegh P, Smith SJ, Scahill RI, *et al.* Epilepsy presenting as AD: neuroimaging, electroclinical features, and response to treatment. *Neurology* 2002; **58**: 298–301.

62 Quality Standards Subcommitte of the American Academy of Neurology. Practice parameter for diagnosis and evaluation of dementia. *Neurology* 1994; **44**: 2203–6/ *Neurology* 2001; **56**: 1143–53.

63 Pijnenburg YA, Sampson EL, Harvey RJ, *et al.* Vulnerability to neuroleptic side effects in frontotemporal lobar degeneration. *Int J Geriatr Psychiatry* 2003; **18**: 67–72.

64 Wolozin B, Kellman W, Ruosseau P, *et al.* Decreased prevalence of Alzheimer disease associated with 3-hydroxy-3-methyglutaryl coenzyme A reductase inhibitors. *Arch Neurol* 2000; **57**: 1439–43.

65 Loscalzo J. Homocysteine and dementias. *N Engl J Med* 2002; **346**: 466–8.

66 Technology and Appraisal Guidance. *Guidance on the use of donepezil, rivastigmine and galantamine for the treatment of Alzheimer's disease.* London: HMSO, 2001: 19.

67 McKeith I, del Ser T, Spano P, *et al.* Efficacy of rivastigmine in dementia with Lewy bodies: a randomised, double-blind, placebo-controlled international study. *Lancet* 2000; **356**: 2031–6.

68 Erkinjuntti T, Kurz A, Gauthier S, *et al.* Efficacy of galantamine in probable vascular dementia and Alzhiemer's disease combined with cerebrovascular disease: a randomised trial. *Lancet* 2002; **359**: 1283–90.

69 Pasquier F, Lebert F, Lavenu I, *et al.* The clinical picture of frontotemporal dementia: diagnosis and follow-up. *Dement Geriatr Cogn Disord* 1999; **10**(suppl 1): 10–14.

70 Wilcock GK. Memantine for the treatment of dementia. *Lancet Neurology* 2003; **2**: 503–5.

71 Schott JM, Simon JE, Fox NC, *et al.* Delineating the sites and progression of in vivo atrophy in multiple system atrophy using fluid-registered MRI. *Mov Disord* 2003; **18**: 955–8.

72 Soliveri P, Monza D, Paridi D, *et al.* Cognitive and magnetic resonance imaging aspects of corticobasal degeneration and progressive supranuclear palsy. *Neurology* 1999; **53**: 502–7.

73 Emre M. Dementia associated with Parkinson's disease. *Lancet Neurology* 2003; **2**: 229–37.

74 Schielke E, Nolte C, Müller W, *et al.* Sarcoidosis presenting as rapidly progressive dementia: clinical and neuropathological evaluation. *J Neurol* 2001; **248**: 522–4.

75 Oktem-Tanor O, Baykan-Kurt B, Gurvit LK, *et al.* Neuropsychological follow-up of 12 patients with neuro-Behçet disease. *J Neurol* 1999; **246**: 113–19.

76 Weber G. Midbrain tumours. In: Vinken PJ, Bruyn GW, eds. *Handbook of clinical neurology.* Amsterdam: North-Holland, 1974; **17**: 620–47.

77 Roos KL. Mycobacterium tuberculosis meningitis and other etiologies of the aseptic meningitis syndrome. *Sem Neurol* 2000; **20**: 329–35.

78 Manzel K, Tranel D, Cooper G. Cognitive and behavioral abnormalities in a case of central nervous system Whipple's disease. *Arch Neurol* 2000; **57**: 399–403.

79 Fallon BA, Nields JA. Lyme disease: a neuropsychiatric illness. *Am J Psychiatry* 1994; **151**: 1571–83.

80 Mawrin C, Lins H, Koenig B, *et al.* Spatial and temporal disease progression of adult-onset subacute sclerosing panencephalitis. *Neurology* 2002; **58**: 1568–71.

81 Krupp LB, Lipton RB, Swerdlow ML, *et al.* Progressive multifocal leukoencephalopathy: clinical and radiographic features. *Ann Neurol* 1985; **17**: 344–9.

82 Ernst A, Zibrak JD. Carbon monoxide poisoning. *N Engl J Med* 1998; **339**: 1603–8.

83 Visvanathan R. Is it truly dementia? *Lancet* 2001; **357**: 684.

84 Caviness JN, Evidente VGH. Cortical myoclonus during lithium exposure. *Arch Neurol* 2003; **60**: 401–4.

85 Moulignier A, Allo S, Zittoun R, *et al*. Recombinant interferon-α-induced chorea and frontal subcortical dementia. *Neurology* 2002; **58**: 328–30.

86 Vigliani MC, Duyckaerts C, Hauw JJ, *et al*. Dementia following treatment of brain tumors with radiotherapy administered alone or in combination with nitrosourea-based chemotherapy: a clinical and pathological study. *J Neurooncol* 1999; **41**: 137–49.

87 Steiner MC, Ward MJ, Ali NJ. Dementia and snoring. *Lancet* 1999; **353**: 204.

88 Jordan BD. Chronic traumatic brain injury associated with boxing. *Semin Neurol* 2000; **20**: 179–85.

89 Rosso SM, Kamphurst W, de Graaf B, *et al*. Familial frontotemporal dementia with ubiquitin-positive inclusions is linked to chromosome 17q21–22. *Brain* 2001; **124**: 1948–57.

90 Kovach MJ, Waggoner B, Leal SM, *et al*. Clinical delineation and localization to chromosome 9p13.3–p12 of a unique dominant disorder in four families: hereditary inclusion body myopathy, Paget disease of bone, and frontotemporal dementia. *Mol Genet Metab* 2001; **74**: 458–75.

91 Gydesen S, Brown JM, Brun A, *et al*. Chromosome 3 linked frontotemporal dementia (FTD-3). *Neurology* 2002; **59**: 1585–94.

92 Hosler BA, Siddique T, Sapp PC, *et al*. Linkage of familial amyotrophic lateral sclerosis with frontotemporal dementia to chromosome 9q21–q22. *JAMA* 2000; **284**: 1664–9.

93 Takahashi H, Ohama E, Naito H, *et al*. Hereditary dentatorubral-pallidoluysian atrophy. *Neurology* 1988; **38**: 1065–70.

94 Rampoldi L, Danek A, Monaco AP. Clinical features and molecular bases of neuroacanthocytosis. *J Mol Med* 2002; **80**: 475–91.

95 Bradshaw CB, Davis RL, Shrimpton AE, *et al*. Cognitive deficits associated with a recently reported familial neurodegenerative disease: familial encephalopathy with neuroserpin inclusion bodies. *Arch Neurol* 2001; **58**: 1429–34.

96 Wills AJ, Sawle GV, Guilbert PR, *et al*. Palatal tremor and cognitive decline in neuroferritinopathy. *J Neurol Neurosurg Psychiatry* 2002; **73**: 86–95.

97 Hayflick SJ, Westaway SK, Levinson B, *et al*. Genetic, clinical, and radiographic delineation of Hallervorden-Spatz syndrome. *N Engl J Med* 2003; **348**: 33–40.

98 Bürk K, Globas C, Bösch S, *et al*. Cognitive deficits in spinocerebellar ataxia type 1, 2, and 3. *J Neurol* 2003; **250**: 207–11.

99 Verrips A, Hoefsloot LH, Steenbergen GC, *et al*. Clinical and molecular genetic characteristics of patients with cerebrotendinous xanthomatosis. *Brain* 2000; **123**: 908–19.

100 Finkelstein JE, Hauser ER, Leonard CO, *et al*. Late-onset ornithine transcarbamylase deficiency in male patients. *J Pediatr* 1990; **117**: 897–902.

101 Mendez MF, Stanley TM, Medel NM, *et al*. The vascular dementia of Fabry's disease. *Dement Geriatr Cogn Disord* 1997; **8**: 252–7.

102 Chavany C, Jendoubi M. Biology and potential strategies for the treatment of GM2 gangliosidoses. *Mol Med Today* 1998; **4**: 158–65.

103 Jardim LB, Giugliani R, Pires RF, *et al*. Protracted course of Krabbe disease in an adult patient bearing a novel mutation. *Arch Neurol* 1999; **56**: 1014–17.

104 Imrie J, Vijayaraghaven S, Whitehouse C, *et al*. Niemann-Pick disease type C in adults. *J Inherit Metab Dis* 2002; **25**: 491–500.

105 Cengiz N, Ozbenli T, Onar M, *et al*. Adult metachromatic leukodystrophy: three cases with normal nerve conduction velocities in a family. *Acta Neurol Scand* 2002; **105**: 454–7.

106 Tuzun E, Baykan B, Gurses C, *et al*. Longterm follow-up of electroencephalographic and clinical findings of a case with Gaucher's disease type 3a. *Seizure* 2000; **9**: 469–72.

107 Nijssen PC, Brusse E, Leyten AC, *et al*. Autosomal dominant adult neuronal ceroid lipofuscinosis: parkinsonism due to both striatal and nigral dysfunction. *Mov Disord* 2002; **17**: 482–7.

108 Palmeri S, Villanova M, Malandrini A, *et al*. Type I sialidosis: a clinical, biochemical and neuroradiological study. *Eur Neurol* 2000; **43**: 88–94.

109 Koeppen AH, Robitaille Y. Pelizaeus-Merzbacher disease. *J Neuropathol Exp Neurol* 2002; **61**: 747–59.

110 Edwin D, Speedie L, Naidu S, *et al*. Cognitive impairment in adult-onset adrenoleukodystrophy. *Mol Chem Neuropathol* 1990; **12**: 167–76.

111 Minassian BA. Progressive myoclonus epilepsy with polyglucosan bodies: Lafora disease. *Adv Neurol* 2002; **89**: 199–210.

112 Klein CM, Bosch EP, Dyck PJ. Probable adult polyglucosan body disease. *Mayo Clin Proc* 2000; **75**: 1327–31.

113 Paloneva J, Autti T, Raininko R, *et al*. CNS manifestations of Nasu-Hakola disease: a frontal dementia with bone cysts. *Neurology* 2001; **56**: 1552–8.

Answers

1. (C) and (D); 2. (D); 3. (A) and (C); 4. (A); 5. (B) and (C).

Chapter Sixteen

Multiple sclerosis: diagnosis and the management of acute relapses

SM Leary, B Porter and AJ Thompson

Multiple sclerosis is an inflammatory demyelinating disease of the central nervous system that may result in a wide range of neurological symptoms and accumulating disability. Its course is unpredictable resulting in a changing pattern of clinical need. Diagnostic criteria for multiple sclerosis require objective evidence for dissemination in space and time. The diagnostic and management process should follow good practice guidelines with the individual at the centre of the process. Appropriate support and information should be available from the time of diagnosis. Continuing education is key in enabling the individual to actively participate in their management. In the event of an acute relapse the individual should have direct access to the most appropriate local service. Provided medical causes have been excluded, steroid therapy to hasten the recovery from the relapse should be considered. Management of an acute relapse should be comprehensive addressing any medical, functional or psychosocial sequelae.

Introduction

Multiple sclerosis affects approximately 85 000 people in the United Kingdom and is the most common cause of neurological disability in young adults. The National Institute for Clinical Excellence (NICE) has recently published management guidelines that highlight the need to improve standards of care offered to people with this condition.[1] Health and social care professionals in both primary and secondary care should be informed of the current evidence-based practice in order to optimise their management of people with multiple sclerosis. People with multiple sclerosis must participate fully in decisions on their care.[2] This review covers both the diagnosis of multiple sclerosis and the management of acute relapses and begins with a brief overview of the condition.

Overview of multiple sclerosis

Multiple sclerosis is characterised by inflammatory, demyelinating lesions scattered throughout the central nervous system (CNS) which occur at different sites and at different times. The exact pathophysiology of multiple sclerosis is not clear but it appears to be autoimmune in nature. The wide distribution of lesions results in a variety of clinical features such as loss of sensation, muscle weakness, visual loss, incoordination, cognitive impairment, fatigue, pain and bladder and bowel disturbance. The course of multiple sclerosis is unpredictable resulting in a changing pattern of need over time. It has relatively little effect on life expectancy and therefore usually has to be managed for many decades.[3]

Multiple sclerosis typically presents between 20 and 40 years of age. Females are more susceptible than males by a factor that approaches 2:1. Race and geography also affect susceptibility to the disease.[4] As a general rule, though with clear exceptions, the risk of multiple sclerosis increases with increased distance from the equator. Migration studies have also suggested that environmental factors in childhood may have an aetiological role.[5]

Types of multiple sclerosis

The natural course of multiple sclerosis is extremely variable with symptoms that may appear, disappear, reappear, or gradually worsen over time. Despite this variability it is possible to recognise broad categories of disease and to classify people according to the course of their disease.[6]

Relapsing Remitting Multiple Sclerosis (RRMS)

This is the most common type of multiple sclerosis; approximately 85% of individuals present with this pattern. RRMS presents with acute or sub-acute onset of neurological symptoms, from which people may recover either completely or partially. Further relapses may then occur at irregular intervals. If recovery from relapses is incomplete people may accrue neurological deficit and disability. A recent study has highlighted the effect of relapses on development of residual deficit; a measurable and sustained increase in disability was seen in up to 42% of patients at follow-up after a relapse.[7]

Secondary Progressive Multiple Sclerosis (SPMS)

Over time RRMS may convert to a disease pattern of gradual progression with accumulating irreversible neurological deficit and disability (SPMS). The proportion of people developing progressive disease increases with length of follow-up. In a Canadian study 41% of people with RRMS entered the secondary progressive phase within 6–10 years of disease onset increasing to 58% between 11 and 15 years after onset.[8] People with SPMS may continue to have superimposed relapses.

Primary Progressive Multiple Sclerosis (PPMS)

PPMS is characterised by progressive disease from onset, with a gradual accumulation of neurological deficit or disability, without relapse or remission, and accounts for approximately 10–15% of multiple sclerosis. The average age of onset, approximately 40 years, is later than in RRMS and relatively more men are affected resulting in an equal male:female ratio.[9] The age of onset and rate of progression is similar to the progressive phase of SPMS.[10]

Progressive Relapsing Multiple Sclerosis (PRMS)

PRMS is defined as progressive disease from onset with superimposed relapses. The progressive disease is predominant and PRMS is considered to be largely

Table 16.1   Diagnostic criteria according to Schumacher *et al.* 1965.[15]

- Age of onset within 10 to 50 years
- Objective neurological signs present on examination
- Neurological symptoms and signs indicative of CNS white matter disease
- Dissemination in space:
  - two or more non-contiguous anatomical areas involved
- Dissemination in time:
  - two or more episodes of worsening lasting at least 24 hours separated by one month or more, or
  - progression over at least six months
- No better explanation by a physician competent in neurology

---

similar to PPMS.[11,12] Approximately 10–15% of people with PPMS will have superimposed relapses.

Disease activity

The activity of disease in multiple sclerosis is also extremely variable ranging from clinically asymptomatic, with only pathological evidence of disease detected incidentally post mortem, to an aggressive course with rapidly accumulating disability. An aggressive or malignant disease course may result from frequent relapses with little or no neurological recovery or from rapid disease progression. Benign multiple sclerosis refers to a disease course with minimal or no disability many years after disease onset. The proportion of people with benign disease is a minority and decreases with length of follow-up. For example, in an Irish study 42% of people had benign disease after 10 years but this had decreased to 34% after 15 years.[13] Although it is recognised that long-standing benign disease can become more aggressive and lead on to severe disability,[8] the longer the duration of multiple sclerosis and the lower the disability, the more likely an individual is to remain stable.[14]

Diagnosis of multiple sclerosis

Diagnostic criteria

Multiple sclerosis remains a clinical diagnosis requiring appropriate expertise to confirm evidence of CNS lesions disseminated in time and space and to exclude other diseases which may give a similar picture. Diagnostic criteria have been developed to improve the certainty of diagnosis. In 1965 Schumacher *et al.* deemed six criteria to be essential in diagnosing multiple sclerosis (*see* Table 16.1).[15]

According to the number of criteria satisfied, the diagnosis was classified as clinically definite, probable or possible multiple sclerosis. Forty years later the clinical principles of these criteria remain valid though modifications have been recommended reflecting the development of diagnostic investigations. In 1983 Poser *et al.* modified the criteria to incorporate paraclinical and laboratory evidence and to extend the age of onset to 59 years.[16] These criteria classified multiple sclerosis as clinically or laboratory-supported definite/probable based on

Table 16.2 Diagnostic tests required for different presentations of multiple sclerosis according to McDonald *et al.* 2001 (detailed criteria for MRI abnormality are defined but are not given here)[17]

- Two or more attacks; objective clinical evidence of 2 or more lesions
  - No additional tests required
- Two or more attacks; objective clinical evidence of 1 lesion
  - Dissemination in space demonstrated by
    MRI (nine or more T2 lesions or one gadolinium enhancing lesion), *or*
    equivocal MRI (two or more lesions) plus positive CSF, *or*
    await further clinical attack implicating a different site
- One attack; objective clinical evidence of 2 or more lesions
  - Dissemination in time demonstrated by
    MRI, *or* second clinical attack
- One attack; objective clinical evidence of 1 lesion (monosymptomatic presentation)
  - Dissemination in space demonstrated by
    MRI, *or* equivocal MRI plus positive CSF, *and*
  - Dissemination in time, demonstrated by
    MRI, *or* second clinical attack
- Insidious neurological progression suggestive of MS
  - Positive CSF, *and*
  - Dissemination in space, demonstrated by
    MRI, *or* abnormal VEP associated with equivocal MRI, and
  - Dissemination in time, demonstrated by
    MRI, *or* continued progression for 1 year

clinical and paraclinical evidence of disseminated lesions and oligoclonal bands in the cerebrospinal fluid (CSF).

The diagnostic criteria have been further revised by McDonald *et al.* in 2001.[17] These criteria still place an emphasis on dissemination of lesions in time and space and incorporate both clinical and paraclinical evidence, notably magnetic resonance imaging (MRI), which is recognised as the most sensitive and specific paraclinical test. MRI criteria have been defined for both dissemination in space and time. Diagnostic criteria have been recommended for different clinical presentations (*see* Table 16.2). If the criteria are fulfilled, the diagnosis is 'multiple sclerosis'; if the criteria are not completely fulfilled, the diagnosis is 'possible multiple sclerosis'; if the criteria are fully explored and not fulfilled, the diagnosis is 'not multiple sclerosis'. The terms clinically and laboratory-supported definite/ probable multiple sclerosis are no longer recommended.

MRI is the investigation of choice but visual evoked potential studies may also provide diagnostic support. Examination of CSF is only required if there is clinical uncertainty. If there are atypical clinical features further investigations may be required to exclude other diseases.

Difficult diagnostic groups

Diagnosis may be straightforward when an individual presents having had two discrete neurological episodes suggestive of multiple sclerosis disseminated in space and time with objective evidence on examination. However, people may present in a number of ways that cause difficulty in diagnosis. Some examples are now discussed.

Monosymptomatic presentation

It is common for people to present after their first episode of neurological symptoms, such as an optic neuritis or a sensory cord episode, with no clinical evidence of dissemination. The revised diagnostic criteria have included criteria for such monosymptomatic presentations. Dissemination in space may often be evident on MRI at initial presentation but dissemination in time cannot be proved if MRI is performed within 3 months of presentation. It is suggested that evidence for dissemination in time may be provided if criteria are fulfilled on delayed or serial MRI. However, if the MRI at presentation shows multiple typical lesions, a more pragmatic approach is to discuss with the individual that the clinical and investigation findings are in keeping with possible multiple sclerosis and if there is a second clinical episode the diagnosis of multiple sclerosis will be confirmed.

Thorough history taking is also important in this situation. During the diagnostic stage it is not unusual for people to recall having had mild neurological symptoms in the past. Such episodes may have not been reported previously as they have recovered quickly or were deemed too trivial to report to a doctor. The significance of previous symptoms has to be evaluated on an individual basis; transient sensory symptoms are not uncommon in the general population but an episode of Lhermittes phenomenon may be highly suggestive of a previous demyelinating episode. Although historical reports are not objective evidence they may raise the suspicion of the diagnosis.

Insidious neurological progression (PPMS)

The onset of PPMS is insidious and there may be a long delay from disease onset to diagnosis. The majority of people with PPMS present with a single progressive symptom, usually a paraparesis implicating the spinal cord and so alternative diagnoses such as spinal cord compression need to be excluded.[18,19] Diagnosis of PPMS has historically been hampered by the lack of specific diagnostic criteria but these have now been developed.[17,20] A diagnosis of PPMS cannot be made on the clinical features alone and more emphasis is put on paraclinical evidence. In particular a definite diagnosis of PPMS cannot be made without demonstrating the presence of oligoclonal bands in the CSF that are not present in paired serum.

Explosive onset

Multiple sclerosis may occasionally have an explosive onset with clinical involvement of multiple areas of the CNS at first presentation. This may be difficult to differentiate from acute disseminated encephalomyelitis (ADEM), a monophasic demyelinating disease of the CNS.[21] ADEM classically occurs following an infection or vaccination but there may be no preceding history and multiple sclerosis may similarly present following an immune trigger. ADEM may be more likely to be associated with headache, fever and drowsiness but encephalopathic presentations of multiple sclerosis also occur especially in children.[22]

MRI in ADEM typically shows extensive multifocal white matter abnormalities but the appearances cannot be reliably differentiated from multiple sclerosis. However, serial MRI demonstrating new lesions is in favour of a diagnosis of multiple sclerosis.[23] CSF examination does not reliably distinguish the diseases and oligoclonal bands may be present in ADEM.

Although establishing a definite diagnosis may not be possible at presentation first-line treatment of the acute episode is the same in both diseases, namely steroids. The diagnosis may become clear with time if the individual has a second episode suggestive of multiple sclerosis and this possibility should be discussed with the individual.

Vague symptoms

A not uncommon scenario is that an individual presents with a history of vague or mild neurological symptoms, often sensory, and is concerned that they have multiple sclerosis. Even if the history is not particularly suggestive of multiple sclerosis and neurological examination is normal, without an alternative explanation for the symptoms the possibility of multiple sclerosis cannot be definitely excluded. There are no clear guidelines for this situation but the decision as to whether to investigate should be made in discussion with the individual. If a decision is made against investigation and the person does later develop multiple sclerosis the delay in diagnosis is unlikely to change long-term outcome. However, if a diagnosis of multiple sclerosis is suspected most people would favour knowing the diagnosis.[24]

Involving the individual in the diagnostic process

People with multiple sclerosis attach great importance to involvement in and clear communication throughout the diagnostic process. The diagnostic phase has been described as a time of anxious waiting.[25] In particular the delay between presenting symptoms, diagnostic tests and receipt of test results is a recurring area of complaint.[26,27]

People with multiple sclerosis want a clear accurate diagnosis, access to appropriate support, information and continuing education at and around the time of diagnosis.[28] The NICE guidelines on multiple sclerosis mirror these principles, making a number of recommendations of good practice (*see* Table 16.3).

Diagnostic models – getting it right from the start

Despite national circulation of guidance documents on standards of care,[1,28] there is currently a wide variation and lack of equity in the services provided throughout the United Kingdom and diagnosis often occurs in a haphazard and unsupported way. This situation may be partly explained by the fact that medical and neurology services are often over-subscribed with long waiting lists for clinics and investigations. There is some evidence that a coordinated diagnostic clinic model facilitates an effective, supportive, efficient and cost-effective structure to manage the diagnostic phase of multiple sclerosis.[29] Such diagnostic models serve as an illustration of how reorganisation, flexibility, team working and forward planning can influence the delivery of care. However, outside of specialist centres the model that is chosen for a diagnostic service will depend on the expertise and resources available locally.

Table 16.3 The diagnostic process. Management of multiple sclerosis in primary and secondary care, NICE 2003.[1]

- An individual who is suspected of having MS should be referred to a specialist neurology service, and seen rapidly within an audited time (will vary according to clinical need but should be no longer than 6 weeks).
- An individual should be informed of the potential diagnosis as soon as a diagnosis of MS is considered likely, before undertaking further investigations.
- Throughout the diagnostic process, the healthcare professional should:
  - find out what and how much information the individual wants to receive;
  - discuss the nature and purpose of all investigations.
- The individual should be seen again after all investigations have been completed (recommended within a further 6 weeks) and the diagnosis confirmed or refuted. If the diagnosis is confirmed the individual should be told the diagnosis by a doctor with specialist knowledge of MS; this will usually be a consultant or an experienced specialist registrar.
- Following diagnosis the individual should be:
  - offered at least one more appointment in the near future (recommended in no longer than 4 weeks) to see wherever possible the doctor who gave the diagnosis;
  - put in touch with a skilled nurse or support worker, ideally with specialist knowledge of MS;
  - offered written information about disease-specific support organisations;
  - offered information about the disease specific to the newly diagnosed.
- Within 6 months of diagnosis, the individual should be offered the opportunity to participate in an educational programme to cover all aspects of MS.

Communication, information and support

People with multiple sclerosis want to be involved in their overall management plan. There is evidence that the quality of communication at the time of diagnosing a chronic disease influences patient health outcomes.[30] Good history taking and discussion of management plans have been observed to have positive effects on emotional health, symptom resolution, general functioning, physiological measures and pain control.[30]

In addition to good communication people with multiple sclerosis require timely, accurate information and support. Within the United Kingdom multiple sclerosis specialist nurses play a vital role in this area, offering one to one educational and supportive sessions.[31] Educational programmes including 'Getting to Grips' courses for the newly diagnosed, and specific workshops for people with secondary or primary progressive disease are also coordinated across the United Kingdom by the Multiple Sclerosis Society.

Multiple sclerosis healthcare professionals also work closely with the voluntary sector to produce educational materials that vary from information booklets, to teaching manuals to help explain the biology of multiple sclerosis,[32] to online decision making aids that help people choose drug treatments.[33] This collaborative approach to management reflects the principles of the NHS expert patient programmes that encourage optimal self-management strategies.[34]

Management of acute relapses

An acute relapse refers to an episode of neurological disturbance, of the kind seen in multiple sclerosis, that lasts for at least 24 hours, and for which there is no other cause such as fever.[17] Typically a relapse evolves over a few days, reaches a plateau and then remits to a variable degree over a few weeks or months. The patient experiencing a relapse has to cope with a relatively sudden onset of neurological symptoms that may be physically and psychologically distressing and functionally and socially incapacitating. In the longer term, incomplete remission from a relapse may result in residual neurological deficit. Management of an acute relapse requires a comprehensive approach addressing its medical, functional and psychosocial effects. Management incorporates education regarding relapses, support in the event of a relapse, treatment to accelerate or improve the recovery from a relapse, and symptomatic treatment and rehabilitation. The other area of management is to reduce the frequency of relapses with disease-modifying therapies such as interferon beta. Disease-modifying therapies are not discussed here but have been reviewed extensively elsewhere.[35,36]

Education and support

Education and support are an ongoing part of management from diagnosis. As discussed earlier, people with multiple sclerosis should be provided with information regarding the disease and its management to enable them to actively participate in their own management. In terms of relapses, individuals should be given information regarding general health factors, such as infection, that may influence the risk of relapse and advised what to do in the event of new symptoms suggestive of a relapse, including how to self-refer into primary or secondary care clinics.

Factors affecting relapse activity

Several general health factors have been proposed to affect relapse activity in multiple sclerosis. Infections may trigger a relapse or exacerbate existing symptoms. Where possible, infections should be anticipated and treated early. An association has been reported between common viral infections and relapse but these are difficult to avoid.[37-39] Infections may occur as a complication of multiple sclerosis, for example urinary tract infections due to retention, and chest infections due to aspiration, so addressing their underlying causes may be preventive.

The possibility that vaccinations may immunologically trigger a relapse has been raised but there is no clear evidence that this is the case. Most vaccines have not been studied prospectively but a double-blind, placebo-controlled trial of influenza vaccine found no effect on relapse rate or disease progression.[40] Particular concern has been expressed regarding hepatitis B vaccination but a large case-crossover study found no increase in risk of relapse following hepatitis B or any other vaccination.[41] Current consensus is that vaccinations are not contraindicated in multiple sclerosis and people with multiple sclerosis should be offered vaccination against influenza.[1,42] However, it should not be forgotten that live vaccines may be contraindicated in individuals on immunosuppressant therapy.

Physical trauma has also been proposed to trigger relapses but a thorough review of the evidence a few years ago did not support a link between physical trauma and relapses.[43] The relationship between psychological stress and relapses has been unclear,[43,44] but a recent prospective study found stressful life events were associated with an increased risk of relapse.[45] A recent meta-analysis also supported an association between stressful life events and subsequent relapses though did not link specific stressors to relapses.[46]

The effect of pregnancy on disease activity is an important concern among young women. A prospective study of pregnancy in multiple sclerosis confirmed that relapse rate declines during pregnancy, especially in the third trimester, increases during the first three months post-partum and then returns to pre-pregnancy rate.[47] In the same study epidural analgesia and breastfeeding did not increase the risk of relapse. There is therefore no medical contraindication to pregnancy in multiple sclerosis.

Assessment of new or increased symptoms

In the event of new or increased symptoms people with multiple sclerosis should be able to identify and contact a professional from their healthcare team who can advise them or direct them to the most appropriate local service. The NICE guidelines recommend that if a person with multiple sclerosis develops new or increased neurological symptoms a formal assessment should be made to determine the diagnosis (*see* Table 16.4).

At the assessment the possibility of any other medical cause for an increase in neurological symptoms must be considered. In particular it is important to exclude an infective cause such as a urinary tract infection, which may be otherwise clinically silent. The possibility of dual neurological pathology, for example, a cord compression mimicking a spinal cord relapse, should also be borne in mind. If the new symptoms are assessed to be unrelated to multiple sclerosis it must still be ensured that the person with multiple sclerosis has access to the appropriate service and treatment.

In developing a service for people with multiple sclerosis it is of key importance that the service is responsive and flexible and so can meet the unpredictable and acute needs of people with multiple sclerosis. As there are often long waiting lists for general neurology/medical clinics this may be difficult. One model to address this problem is a specialist multiple sclerosis relapse clinic, which is specifically set up to respond to and assess and manage acute episodes.

Table 16.4 Assessment of new or increased symptoms. Management of multiple sclerosis in primary and secondary care, NICE 2003.[1]

- If an individual has a relatively sudden increase in neurological symptoms or disability, or develops new neurological symptoms, a formal assessment should be made to determine the diagnosis (reason for change).
- This diagnostic assessment should:
  - Be undertaken within a time appropriate to the clinical presentation;
  - Consider the presence of an acute infective cause;
  - Involve a GP or acute medical/neurological services.
- Further neurological investigation should not be undertaken unless the diagnosis of MS itself is in doubt.

Treatment of acute relapses

If an acute episode of neurological symptoms is assessed to be a relapse of multiple sclerosis treatment to hasten the recovery from the relapse should be considered. The only recommended treatment is steroid therapy. NICE guidelines recommend that steroid therapy should be offered if the episode is sufficient to cause distressing symptoms or an increased limitation on activities.

Evidence base for steroid therapy

There is good evidence that steroid therapy accelerates the recovery from relapse. The exact mode of action of steroids in multiple sclerosis is unclear. However, there are several potential modes of action, which include reducing oedema, stabilising the blood-brain barrier, decreasing pro-inflammatory cytokines and inducing T-cell apoptosis.[48] Efficacy was demonstrated in early studies using intramuscular adrenocorticotropic hormone (ACTH) though this practice is now discontinued. Intravenous methylprednisolone has been demonstrated to accelerate recovery rate,[49,50] and to be as effective as ACTH.[51,52]

The comparative efficacy of intravenous and oral steroids has been more controversial. The largest study to date was a randomised, placebo-controlled study of intravenous methylprednisolone, followed by oral prednisone, and oral prednisone alone which was carried out in acute optic neuritis.[53] In the intravenous steroid group visual recovery was accelerated but there was no long-term benefit to vision. In the oral prednisone group there was no improvement in visual outcome and there was an increased rate of new attacks of optic neuritis. At two years there was a reduction in the rate of development of multiple sclerosis in the intravenous group but this was not sustained at the three year follow-up.[54] Other studies have shown no clear advantage of intravenous over oral methylprednisolone in acute relapses.[55,56] The choice of steroid therapy remains variable among neurologists although the most popular regime is an infusion of 1 g daily over three days.[57] NICE guidelines recommend either intravenous methylprednisolone, 500 mg–1 g daily, or high-dose oral methylprednisolone, 500 mg–2 g daily, for between 3 and 5 days. To date steroid therapy has only been definitively proven to hasten the recovery from relapses. The effect on long-term outcome has not been established.[58]

There has been debate as to the optimal location for the administration of intravenous steroid therapy. Intravenous steroids may be administered as a hospital inpatient, in an outpatient clinic or at home. Factors that may influence the choice of location include cost-effectiveness, nursing dependency and patient preference. In a Canadian study both outpatient and at home treatment were found to be more cost-effective than inpatient treatment.[59] A study of outpatient versus home treatment in the United Kingdom is currently underway.[60]

Risks of steroid therapy

The potential benefits and risks should be explained to an individual when considering steroid therapy. It must be emphasised that steroids do have side effects though their incidence is relatively low. In the short term, complications from intravenous methylprednisolone include disturbance of taste, facial flushing, insomnia, psychiatric disturbance, exacerbation of acne and transient hyperglycaemia and hypertension.[61] Infection may be exacerbated and should be excluded before commencing steroid therapy; urinalysis to exclude a urinary tract infection should be performed routinely. Gastrointestinal disturbance, such as peptic ulceration, may be exacerbated and it is sensible to screen for a history of other risk factors such as use of non-steroidal anti-inflammatory drugs or excess alcohol intake. The long-term complications of steroid therapy are generally not a problem with intermittent courses of intravenous steroids but may be more likely to occur with oral steroids that are more susceptible to abuse. Aseptic bone necrosis has been reported rarely. There is no clear evidence on how often it is acceptable to treat with intravenous steroids but it is recommended not to have more than three courses a year.[1]

Other therapies

Currently no other immuno-modulating therapies are recommended for the treatment of acute relapses. A small randomised trial of plasma exchange in patients with acute severe neurological deficits due to demyelinating diseases, that had not responded to steroid therapy, resulted in improvement in some patients.[62] Plasma exchange may be considered in the event of a catastrophic acute relapse.

Comprehensive management

Management of acute relapses should not just be limited to steroid therapy but should be comprehensive, addressing all aspects of the relapse. Practical support-ive measures, such as the provision of care or equipment, may be essential and should not be forgotten. Symptomatic treatment for new symptoms from a relapse may sometimes be required. If a relapse is improving spontaneously or with steroids, the duration of symptoms may be too short to warrant symptomatic treatment. However, if symptoms are distressing or not resolving then treatment may be required. For example, trigeminal neuralgia due to an acute relapse may be very distressing even for a short period of time but may be alleviated with medication such as carbamazepine. Symptomatic treatments are not discussed further here but are reviewed elsewhere.[63]

Functional recovery from a relapse may be facilitated by multidisciplinary input from neurological rehabilitation services. This input should run in parallel with any medical treatment and depending on need may be on an outpatient or inpatient basis. A recent randomised controlled trial found a multidisciplinary rehabilitation approach to be superior to a standard ward routine in people with multiple sclerosis receiving intravenous steroid therapy.[64] Inpatient rehabilitation has also been shown to be useful in relapsing remitting multiple sclerosis, particularly in people with incomplete recovery from relapses with moderate to severe disability.[65]

Conclusion

Multiple sclerosis is an unpredictable disease that may cause significant neuro-logical deficit and disability. The diagnostic stage is an anxious time for the individual and the diagnostic process should be rapid and adhere to good practice guidelines. Appropriate support and information should be provided from the time of diagnosis. Education should be an ongoing part of management with an emphasis on self-management. Due to the unpredictable nature of relapses, healthcare services should be flexible and responsive to meet acute needs. Management of acute relapses requires a comprehensive approach addressing medical, functional and psychosocial aspects of the relapse. Although historically management has often been haphazard, the introduction of clinical guidelines and the development of specialist clinical resources aims to standardise and optimise management across the United Kingdom.

References

1 National Institute for Clinical Excellence. Management of multiple sclerosis in primary and secondary care. *NICE Guideline* 2003.

2 Federation of Royal Colleges of Physicians of the UK. *Good medical practice for physicians.* London: Royal College of Physicians 2004.

3 Sadovnick AD, Ebers GC, Wilson RW, *et al.* Life expectancy in patients attending multiple sclerosis clinics. *Neurology* 1992; **42**: 991–4.

4 Sadovnick AD, Ebers GC. Epidemiology of multiple sclerosis: A critical overview. *Can J Neurol Sci* 1993; **20**: 17–29.

5 Dean G, Kurtzke JF. On the risk of multiple sclerosis according to the age at immigration to South Africa. *Br Med J* 1971; **3**: 725–9.

6 Lublin FD, Reingold SC. Defining the clinical course of multiple sclerosis: results of an international survey. National Multiple Sclerosis Society (USA) Advisory Committee on Clinical Trials of New Agents in Multiple Sclerosis. *Neurology* 1996; **46**: 907–11.

7 Lublin FD, Baier M, Cutter G. Effect of relapses on development of residual deficit in multiple sclerosis. *Neurology* 2003; **61**: 1528–32.

8 Weinshenker BG, Bass B, Rice GPA. The natural history of multiple sclerosis: a geographically based study. 1. Clinical course and disability. *Brain* 1989; **112**: 133–46.

9 Thompson AJ, Polman CH, Miller DH, *et al.* Primary progressive multiple sclerosis. *Brain* 1997; **120**: 1085–96.

10 Runmarker B, Andersen O. Prognostic factors in a multiple sclerosis incidence cohort with twenty-five years of follow-up. *Brain* 1993; **116**: 117–34.

11 Kremenchutzky M, Cottrell D, Rice G. The natural history of multiple sclerosis: a geographically based study. 7. Progressive-relapsing and relapsing-progressive multiple sclerosis: a re-evaluation. *Brain* 1999; **122**: 1941–50.

12 Andersson PB, Waubant E, Gee L, *et al.* Multiple sclerosis that is progressive from the time of onset: clinical characteristics and progression of disability. *Arch Neurol* 1999; **56**: 1138–42.

13 Thompson AJ, Hutchinson M, Brazil J, *et al.* A clinical and laboratory study of benign multiple sclerosis. *Q J Med* 1986; **58**: 69–80.

14 Pittock SJ, McClelland RL, Mayr WT, *et al.* Clinical implications of benign multiple sclerosis: a 20-year population-based follow-up study. *Ann Neurol* 2004; **56**: 303–6.

15 Schumacher GA, Beebe G, Kibler RF, *et al.* Problems of experimental trials of therapy in multiple sclerosis: report by the panel on the evaluation of experimental trials of therapy in multiple sclerosis. *Ann NY Acad Sci* 1965; **122**: 552–68.

16 Poser CM, Paty DW, Scheinberg L, *et al.* New diagnostic criteria for multiple sclerosis: Guidelines for research protocols. *Ann Neurol* 1983; **13**: 227–31.

17 McDonald WI, Compston A, Edan G, *et al.* Recommended diagnostic criteria for multiple sclerosis: guidelines from the international panel on the diagnosis of multiple sclerosis. *Ann Neurol* 2001; **50**: 121–7.

18 McDonnell GV, Hawkins SA. Clinical study of primary progressive multiple sclerosis in Northern Ireland, UK. *J Neurol Neurosurg Psychiatry* 1998; **64**: 451–4.

19 Stevenson VL, Miller DH, Rovaris M, *et al.* Primary progressive multiple sclerosis: a clinical and MRI cross sectional study. *Neurology* 1999; **52**: 839–45.

20 Thompson AJ, Montalban X, Barkhof F, *et al.* Diagnostic criteria for primary progressive multiple sclerosis: a position paper. *Ann Neurol* 2000; **47**: 831–5.

21 Garg RK. Acute disseminated encephalomyelitis. *Postgrad Med J* 2003; **79**: 11–17.

22 Matthews B. Differential diagnosis of multiple sclerosis and related disorders. In: Compston A, Ebers G, Lassmann H, *et al.* eds. *McAlpine's multiple sclerosis*. 3rd edn. London: Churchill Livingstone, 1998: 223–250.

23 Kesselring J, Miller DH, Robb SA, *et al.* Acute disseminated encephalomyelitis. MRI findings and the distinction from multiple sclerosis. *Brain* 1990; **113**: 291–302.

24 Elian M, Dean G. To tell or not to tell the diagnosis of multiple sclerosis. *Lancet* 1985; **2**: 27–8.

25 Koopman W, Schweitzer A. The journey to multiple sclerosis: a qualitative study. *J Neurosci Nurs* 1999; **31**: 17–26.

26 Robinson I. The context and consequences of communicating the diagnosis of multiple sclerosis: some brief findings from a survey of 900 patients. In: Wietholer H, *et al.* eds. *Current Concepts in Multiple Sclerosis*. New York: Elsevier 1991.

27 Robinson I, *et al. The views of people with MS about their needs*. Brunel MS Research Unit 1996.

28 Freeman J, Johnson J, Rollinson S, *et al. Standards of healthcare for people with multiple sclerosis*. Multiple Sclerosis Society of Great Britain and Northern Ireland and The National Hospital for Neurology and Neurosurgery 1997.

29 Porter B, Keenan E, Record E, *et al.* Diagnosis of MS: a comparison of three different clinical settings. *Mult Scler* 2003; **9**: 431–9.

30 Stewart MA. Effective physician-patient communication and health outcomes: a review. *CMAJ* 1995; **152**: 1423–33.

31 MS Trust, UKMSSNA, RCN. *Specialist nursing in MS – the way forward: the key elements for developing MS specialist nurse services in the UK*. MS Trust, Letchworth 2001.

32 Multiple Sclerosis Society. *Helping you explain MS: a teaching resource for healthcare professionals*. London: MS Society 2004.

33 Medicines Partnership. Multiple sclerosis decisions. An independent aid to your decision. www.msdecisions.org.uk 2004.

34 Lorig KR, Holman H. Self-management education: history, definition, outcomes, and mechanisms. *Ann Behav Med* 2003; **26**: 1–7.

35 Kieseier BC, Hartung HP. Current disease-modifying therapies in multiple sclerosis. *Semin Neurol* 2003; **23**: 133–46.

36 Khan O, Zabad R, Caon C, *et al.* Comparative assessment of immunomodulating therapies for relapsing-remitting multiple sclerosis. *CNS Drugs* 2002; **16**: 563–78.

37 Sibley WA, Bamford CR, Clark K. Clinical viral infections and multiple sclerosis. *Lancet* 1985; **1**: 1313–15.

38 Andersen O, Lygner PE, Bergstrom T, *et al.* Viral infections trigger multiple sclerosis relapses: a prospective seroepidemiological study. *J Neurol* 1993; **240**: 417–22.

39 Buljevac D, Flach HZ, Hop WCJ, *et al.* Prospective study on the relationship between infections and multiple sclerosis exacerbations. *Brain* 2002; **125**: 952–60.

40 Miller AE, Morgante LA, Buchwald LY, *et al.* A multicentre, randomised, double-blind, placebo controlled trial of influenza immunisation in multiple sclerosis. *Neurology* 1997; **48**: 312–14.

41 Confavreux C, Suissa S, Saddier P, *et al.* Vaccinations and the risk of relapse in multiple sclerosis. Vaccines in Multiple Sclerosis Study Group. *N Eng J Med* 2001; **344**: 319–26.

42 Rutschmann OT, McCrory DC, Matchar DB; Immunization Panel of the Multiple

Sclerosis Council for Clinical Practice Guidelines. Immunization and MS: a summary of published evidence and recommendations. *Neurology* 2002; **59**: 1837–43.

43 Goodin DS, Ebers GC, Johnson KP, *et al*. The relationship of MS to physical trauma and psychological stress. Report of the Therapeutic and Technology Assessment Subcommittee of the American Academy of Neurology. *Neurology* 1999; **52**: 1737–45.

44 Mohr DC, Goodkin DE, Bacchetti P, *et al*. Psychological stress and the subsequent appearance of new brain lesions in MS. *Neurology* 2000; **55**: 55–61.

45 Buljevac D, Hop WC, Reedeker W, *et al*. Self reported stressful life events and exacerbations in multiple sclerosis: prospective study. *BMJ* 2003; **327**: 646.

46 Mohr DC, Hart SL, Julian L, *et al*. Association between stressful life events and exacerbation in multiple sclerosis: a meta-analysis. *BMJ* 2004; **328**: 731.

47 Confavreux C, Hutchinson M, Hours MM, *et al*. Rate of pregnancy-related relapse in multiple sclerosis. Pregnancy in Multiple Sclerosis Group. *N Eng J Med* 1998; **339**: 285–91.

48 Gold R, Buttgereit F, Toyka KV. Mechanism of action of glucocorticosteroid hormones: possible implications for therapy of neuroimmunological disorders. *J Neuroimmunol* 2001; **117**: 1–8.

49 Buckley C, Kennard C, Swash M. Treatment of acute exacerbations of multiple sclerosis with intravenous methyl-prednisolone. *J Neurol Neurosurg Psychiatry* 1982; **45**: 179–80.

50 Milligan NM, Newcombe R, Compston DA. A double-blind controlled trial of high dose methylprednisolone in patients with multiple sclerosis: 1. Clinical effects. *J Neurol Neurosurg Psychiatry* 1987; **50**: 511–16.

51 Barnes MP, Bateman DE, Cleland PG, *et al*. Intravenous methylprednisolone for multiple sclerosis in relapse. *J Neurol Neurosurg Psychiatry* 1985; **48**: 157–9.

52 Thompson AJ, Kennard C, Swash M, *et al*. Relative efficacy of intravenous methyl-prednisolone and ACTH in the treatment of acute relapse in MS. *Neurology* 1989; **39**: 969–71.

53 Beck RW, Cleary PA, Trobe JD, *et al*. The effect of corticosteroids for acute optic neuritis on the subsequent development of multiple sclerosis. *N Eng J Med* 1993; **329**: 1764–9.

54 Beck RW. The optic neuritis treatment trial: three-year follow-up results. *Arch Ophthalmol* 1995; **113**: 136–7.

55 Alam SM, Kyriakides T, Lawden M, *et al*. Methylprednisolone in multiple sclerosis: a comparison of oral with intravenous therapy at equivalent high dose. *J Neurol Neurosurg Psychiatry* 1993; **56**: 1219–20.

56 Barnes D, Hughes RA, Morris RW, *et al*. Randomised trial of oral and intravenous methylprednisolone in acute relapse of multiple sclerosis. *Lancet* 1997; **349**: 902–6.

57 Tremlett HL, Luscombe DK, Wiles CM. Use of corticosteroids in multiple sclerosis by consultant neurologists in the United Kingdom. *J Neurol Neurosurg Psychiatry* 1998; **65**: 362–5.

58 Filippini G, Brusaferri F, Sibley WA, *et al*. Corticosteroids for acute exacerbations in multiple sclerosis. *Cochrane Database Syst Rev* 2000; **4**: CD001331.

59 Robson LS, Bain C, Beck S, *et al*. Cost analysis of methylprednisolone treatment of multiple sclerosis patients. *Can J Neurol Sci* 1998; **25**: 222–9.

60 Riazi A, Hobart JC, Porter B, *et al*. Developing a measure of patients' experiences of relapse management in multiple sclerosis [abstract]. *Mult Scler* 2003; 9(suppl 1): S152.

61 Lyons PR, Newman PK, Saunders M. Methylprednisolone therapy in multiple sclerosis: a profile of adverse effects. *J Neurol Neurosurg Psychiatry* 1988; **51**: 285–7.

62 Weinshenker BG, O'Brien PC, Petterson TM, *et al*. A randomized trial of plasma exchange in acute central nervous system inflammatory demyelinating disease. *Ann Neurol* 1999; **46**: 878–86.

63 Thompson AJ. Symptomatic management and rehabilitation in multiple sclerosis. *J Neurol Neurosurg Psychiatry* 2001; 71(suppl 2): 22–7.

64 Craig J, Young CA, Ennis M, *et al.* A randomised controlled trial comparing rehabilitation against standard therapy in multiple sclerosis patients receiving intravenous steroid treatment. *J Neurol Neurosurg Psychiatry* 2003; **74**: 1225–30.

65 Liu C, Playford ED, Thompson AJ. Does neurorehabilitation have a role in relapsing-remitting multiple sclerosis. *J Neurol* 2003; **250**: 1214–18.

Key references

1 National Institute for Clinical Excellence. Management of multiple sclerosis in primary and secondary care. *NICE Guideline* 2003.

2 McDonald WI, Compston A, Edan G, *et al.* Recommended diagnostic criteria for multiple sclerosis: guidelines from the international panel on the diagnosis of multiple sclerosis. *Ann Neurol* 2001; **50**: 121–7.

3 Medicines Partnership. Multiple sclerosis decisions. An independent aid to your decision. www.msdecisions.org.uk 2004.

4 Filippini G, Brusaferri F, Sibley WA, *et al.* Corticosteroids for acute exacerbations in multiple sclerosis. *Cochrane Database Syst Rev* 2000; **4**: CD001331.

5 Craig J, Young CA, Ennis M, *et al.* A randomised controlled trial comparing rehabilitation against standard therapy in multiple sclerosis patients receiving intravenous steroid treatment. *J Neurol Neurosurg Psychiatry* 2003; **74**: 1225–30.

Part 4

Stroke

Migraine, memory loss, and 'multiple sclerosis': neurological features of the antiphospholipid (Hughes') syndrome

GRV Hughes

The antiphospholipid syndrome (APS, Hughes' syndrome), first described in 1983, is a prothrombotic disease in which neurological events feature prominently. Strokes, transient ischaemic attacks, and headaches (including migraine) are important complications. However, it is clear that other neurological symptoms, including diplopia, memory loss, ataxia, and 'multiple sclerosis-like' features are common. A notable feature of Hughes' syndrome is the clinical response to anticoagulants; features such as headache and memory loss often improving dramatically with appropriate warfarin dosage. APS may well become recognised as an important (and potentially treatable) cause of neurological disease.

It is now recognised that antiphospholipid syndrome (APS) is a major neurological disease.[1] The syndrome, first described in 1983, is characterised by recurrent thrombosis (both venous and arterial), recurrent miscarriage, neurological disease, including stroke, and the presence of circulating antibodies against phospholipids.[2]

Our early studies focused on lupus, but we recognised that the syndrome was just as prevalent outside lupus and called this syndrome the antiphospholipid syndrome. The title is not strictly correct – the antibodies are in fact directed against phospholipids and proteins.

The syndrome is now recognised as a common and important prothrombotic condition with ramifications into almost all spheres of medicine, surgery, and obstetrics.

While our earliest descriptions highlighted the neurological aspects of the syndrome (strokes, chorea, myelopathy, headaches, memory loss, and dementia),[3,4] the full impact of the syndrome on neurology is now becoming more widely recognised.

Clinical features

This short review addresses these nervous system features, their pathogenesis, and their management.

Headache and migraine

Recently, we set up a patients' website on APS (www.hughes-syndrome.org). In the first week of operation we received over 20 000 hits. Far and away the commonest symptom reported was headache: not evidence-based medicine perhaps, but a pointer to the importance of this symptom.[5]

The history is remarkably similar in many patients with teenage headaches that are frequently migrainous – often premenstrual – often disappearing for 10–20 years only to return in the 30s or 40s. There is, significantly, a strong family history of headaches or of migraine in many of our patients, pointing to genetic influences. In some patients the headaches are accompanied by visual or speech disturbance, or by transient ischaemic attacks.

It is my view that antiphospholipid antibody testing should be among the armamentarium of those investigating migraine or recurrent headache.[6]

Memory loss

All those dealing with large numbers of patients with the syndrome recognise memory loss as possibly the most important feature. Unfortunately, as yet, there have been few formal psychometric studies of these patients – for example, before and after anticoagulation treatment is started.

In some patients, the disease, if untreated, progresses to widespread brain infarction, grossly abnormal magnetic resonance images and, ultimately, multi-infarct dementia.

In the majority of patients, the memory loss is less extreme – though sufficiently frightening for the patient to worry about the possibility of Alzheimer's disease.[7] It is this aspect of the syndrome which – like headaches – often improves when anticoagulation is started.

Epilepsy

Seizures are a feature of APS: indeed in a patient with lupus presenting with seizures, APS is the most likely underlying pathology – an observation with therapeutic implications.

All ages are affected, and all forms of epilepsy are seen, as are subclinical (abnormal electroencephalogram) forms. The association of antiphospholipid antibody with epilepsy, first reported in 1985,[8] may be of significant importance in the investigation of seizures in general.[9]

Box 17.1　A typical scenario

A 39 year old woman complained of headaches, fatigue, and memory loss. She was concerned about a possible diagnosis of Alzheimer's disease.

Two years earlier, she had suffered from similar headaches, associated with gait disturbance and ataxia. She had been investigated for multiple sclerosis but brain magnetic resonance imaging had been normal. Her past history included a strong teenage tendency to headaches, often migrainous. In her 20s she had been investigated for infertility, but on two occasions had conceived only to suffer a miscarriage at three months. At the age of 35 she had a successful pregnancy. In view of the possible diagnosis of APS (Hughes' syndrome), blood tests for antiphospholipid antibodies were ordered and found to be strongly positive. She was treated initially with aspirin 75 mg daily, with moderate though incomplete resolution of the headaches. Ultimately, in view of the known prothrombotic nature of APS, and especially its neurological and obstetric sequlae, the patient was anti-coagulated with warfarin. Not only did this treatment result in disappearance of the headaches, but the patient noted a marked improvement in memory. Interestingly, these two major symptoms returned whenever the international normalised ratio (INR) fell below 2.5.

Stroke

The commonest serious complication of APS is stroke. Indeed, the syndrome is becoming recognised as a major, and potentially preventable, cause of stroke. It has been estimated that up to one in five of all young (under 45) strokes are associated with Hughes' syndrome, although all ages can be affected. The clinical spectrum ranges from transient ischaemic attacks and focal lesions – such as amaurosis fugax – to widespread cerebral infarction, ataxia, bladder, and gait disturbance and – in extreme cases – multi-infarct dementia.

More than anything else, it is this propensity to (arterial) stroke which marks out Hughes' syndrome from the other less serious coagulopathies such as factor V Leiden deficiency.

Myelopathy

Transverse myelopathy is a rare but well recognised feature of APS. It is some-times associated with optic nerve ischaemia (Devic's disease). The pathology of the myelopathy is poorly understood. However, some interesting observations have come from the mouse model of APS. Some of these animals which develop an APS-like disease became paraplegic. Histology of the spinal cord in these animals showed vessel thrombosis.[10] These observations might be taken to support the suggestion that anticoagulation may have to be considered in addition to the more conventional steroid and immunosuppressive regimens generally given to some lupus patients with myelopathy, for example.

Multiple sclerosis

Not surprisingly, a number of patients with APS have carried a working diagnosis of 'multiple sclerosis'. In a recent study from our unit, 28 APS patients were reviewed in whom an original diagnosis of multiple sclerosis had been made.[11]

Some interesting lessons were learnt. Firstly, differential diagnosis was difficult – in this particular study the magnetic resonance imaging did not clearly distinguish the two conditions. Secondly, with hindsight, there had been clues to the underlying diagnosis, notably recurrent headaches, previous thrombosis, or recurrent miscarriage. Thirdly, and perhaps most significantly of all, in the majority of the patients ultimately correctly diagnosed and appropriately anti-coagulated, there were no further neurological events.

Clearly, there will be many similar studies to come. However, it seems probable that a small percentage of patients diagnosed with multiple sclerosis do in fact have Hughes' syndrome, a condition with totally different treatment and prognosis.

Chorea

Our original studies in 1983 included chorea. Although rare, this feature has been strongly associated with the presence of antiphospholipid antibodies – indeed, the combination in some APS patients of joint pains, heart murmurs, and chorea has led, not unexpectedly, to a label of 'rheumatic fever'. Although the precise pathophysiology of the chorea is unclear, an interesting clinical observation has been made that in a small number of patients, the chorea has ceased with the institution of anticoagulants.

Neuropathy

Possibly one of the more surprising findings has been the association in some patients between antiphospholipid antibodies and neuropathy, both peripheral and cranial. In classical lupus, peripheral neuropathy is relatively uncommon, and larger numbers will be required before this possible association can be confirmed.

Behavioural disorders

A number of cases of frontal lobe ischaemia, with its attendant behavioural disorder, have been seen (this author was referred one 3 year old boy with an aggressive behavioural disorder found to be associated with multiple cerebral infarcts). To date there have been surprisingly few studies detailing the neuro-psychiatric manifestations of APS.

Treatment

Anticoagulation is required. Current experience shows that antiphospholipid antibodies constitute a significant risk for thrombosis, including stroke. For example, in our clinic, in a 10 year retrospective analysis, no fewer than 50% of those individuals (mainly lupus patients or women with recurrent miscarriage) with positive antibodies in 1985 had developed thrombosis by 1995.[12]

A more difficult decision is whether to use aspirin alone or to anticoagulate with warfarin. Most data currently available point to the superiority of warfarin if there has been clear-cut cerebral ischaemia.

Khamashta *et al.* analysed APS patients over a 10 year period.[13] Of those treated with aspirin alone, over half developed further thrombosis. Likewise, in those treated with warfarin to an INR of less than 3, one half developed further thrombosis. Only in those maintained at an INR of 3 or over was there a significant 10 year benefit.

Our study had two possible weaknesses. Firstly, it was retrospective. Secondly, it was directed mainly to patients with arterial rather than venous thrombosis – it could be argued that subsets of patients with venous thrombosis alone might require less aggressive anticoagulation.

One point, however, is clear. The danger of thrombosis and stroke in these patients far outweighs the risks of anticoagulant induced bleeding. The traditional fear of cerebral haemorrhage has, almost certainly, resulted in the undertreatment of many patients with APS.

Finally, what of the 'non-thrombotic' neurological features? What of the patient with severe, recurrent headaches who has antiphospholipid antibodies but who has not had a previous thrombosis. It is a common observation that warfarin treatment when finally given (for example, for a deep vein thrombosis) results in dramatic improvement in headache. Recently, we have introduced a 'clinical trial' of heparin in this situation. A two week trial of self administered heparin (for example, Fragmin 5000 units daily) is both safe, and, in our preliminary studies, has provided a clear indication (for example, immediate disappearance of the headaches) as to whether anticoagulation might be suitable.[5,14] We are involved in a prospective controlled trial of this treatment in APS associated headache and migraine.

Research and speculation

Epidemiology

APS (Hughes' syndrome) may well prove to be a much more common neurological diagnosis than hitherto realised. Multicentre studies are now in progress in migraine, multiple sclerosis, memory loss, epilepsy, and stroke clinics. The observation that some patients have strong family histories of APS features (especially migraine) suggests that genetic studies should broaden the clinical spectrum beyond 'classical' cases.

Why the brain?

The 20 year experience of the syndrome has shown that the central nervous system appears to be particularly at risk. The reasons (if this observation proves correct) are uncertain. However, interactions between brain and clotting processes have a long history.

The coagulation mechanism within the central nervous system has clear differences from that found in other organs. For example, the brain endothelium expresses little thrombomodulin, unlike other endothelial surfaces. While some experimental work has suggested that antiphospholipid antibodies may have direct antineuronal ties, at the present time the available evidence suggests that the major underlying mechanism in the cerebral features of Hughes' syndrome is either vascular thrombosis or sludging.

Future trends

As imaging techniques improve, so presumably will the diagnostic yield. Conventional magnetic resonance imaging may be normal in some cases of classical APS (as in the case presented at the beginning of this review).

The standard blood tests – anticardiolipin and lupus anticoagulant – are reasonably standardised internationally, but do have limitations. To date, the addition of other tests such as IgA anticardiolipin, anti-β2 GP1, antiprothrombin, and antiphosphatidyl serine, for example, have not added much in the way of further clinical definition.[15]

Health economics

The links between APS and stroke, migraine, and epilepsy are well established. The links between APS and memory loss and between APS and multiple sclerosis are recognised but require further validation. In any event the diagnosis of this prothrombotic condition, and its response to anticoagulation, has major therapeutic and economic implications.

Up to one in five of all strokes in the under 45 year olds are associated with APS and are potentially preventable. The economic cost of strokes per annum in the UK has been estimated at £2.3 billion and in the USA at £23 billion. More frequent and earlier diagnosis of APS and precise anticoagulant therapy could have an impact on these costs, both economic and human.

Acknowledgement

This review is based on a lecture given at the 6th European Lupus Congress, May 2002.

References

1 Narvarreta MG, Boey RL, Levine SR. Cerebral disease in the antiphospholipid syndrome. In: Khamashta MA, ed. *Hughes syndrome: antiphospholipid syndrome*. London: Springer-Verlag, 2000: 43–58.

2 Hughes GRV. Thrombosis, abortion, cerebral disease and the lupus anticoagulant. *BMJ* 1983; **287**: 1088–9.

3 Khamashta MA. Hughes syndrome: history. In: Khamashta MA, ed. *Hughes syndrome: antiphospholipid syndrome*. London: Springer-Verlag, 2000: 3–7.

4 Harris EN, Gharavi AE, Asherson RA, *et al*. Cerebral infarction in systemic lupus. Association with anticardiolipin antibodies. *Clin Exp Rheumatol* 1984; **2**: 47–51.

5 Cuadrado MJ, Khamashta MA, Hughes GRV. Sticky blood and headache. *Lupus* 2001; 10: 392–3.

6 Cuadrado MJ, Khamashta MA, Hughes GRV. Migraine and stroke in young women. *Q J Med* 2002; **93**: 317–19.

7 Hughes GRV. Off the beaten track: a clinician's view. In: Khamashta MA, ed. *Hughes syndrome: the antiphospholipid syndrome*. London: Springer-Verlag, 2000: 105–10.

8 Mackworth-Young CG, Hughes GRV. Epilepsy: an early symptom of SLE. *J Neurol Neurosurg Psychiatry* 1985; **48**: 185.

9 Peltola JT, Haapala A, Isojarvi JI, *et al*. Antiphospholipid and antinuclear antibodies in patients with epilepsy or new-onset seizure disorders. *Am J Med* 2000; **109**: 712–17.

10 Blank M, Krause I, Shoenfeld Y. The contribution of experimental models to our understanding of etiology, pathogenesis and novel therapies in the antiphospholipid syndrome. In: Khamashta MA, ed. *Hughes syndrome: antiphospholipid syndrome*. London: Springer-Verlag, 2000: 379–90.

11 Cuadrado MJ, Khamashta MA, Ballesteros A, *et al*. Can Hughes (antiphospholipid) syndrome be distinguished from multiple sclerosis? Analysis of 27 patients and review of the literature. *Medicine (Baltimore)* 2002; **79**: 57–68.

12 Shah MN, Khamashta MA, Atsumi T, *et al*. Outcome of patients with anticardiolipin antibodies: a ten year follow-up of 52 patients. *Lupus* 1998; 7: 3–6.

13 Khamashta MA, Cuadrado MJ, Mujic F, *et al.* The management of thrombosis in the antiphospholipid antibody syndrome. *N Engl J Med* 1995; **332**: 993–7.

14 Cuadrado MJ, Khamashta MA, D'Cruz D, *et al.* Migraine in Hughes syndrome – heparin as a therapeutic trial. *Q J Med* 2001; **94**: 114–15.

15 Bertolaccini ML, Atsumi T, Escudero A, *et al.* The value of IgA antiphospholipid testing for the diagnosis of antiphospholipid (Hughes) syndrome in SLE. *J Rheumatol* 2001; **28**: 2637–43.

Chapter Eighteen

Chronic subdural haematoma in the elderly

V Adhiyaman, M Asghar, KN Ganeshram and BK Bhowmick

Chronic subdural haematoma is predominantly a disease of the elderly. It usually follows a minor trauma. A history of direct trauma to the head is absent in up to half the cases. The common manifestations are altered mental state and focal neurological deficit. Neurological state at the time of diagnosis is the most important prognostic factor. Morbidity and mortality is higher in the elderly but outcome is good in patients who undergo neurosurgical intervention.

Chronic subdural haematoma (CSDH) is an encapsulated collection of old blood, mostly or totally liquefied and located between the dura mater and arachnoid. It was first described by Virchow in 1857 as 'pachymeningitis haemorrhagica interna'. Later Trotter put forward the theory of trauma to the bridging veins as a cause of what he named 'subdural haemorrhagic cyst'. Since then trauma has been recognised as an important factor in the development of CSDH. CSDH should be differentiated from acute subdural haematoma. Acute subdural haematomas generally occur in younger adults, after a major trauma, often associated with structural brain injury, and present within 72 hours. In contrast, CSDHs often occur in the elderly after a trivial injury without any damage to the underlying brain and usually there is a period of weeks to months before it becomes clinically evident. It has a peak incidence in the sixth and seventh decade of life. Fogelholm and Waltimo estimated an incidence of 1.72/100 000 per year, the incidence increasing steeply with advancing age up to 7.35/100 000 per year in the age group 70–79.[1] This incidence is expected to rise further due to the continuing growth of the older population.

Risk factors

It has long been recognised that the elderly are more likely to develop subdural haematoma, particularly from minor trauma. Generalised cerebral atrophy and increased venous fragility associated with ageing are the major predisposing factors. With ageing, the mass of the brain decreases leading to an increase in the space between the brain and the skull from 6% to 11% of the total intracranial space. This causes stretching of the bridging veins and the greater movement of the brain within the cranium makes these veins vulnerable to trauma.[2,3]

275

Trauma is an important factor in the development of CSDH. However, a history of head injury (direct trauma) is absent in about 30–50% of the cases. Indirect trauma seems to be more important. About half the patients have a history of fall but without hitting their head on the ground.[4,5] In many situations the trauma is so trivial that it is forgotten. Other predisposing factors include anticoagulation, alcoholism, epilepsy, bleeding diathesis, low intracranial pressure secondary to dehydration or after the removal of cerebrospinal fluid, and receiving renal dialysis, presumably due to platelet dysfunction.[3] As many as 24% of patients with CSDH are on warfarin or an antiplatelet drug;[6] 5–10% have a history of alcoholism and epilepsy.

Box 18.1 Risk factors

- Advancing age.
- Fall.
- Head injury.
- Anticoagulants/antiplatelet drugs.
- Bleeding diatheses.
- Alcohol.
- Epilepsy.
- Low intracranial pressure.
- Haemodialysis.

Pathophysiology

The initial trauma to the bridging veins results in haemorrhage in to the subdural space. A day after the haemorrhage, the outer surface of the haematoma is covered by a thin layer of fibrin and fibroblasts. Migration and proliferation of the fibroblasts leads to formation of a membrane over the clot by the fourth day. The outer membrane progressively enlarges and the fibroblasts invade the haematoma and form a thin membrane during the next two weeks.[7] Liquefaction of the haematoma occurs due to the presence of phagocytes. Then the haematoma may either resorb spontaneously or slowly increase in size resulting in a CSDH.

Two major theories have been proposed to explain the growth of a CSDH – namely, the osmotic theory and the theory of recurrent bleeding from the haematoma capsule. Osmotic theory was based on the hypothesis that the liquefaction of the haematoma increases the protein content and oncotic pressure in the encapsulated fluid. This attracts fluid from the neighbouring vessels into the cavity due to osmotic pressure gradient across the semipermeable membrane (haematoma capsule).[8] However, this theory was disproved by Weir, who demonstrated that the osmolality of the haematoma fluid was identical to that of blood and cerebrospinal fluid.[9]

Recurrent bleeding from the haematoma capsule is the proved and more widely accepted theory. The haematoma capsule has been shown to have abnormal and dilated blood vessels, the source of haemorrhage.[10] This theory was supported by the study done by Ito *et al.* They administered ^{51}Cr-labelled red cells intravenously six to 24 hours before the evacuation of haematoma and demonstrated that it contained 0.2–28% of fresh blood.[11] Also increased fibrinolytic activity and coagulation abnormalities have been demonstrated within the CSDH. This may also play a part in the expansion of CSDH.[3]

The intracranial pressure is usually normal or only slightly increased. The atrophied brain and lack of tamponading effect contributes to the gradual expansion of CSDH. The nature of the subdural collection may vary between watery, altered blood and fresh blood clots, depending on the age of the CSDH and the frequency of recurrent haemorrhages. Onset of symptoms may be delayed by weeks or even months. Because of the many ways in which CSDH can present, it has been described as 'the great neurological imitator'.[12]

Common presentations

Altered mental state

The most common presentation in the elderly (50–70%) is altered mental state.[12–14] It may manifest as varying degrees of confusion, drowsiness, or coma. Acute delirium may be very difficult to differentiate from behavioural or psychotic symptoms. Some patients are even considered to be suffering from major psychiatric illness because of depressive and paranoid symptoms. Also the diagnosis may be very easy to miss in patients with psychiatric or neurological illnesses in whom any change in behaviour or functional state is usually attributed to their pre-existing illness.[15] In the era before computed tomography, a post-mortem study on 200 psychiatric patients revealed 14 subdural haematomas of which only one had been diagnosed in life.[16]

Focal neurological deficit

Hemiparesis was found in 58% of cases in one series.[13] Weakness of the limbs is usually mild but drowsiness is out of proportion to the degree of neurological deficit. Mostly the deficit is contralateral but there are reports of ipsilateral symptoms. Direct pressure on the cerebral hemisphere is thought to be the underlying mechanism. Fluctuating neurological symptoms are uncommon and usually the symptoms start insidiously and progress gradually.[5,13]

Headache

The incidence of headache varies in different studies ranging from 14% to 80%.[6,17] It is less common in the elderly when compared with a younger patient.[17] It is partly due to the large available intracranial space for the haematoma to accommodate before creating pressure on the adjacent brain. Another reason is the earlier onset of confusion, which attracts medical attention before the development of headache in the elderly.

Falls

Interestingly, falls have been reported to be a very common presenting symptom (74%) in a recent prospective study involving 43 elderly patients.[6] It is a well-known fact that recurrent fall is a significant risk factor for CSDH. Development of

CSDH may lead to recurrent falls or increase the frequency of falls due to altered mental state, neurological deficits, and postural disturbances.

Seizures

Epilepsy is traditionally thought to be a rare presentation, even though it has been reported in up to 6% of cases as an initial symptom.[13] In patients with known epilepsy increasing frequency of seizures has been noted with the development of CSDH. Simple partial seizure has been reported as a sole manifestation of CSDH, and this could be easily mistaken for a transient ischaemic attack.[18] Seizures usually occur in the presence of a large haematoma associated with focal neurological deficit.

Transient neurological deficits

Transient neurological deficits (TND) do not always imply cerebral ischaemia. The incidence of CSDH presenting with TND varies from 1% to 12%.[19] The most common symptom is disturbance in language and the most frequent sign is hemiplegia or hemisensory deficit. An interesting case of intermittent paraparesis due to bilateral CSDH resolving completely after drainage has been reported.[20] The mechanisms proposed to explain TND in CSDH are intermittent mechanical pressure on the neighbouring vessels, transient increase in parenchymal swelling causing vascular displacement and ischaemia, small repeated haemorrhages in the subdural space, seizure activity with postictal deficits, and spreading cortical depression.[21,22]

Atypical (uncommon) presentations

Isolated neurological deficits

Patients presenting with vertigo and nystagmus, upward gaze palsy, and isolated oculomotor palsy due to CSDH have been reported.[23–25] Increased intracranial pressure causing uncal herniation and stretching of cranial nerves was thought to be the mechanism involved.

Extrapyramidal syndromes

CSDH causing parkinsonian symptoms is a well recognised phenomenon.[26] In a review of 20 cases the haematoma was found to be bilateral in nine and marked improvements were seen in most patients after surgical drainage. Reversible akinetic-rigid syndrome due to bilateral CSDH with complete resolution after surgery has also been reported.[27] The mechanisms suggested are pressure on the basal ganglia, compression of midbrain, and circulatory disturbances in the basal ganglia caused by displacement and compression of anterior choroidal artery.

Rare neurological syndromes

Gerstmann's syndrome (right-left disorientation, finger agnosia, agraphia, and acalculia) and progressive quadriparesis due to CSDH has been reported in the literature.[28,29] These patients made a good recovery after the evacuation of haematoma.

Ease of falling

'Ease of falling' syndrome refers to acute onset contralateral postural deficit secondary to a lesion in the basal ganglia. It is usually associated with small ischaemic lesions. The falls are contralateral slow tilting motion either laterally or diagonally backwards. The patient shows a lack of awareness and does not make postural adjustments to avoid the fall. Wali has described a case of subdural haematoma presenting as 'ease of falling' syndrome which resolved completely after treatment.[30]

Box 18.2   Presentations of CSDH

Common presentations
- Altered mental state.
- Focal neurological deficit.
- Headache.
- Falls.
- Seizures.
- Transient neurological deficits.

Atypical presentations
- Isolated neurological deficits.
- Extrapyramidal syndromes.
- Rare neurological syndromes.
- Ease of falling.

Diagnosis

The diagnosis of a CSDH is not usually suspected at the time of initial presentation in majority of cases. In a series of 194 cases (in 1979), CSDH was suspected only in 28% of patients.[13] Other suspected diagnoses at the time of presentation include tumour (27%), subarachnoid haemorrhage (10%), and cerebrovascular accident (6%). However, in our recent study involving 40 patients (unpublished data), cerebrovascular accident was the most common initial diagnosis (48%) followed by CSDH (20%) and others including tumour (32%).

The most important step in the diagnosis of CSDH is a high index of suspicion. It should be considered in any patient with or without a history of trauma presenting with:

1 a change in mental status or worsening of pre-existent neurological or psychological illness
2 focal neurological deficit and
3 headache with or without focal neurological deficit.

Computed tomography of the brain should be strongly considered in these patients to exclude a CSDH.

In the era before computed tomography, the diagnosis was usually made by angiography or diagnostic burr holes. The advent of computed tomography has made a major impact on the radiological diagnosis of CSDH and nowadays most of the cases are diagnosed on cranial computed tomography. A CSDH is a dynamic lesion and its appearance on computed tomography is dependent on its age (*see* Figures 18.1 and 18.2). Soon after a haemorrhage (acute phase), the haematoma looks hyperdense when compared with the normal brain, due to the presence of fresh blood. During the next few weeks (subacute phase) resolution occurs due to fibrinolysis so the haematoma appears isodense. After about four weeks (chronic phase) it appears hypodense due to the resorption of fluid.[2] However, repeated microhaemorrhages into a CSDH can increase the density, giving rise to a heterogeneous or a hyperdense picture. So classification of CSDH based on the appearance on computed tomography is far from reliable.[31]

Hyperdense haematoma can be readily recognised but an isodense haematoma may be difficult to visualise on the computed tomogram. A specific finding is the displacement of the brain parenchyma away from the skull and the usual convex border appears flattened or even concave. Also several other indirect features due to the displacement of the brain – for example, effacement of the sulci, compression of the ipsilateral ventricle leading to midline shift, deformity of the normal ventricular anatomy, and obliteration of the basal cisterns – could aid in the diagnosis. Bilateral haematomas may lead to medial compression of both ventricles resulting in a narrow, slit-like elongated ventricle (so called 'squeezed ventricle' or 'rabbit's ears'). If in doubt, a contrast computed tomogram may show displacement of cortical vessels and a delayed scan may reveal accumulation of contrast material in the subdural collection.[2,32,33]

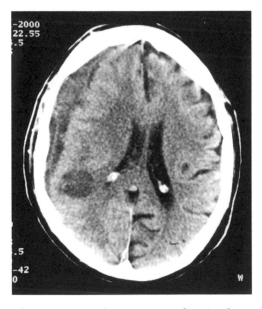

Figure 18.1 Computed tomogram without contrast showing large right CSDH extending from the frontal lobe to the parietal lobe with blood in the lateral ventricles. There is mass effect with effacement of the sulci, compression of the cerebral hemisphere and midline shift to the left.

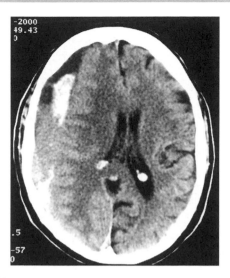

Figure 18.2 Computed tomogram with contrast reveals recent haemorrhage giving a non-homogenous appearance of CSDH in the same patient.

However, magnetic resonance imaging (MRI) scan may be required in patients with isodense haematoma without midline shift and in identifying small collections at the vertex, base of the skull, and in the posterior fossa.[34-36] It has been clearly shown that MRI is better than computed tomography in identifying small and transversely oriented collections where the computed tomogram has failed to identify a collection in as much as 80% of cases.[37] Even though some of these lesions may not need surgical intervention, they have significant therapeutic implications such as prevention of anticoagulation in these patients.

Even though MRI has advantages, computed tomography remains the procedure of choice in the acute setting because of shorter examination time, which is important in acutely ill patients, reliability in identifying other parenchymal lesions, no magnetic interference (especially in patients on life support machines) and the ready availability.

Box 18.3   Diagnosis of CSDH should be suspected if there is:

- Change in mental state.
- Worsening of pre-existent neurological/psychological illness.
- Focal neurological deficit.
- Headache.

Management

Treatment of CSDH is by surgical evacuation, although small haematomas may resolve spontaneously.[38] A recent study has shown that 23% of the patients did not warrant surgery because the haematoma was small.[6] Patients treated conservatively should be carefully monitored and the scan should be repeated if there is a clinical deterioration. Some studies have shown that concurrent use of high dose steroids accelerates the resolution of subdural collection.[39] But these studies were done in the 1970s involving a small number of patients and there is no strong evidence to advocate the routine use of steroids in CSDH.

The commonly followed surgical procedures include drainage by twist drill/ burr hole craniostomy or craniotomy. Twist drill trephination was associated with lower mortality rate, reoperation rate, and duration of inpatient stay compared with burr hole craniostomy.[40] Craniotomy is usually reserved for those patients in whom there is reaccumulation with recurrence of symptoms or where there is a solid haematoma. Recently Reinges and colleagues have described a less invasive bedside technique for treating CSDH.[41] They performed twist drill craniostomy under local anaesthesia and drained the fluid through a cannula by gravity. The procedure was repeated if reaccumulation occurred and it was done up to five times in unilateral haematoma and up to 10 times in bilateral haematoma. If there was no improvement, insufficient evacuation or development of subdural empyema, they proceeded to burr hole evacuation or craniotomy (9% of patients). With very low complication rates and good results, they recommend this minimally invasive procedure especially for severely ill patients. However, wider acceptance of this treatment remains to be seen.[42]

Complications

The following complications are encountered in addition to the usual post-operative problems such as infection and inappropriate secretion of antidiuretic hormone.

Recurrence

Reaccumulation of the haematoma is the most common postoperative problem. Residual fluid can be detected on computed tomography in as many as 80% of the patients, a majority of them asymptomatic and clinically insignificant. Symptomatic recurrence has been noted in 8–37% of postoperative patients.[3] It usually occurs in 4 days to 4 weeks with an average interval of 12 days. Clinical deterioration with radiological evidence brings attention to this condition. It is more common in the elderly and inadequate expansion of the brain following the evacuation of the haematoma is thought to play a part.

Seizures

Around 11% of patients develop seizures after surgery. Patients with a previous history of epilepsy are at particular risk to develop postoperative seizures. It has been recommended that prophylactic anticonvulsants should be started pre-operatively and continued for six months.[14]

Tension pneumocephalus

Development of tension pneumocephalus after burr hole evacuation of CSDH is a rare postoperative complication. The chronically compressed brain is thought to contribute to the ingression of intracranial air. The slow re-expansion of the brain and trapped subdural air leads to increase in intracranial pressure leading to neurological deterioration. This complication has been reported in as many as 8% of patients after surgical intervention.[43] Craniostomy and aspiration is the usual treatment.

Prognosis

The morbidity and mortality in CSDH varies widely in the literature. The overall in-hospital mortality during index admission was found to be 15.6% for patients with CSDH in a large series involving 157 patients.[5] However, the outcome is good in patients who undergo neurosurgical intervention where the morbidity and mortality after surgery is around 16% and 6.5% respectively.[44] The significant difference is due to the fact that critically ill patients are not considered fit for surgery resulting in a higher overall mortality.

In a recent prospective study of 43 patients, only 16 (37%) were able to undergo surgical intervention, four were too ill, and one died soon after the scan. The rest of the patients were treated conservatively for either the haematoma was small (10 patients) or for other reasons not clearly identified in the study.[6] Six month mortality was 31% (13 patients) of which only one death occurred in the operated group. In patients who died, CSDH was the direct cause of death in half and the rest were due to underlying disease.

Neurological status at the time of diagnosis is the most significant prognostic factor.[5] The influence of age on the morbidity and mortality is controversial and several studies have shown no relationship with age.[2] However in a multivariate model, increasing age was significantly associated with mortality, but its contribution was small compared with the level of consciousness.[5] In general, morbidity and mortality increase with advancing age and a major contributing factor to a poorer prognosis is frailty and the presence of multiple concomitant medical problems.[2,44]

Box 18.4   Key references

- Jones S, Kafetz K. A prospective study of chronic subdural haematomas in elderly patients. *Age Ageing* 1999; **28**: 519–21.
- Rozzelle CJ, Wofford JL, Branch CL. Predictors of hospital mortality in older patients with subdural haematoma. *J Am Geriatr Soc* 1995; **43**: 240–4.
- Traynelis VC. Chronic subdural haematoma in the elderly. *Clin Geriatr Med* 1991; **7**: 583–98.
- Luxon LM, Harrison MJG. Chronic subdural haematoma. *Q J Med* 1979; **189**: 43–53.
- Cameron MM. Chronic subdural haematoma: a review of 114 cases. *J Neurol Neurosurg Psychiatry* 1978; **41**: 834–9.

Questions

True/false – answers can be found at the end of 'References'.
1.   The following are risk factors for CSDH:
(A) Advancing age.
(B) Antidepressants.

(C) Aspirin.
(D) Falls.

2. The following statements are true in CSDH:
(A) Occurs after a trivial injury.
(B) Associated with brain contusion and damage.
(C) Evident soon after injury.
(D) Mechanism involves trauma to the bridging veins.

3. The common presenting features of CSDH in the elderly are:
(A) Fluctuating neurological weakness.
(B) Drowsiness.
(C) Headache.
(D) Falls.

4. The uncommon manifestations of CSDH are:
(A) Diplopia.
(B) Ataxia.
(C) Parkinson's disease.
(D) Transient ischaemic attack.

5. The diagnosis of CSDH should be suspected in patients with:
(A) Increasing confusion.
(B) Recurrent falls.
(C) Neurological deficit.
(D) Rapidly worsening extrapyramidal symptoms.

6. The important prognostic factors are:
(A) Age.
(B) Clinical picture at the time of diagnosis.
(C) Coexistent medical problems.
(D) Bilateral haematoma.

References

1 Fogelholm R, Waltimo O. Epidemiology of chronic subdural haematoma. *Acta Neurochir* 1975; **32**: 247–50.
2 Ellis GL. Subdural haematoma in the elderly. *Emerg Med Clin North Am* 1990; **8**: 281–94.
3 Traynelis VC. Chronic subdural haematoma in the elderly. *Clin Geriatr Med* 1991; **7**: 583–98.
4 Feldman RG, Pincus JH, McEntee WJ. Cerebrovascular accident or subdural fluid collection? *Arch Intern Med* 1963; **112**: 966–76.
5 Rozzelle CJ, Wofford JL, Branch CL. Predictors of hospital mortality in older patients with subdural haematoma. *J Am Geriatr Soc* 1995; **43**: 240–4.
6 Jones S, Kafetz K. A prospective study of chronic subdural haematomas in elderly patients. *Age Ageing* 1999; **28**: 519–21.
7 Munro D, Merritt HH. Surgical pathology of subdural haematoma: based on a study of one hundred and five cases. *Arch Neurol Psych* 1936; **35**: 64–78.
8 Gardner WJ. Traumatic subdural haematoma with particular reference to the latent interval. *Arch Neurol Psych* 1932; **27**: 847–58.

9 Weir B. The osmolality of subdural haematoma fluid. *J Neurosurg* 1971; **34**: 528–33.

10 Sato S, Suzuki J. Ultrastructural observations of the capsule of chronic subdural haematoma in various clinical stages. *J Neurosurg* 1975; **43**: 569–78.

11 Ito H, Yamamoto S, Saito K, *et al*. Quantitative estimation of haemorrhage in chronic subdural haematoma using the ^{51}Cr erythrocyte labeling method. *J Neurosurg* 1987; **66**: 862–64.

12 Potter JF, Fruin AH. Chronic subdural haematoma – 'the great imitator'. *Geriatrics* 1977; **32**: 61–6.

13 Luxon LM, Harrison MJG. Chronic subdural haematoma. *Q J Med* 1979; **189**: 43–53.

14 Cameron MM. Chronic subdural haematoma: a review of 114 cases. *J Neurol Neurosurg Psychiatry* 1978; **41**: 834–9.

15 Henderson MJ. A difficult psychiatric patient. *Postgrad Med J* 2000; **76**: 585, 590–1.

16 Cole G. Intracranial space occupying lesions in mental hospital patients: necropsy study. *J Neurol Neurosurg Psychiatry* 1978; **41**: 730–6.

17 Fogelholm R, Heiskanen O, Waltimo O. Chronic subdural haematoma in adults; influence of patient's age on symptoms, signs, and thickness of hematoma. *J Neurosurg* 1975; **42**: 43–6.

18 Hilt DC, Alexander GE. Jacksonian somatosensory seizures as the sole manifestation of chronic subdural hematoma. *Arch Neurol* 1982; **39**: 786.

19 Moster ML, Johnston DE, Reinmuth OM. Chronic subdural haematoma with transient neurologic deficits: a review of 15 cases. *Ann Neurol* 1983; **14**: 539–42.

20 Schaller B, Radziwill AJ, Wasner M, *et al*. Intermittent paraparesis as manifestation of chronic subdural haematoma [German]. *Schweiz Med Wochenschr* 1999; **129**: 1067–72.

21 Melamed E, Lavy S, Reches A, *et al*. Chronic subdural hematoma simulating transient cerebral ischemic attacks. *J Neurosurg* 1975; **42**: 101–3.

22 Welsh JE, Tyson GW, Winn HR, *et al*. Chronic subdural hematoma presenting as transient neurologic deficits. *Stroke* 1979; **10**: 564–7.

23 Ashkenazi E, Pomeranz S. Nystagmus as the presentation of tentorial incisure subdural haematoma. *J Neurol Neurosurg Psychiatry* 1994; **57**: 830–1.

24 Phookan G, Cameron M. Bilateral chronic subdural haematoma: an unusual presentation with isolated oculomotor nerve palsy (letter). *J Neurol Neurosurg Psychiatry* 1994; **57**: 1146.

25 Sandyk R. Isolated failure of upward gaze as a sign of chronic subdural haematoma (letter). *S Afr Med J* 1982; **61**: 32.

26 Sunada I, Inoue T, Tamura K, *et al*. Parkinsonism due to chronic subdural haematoma. *Neurol Med Chir (Tokyo)* 1996; **36**: 99–101.

27 Abdulla AJJ, Pearce VR. Reversible akinetic-rigid syndrome due to bilateral subdural haematomas (letter). *Age Ageing* 1999; **28**: 582–3.

28 Maeshima S, Okumura Y, Nakai K, *et al*. Gerstmann's syndrome associated with chronic subdural haematoma. *Brain Inj* 1998; **12**: 697–701.

29 Lesoin F, Destee A, Jomin M, *et al*. Quadriparesis as an unusual manifestation of chronic subdural haematoma. *J Neurol Neurosurg Psychiatry* 1983; **46**: 783–5.

30 Wali GM. 'Ease of falling' syndrome associated with subdural haematoma (letter). *J Neurol Neurosurg Psychiatry* 1994; **57**: 1144–5.

31 Lee K, Bae W, Bae H, *et al*. The computed tomographic attenuation and the age of subdural haematomas. *J Korean Med Sci* 1997; **12**: 353–9.

32 Karasawa H, Tomita S, Suzuki S. Chronic subdural haematomas: time density curve and iodine concentrations in enhanced CT. *Neuroradiology* 1987; **29**: 36–9.

33 Kim KS, Hemmati M, Weinberg P. Computed tomography in isodense subdural haematoma. *Radiology* 1978; **128**: 71–4.

34 Hosoda K, Tamaki N, Masumura M, *et al*. Magnetic resonance images of chronic subdural hematoma. *J Neurosurg* 1987; **67**: 677–83.

35 Snow RB, Zimmerman RD, Gandy SE, *et al*. Comparison of magnetic resonance imaging and computed tomography in the evaluation of head injury. *Neurosurgery* 1986; **18**: 45–52.

36 Han J, Kaufman B, Alfidi RJ, *et al*. Head trauma evaluated by magnetic resonance and computed tomography: a comparison. *Radiology* 1984; **150**: 71–7.

37 Kelly AB, Zimmerman RD, Snow RB, *et al*. Head trauma: comparison of MR and CT experience in 100 patients. *Am J Neuroradiol* 1988; **9**: 699–708.

38 Naganuma H, Fukamachi A, Kawakami M, *et al*. Spontaneous resolution of chronic subdural hematomas. *Neurosurgery* 1986; **19**: 794–8.

39 Bender MB, Christoff N. Nonsurgical treatment of subdural hematomas. *Arch Neurol* 1974; **31**: 73–9.

40 Smely C, Madlinger A, Scheremet R. Chronic subdural haematoma – a comparison between two different treatment modalities. *Acta Neurochir (Wien)* 1997; **139**: 818–26.

41 Reinges MHT, Hasselberg I, Rhode V, *et al*. Prospective analysis of bedside percutaneous tapping for the treatment of chronic subdural haematoma in adults. *J Neurol Neurosurg Psychiatry* 2000; **69**: 40–7.

42 Maurice-Williams RS. Bedside treatment of chronic subdural haematoma? *Lancet* 2001; **357**: 1308–9.

43 Sharma BS, Tewari MK, Khosla VK, *et al*. Tension pneumocephalus following evacuation chronic subdural haematoma. *Br J Neurosurg* 1989; **3**: 381–7.

44 Van Havenberg T, van Calenbergh F, Goffin J, *et al*. Outcome of chronic subdural haematoma: analysis of prognostic factors. *Br J Neurosurg* 1996; **10**: 35–9.

Answers

T= True/F = False
1 (A) T, (B) F, (C) T, (D) T
2 (A) T, (B) F, (C) F, (D) T
3 (A) F, (B) T, (C) T, (D) T
4 (A) T, (B) T, (C) T, (D) F
5 (A) T, (B) T, (C) T, (D) T
6 (A) T, (B) T, (C) T, (D) F

Chapter Nineteen

Management of stroke

R McGovern and AG Rudd

This article outlines the current evidence-based practice for stroke care. It outlines many of the recommendations in the National Clinical Guidelines for Stroke published by the Royal College of Physicians. It also covers all aspects of multidisciplinary stroke care from initial assessment and acute treatment to rehabilitation strategies and management of complications. The article concludes with an examination of the latest evidence for secondary prevention of cerebrovascular disease.

The profile of stroke care in the UK is increasing with several factors contributing to the change. Firstly, in March 2000, the Royal College of Physicians published its National Clinical Guidelines for Stroke.[1] The stimulus for the guidelines came from evidence provided by National Sentinel Audit of Stroke[2] and a Clinical Standards Advisory Group report,[3] confirming suboptimal stroke care.

The second contributing factor is renewed government awareness of the importance of stroke given that stroke is the third highest cause of death in the UK, is the biggest single cause of major disability, and uses 4% of the total annual NHS expenditure. The first government initiative came in 1999, when the Department of Health published *Saving Lives: Our Healthier Nation*.[4] The government made reduction in death from coronary heart disease and stroke in people aged less than 75 years one of the four priority areas and set a target to reduce death in this area by 40% between 1997 and 2010. This was followed by the National Service Framework for Older People in 2001, which included a section dedicated to stroke management (standard 5).[5] This standard, when implemented, will ensure that stroke patients have prompt access to diagnostic services, are treated by a specialist stroke service, and participate in a multidisciplinary rehabilitation programme.

The final factor is the growing evidence base, built up particularly over the last decade, which informs all aspects of stroke care from acute treatment to long-term rehabilitation.

Royal College of Physicians' Guidelines

Many of the recommendations made in this article are derived from the National Clinical Guidelines for Stroke published by the Royal College of Physicians (London) in March 2000 and updated in February 2002. The guidelines cover the management of patients with acute stroke from onset, through rehabilitation, to the longer term. They are evidence-based and each recommendation is accompanied by both a level of evidence (Ia–IV) and grade of recommendation (A–C) (*see* Table 19.1).

They are available in book format from the Royal College of Physicians and can be downloaded from the college's home page at www.rcplondon.ac.uk. The Scottish Intercollegiate Guidelines Network has also published guidelines on specific aspects of stroke care and these are currently being updated with the expectation that they will be available within the next 12 months on www.sign.ac.uk.[6]

Diagnosis

The World Health Organization (WHO) definition (1978) defines stroke as a clinical syndrome typified by rapidly developing signs of focal or global disturbance of cerebral functions, lasting more than 24 hours or leading to death, with no apparent causes other than of vascular origin. A senior clinician should review all patients admitted with presumed stroke to clinically confirm diagnosis (B).[7] Care is needed in younger stroke patients (age <45) or if there is any unusual feature such as unexplained fever, severe headache, or gradual progression of signs. The consensus guidelines and the National Service Framework state that brain imaging should be undertaken within 48 hours of stroke; however, imaging should be undertaken urgently in the following situations – depressed level of consciousness, fluctuating symptoms, papilloedema, neck stiffness, fever, severe headache, previous trauma, anticoagulant treatment, or bleeding diathesis (B).[1]

How should care be delivered?

Trials of stroke units have compared conventional care with a variety of services labelled as 'stroke units'. There are, however, certain features that all these services have in common. The stroke service should be centred in a hospital-based stroke unit. It should be staffed by a multidisciplinary team with expertise in stroke care and rehabilitation (A).[8] The team should work to agreed protocols for common problems (A)[9] and provide educational programmes for staff, patients, and carers (A).[10] The Royal College of Physicians' guidelines strongly recom-

Table 19.1 Type of evidence and grade of recommendation from Royal College of Physicians' guidelines

Type of evidence	Grade of recommendation
Meta-analyses of randomised controlled trials *or* at least one RCT	A
Well designed controlled study but without randomisation *or* well designed quasiexperimental study *or* well designed descriptive study	B
Expert committee reports, opinions *and/or* experience of respected authorities	C

RCT, randomised controlled trial.

mended that the WHO's international classification of impairments, disabilities, and handicaps terminology be used.

Where should care be delivered?

All patients with stroke should be admitted to hospital (A) unless they present late and have few or no residual symptoms. The evidence for organised inpatient (stroke unit) stroke care is robust and the Stroke Unit Trialists' Collaboration showed that compared with alternatives, stroke unit care showed reductions in the odds of death recorded at follow-up (odds ratio (OR) 0.86; 95% confidence interval (CI) 0.71 to 0.94; p=0.005). The odds of death or institutionalised care and death or dependencies were also significantly reduced. Outcomes were independent of patient age, sex, and stroke severity and appeared to be better in stroke units based in a geographically discrete ward. There was no indication that organised stroke unit care resulted in increased hospital stay[8] and it is likely to be cost saving. Stroke units have also been shown to be superior to other forms of organised stroke care. In a study where patients were randomly assigned to stroke unit care, general wards with stroke team support, or domiciliary stroke care, mortality and institutionalisation rates at one year were lower in patients who received care on the stroke ward.[11] The benefits of stroke unit care have been shown to persist at 10 years after initial stroke.[12]

Early supported discharge from hospital to a specialist rehabilitation team providing care in the patient's own home has been shown to be feasible for selected patients, with clinical outcomes at one year similar for the early discharge group and those who remained in hospital (A).[13,14] The early discharge group showed increased satisfaction with hospital care and reductions in use of hospital beds were achieved. The guidelines state that specialist stroke services can be delivered to patients after the acute phase, equally effectively in hospital or in the community provided that the patient can transfer from bed to chair before going home and that they continue to be seen by a specialised multidisciplinary stroke team (A).

There is currently no evidence from clinical trials to support a radical shift in the care of acute stroke patients from hospital-based care.[15] Patients should only be managed at home if acute assessment guidelines can be adhered to and the services organised for home are flexible, and part of a specialist stroke service (A). The guidelines do allow for the management of some patients in the community, particularly those with transient ischaemia attacks (TIAs) and strokes with good recovery. The consensus was that these patients could be managed at home provided they had access to a neurovascular clinic within two weeks (C). More than one TIA within a short period (crescendo TIA) requires admission to hospital (C). The guidelines are not prescriptive in defining a short period but the authors consider that recurrent TIAs within one week merit admission.

Carers and families

Patients and carers want to be looked after by knowledgeable staff, who understand the full range of their needs after a stroke. Unfortunately the diagnosis and management plan are not always explained in a manner that all patients and carers can comprehend and recall.[16] The guidelines recommend that families are involved in the decision making process and have input into future plans for the patient (C). A separate version of the National Clinical Guidelines, available through the Stroke Association, has been produced for patients and their carers setting out the standards that a patient should expect to receive during the course of their illness.

Caring for a stroke patient can be very difficult and emotional distress is seen in 55% of caregivers at six months after stroke.[17] Caregivers are more likely to be depressed if the patients are severely dependent or emotionally distressed themselves. The stroke team must be alert to recognising carer stress and helping carers in this difficult situation (B). Disseminating information about the nature of stroke and on relevant local and national services improves patient and carer knowledge (A).[18] The introduction of stroke family support workers has been shown to significantly increase social activities and quality of life for carers[19] and to improve patients' and carers' satisfaction in terms of communication and support.[20] Family support workers have not been shown to improve patient outcomes in term of disability, handicap, and quality of life.[19]

Acute intervention

A large number of trials have been conducted on the use of pharmacological agents in the acute phase of stroke. Few have yielded positive results despite promising data from animal models. There is insufficient evidence to support the use of any neuroprotective agents, prostacyclin analogues or methylxanthines (vasodilators), steroids, or osmostic diuretics to reduce oedema.

Patients with acute ischaemic stroke should receive aspirin (160–300 mg) as soon as possible after stroke if a diagnosis of haemorrhage is considered unlikely (A). Ideally brain imaging to rule out haemorrhage should be performed before starting aspirin. This evidence comes from two large randomised controlled trials, the International Stroke Trial (IST) and Chinese Acute Stroke Trial (CAST) involving a total of 40 000 patients. Combining data from both trials gives a significant decrease in death and dependency at six months (OR 0.94; 95% CI 0.91 to 0.98), which in absolute terms translates to 13 more patients who were alive and independent at six months for every 1000 patients treated. The increase in symptomatic intracranial haemorrhages (two per 1000 patients) is offset by the reduction in recurrences (seven per 1000 patients treated) (A).[21]

Perhaps the most exciting acute pharmacological intervention is thrombolysis. It is associated with an increase in symptomatic intracranial haemorrhages but disability is reduced in survivors. A meta-analyses of thrombolysis in acute stroke reveals that for every 1000 patients treated with thrombolysis, 44 avoided death or dependency.[22] The most promising agent is recombinant tissue plasminogen activator (rt-PA) administered intravenously within three hours of stroke onset. As compared with placebo, patients treated with rt-PA were at least 30% more likely to have minimal or no disability at three months (A).[23] However, some authors have challenged conclusions drawn from the NINDS Stroke Study Group[24] and questioned the wisdom of expanding a thrombolysis programme based on the results of one relatively small trial.[25] Information on thrombolysis is based on only 5000 patients and further knowledge on patient selection in terms of stroke severity, stroke subtype, concomitant use of antithrombotic drugs, and computed tomogram appearance is still needed. A measured approach is reflected in the Royal College of Physicians' guidelines, which state that use of thrombolysis should be restricted to a specialist centre with appropriate experience.

If the use of thrombolysis does become widely accepted in the UK there will need to be a dramatic change in the organisation of stroke services, such that they are able to deliver patients to specialist units capable of giving the drug within three hours of the onset of symptoms, having already had brain imaging and detailed clinical assessment. While thrombolysis is only ever likely to be given to a small proportion of stroke sufferers the improvements in acute stroke care that result from establishing services that are capable of giving the drug will, in the view of the authors, result in reductions in mortality and morbidity in the stroke population as a whole.

Immediate anticoagulant therapy in patients with acute ischaemic stroke is not associated with net short or long-term benefit. Although acute anticoagulant therapy is associated with about nine fewer recurrent ischaemic strokes and four fewer pulmonary emboli per 1000 patients treated, the benefit is offset with a similar sized nine per 1000 increase in symptomatic intracranial haemorrhages.[26] While there is evidence for the secondary prevention of ischaemic stroke by anticoagulating patients in atrial fibrillation,[27] immediate anticoagulation of patients with ischaemic stroke and atrial fibrillation is not beneficial.[28] The Royal College of Physicians' consensus guidelines recommend that anticoagulation should not be started until 14 days after the acute event (A).

There is evidence for acute anticoagulation in the specific stroke syndrome of cerebral venous thrombosis[29] but insufficient evidence to advise on the use of anticoagulants in other subgroups of patients such as those with vertebral occlusion or large vessel dissection. It is unlikely that such evidence will ever be sufficient, given the rarity of the conditions. The practice of the authors is currently to anticoagulate patients with dissection and those with progressive ischaemic lesions in the posterior circulation.

There have been few trials of the effect of careful maintenance of normal physiology in the acute phase of stroke. The evidence for acute lowering of blood pressure, body temperature, or administration of hyperosmolar agents such as mannitol and glycerol to reduce brain oedema is not robust enough for recommendation. However, the guidelines state it is important to keep physiological variables such as hydration, temperature, nutrition, and oxygenation within normal range in the acute phase of stroke (C). This may be achieved in an acute stroke unit. Such units are still uncommon in the UK but are well developed elsewhere in Europe. This difference may explain the comparatively better survival and impairment outcomes seen in some European centres.[30]

The guidelines are not prescriptive in detailing investigations of patients after stroke but a pragmatic approach is outlined on p 266 in *Stroke: A Practical Guide to Management* by Warlow *et al.*[31]

Rehabilitation

There is no evidence to support selection criteria for more active rehabilitation or admission to a stroke unit. If anything, those with more severe stroke have the most to gain from admission.[8] The first step in the rehabilitation of the stroke patient begins with assessment of disability. Assessment is effective in rehabilitation when, as happens in a stroke unit, it is linked to later management (A).[32] The guidelines recommend that assessments and measures with proved reliability and validity are used and that patients are assessed at appropriate intervals (C). In practical terms this requires prompt assessment of the patient's consciousness level, swallowing, nutritional status, cognition, and moving and handling needs on the stroke unit.

Dysphagia occurs in about 45% of all stroke patients admitted to hospital. It is associated with more severe strokes and with a worse outcome. Dysphagia management involving an initial swallow screen, diet modification, and compensatory swallowing techniques reduces the risk of aspiration pneumonia.[33] Patient and family instruction in the management of dysphagia has been shown to be as effective as daily therapist input,[34] although this needs to confirmed in a larger study.

Malnutrition is also common and is seen in 30% of patients one week after stroke. Routine oral or enteral protein supplementation improves nutritional indices but there is no evidence that it affects outcome.[35] In the dysphagic patient, enteral nutrition can be supplied by either nasogastric tube or percutaneous endoscopic gastrostomy. There is some evidence that percutaneous endoscopic gastrostomy feeding is superior to nasogastric feeding,[36] but its insertion requires an invasive procedure. Questions concerning the most effective nutritional route as well as the timing of nutritional intervention after stroke are being addressed in a large randomised controlled trial, the FOOD trial. Information is available at www.dcn.ed.ac.uk/food.

Stroke can affect communication and speech in a variety of ways, including impaired motor speech production (dysarthria), impaired language skills (dysphasia), and impaired planning and execution of motor speech (articulatory dyspraxia). Deficits can be subtle and every patient with a communication difficulty needs to be assessed by a speech and language therapist. Speech therapy input is effective at improving communication,[37] with short, intensive courses of speech therapy lasting 4–8 weeks proving most beneficial (B).[38]

A physiotherapist with expertise in neurodisability should coordinate treatment to improve movement performance of patients with stroke (C). The effectiveness of motor and strength rehabilitation is being underpinned by new evidence-based strategies. Task specific training, such as reaching for coins, improves the reaching ability of the impaired limb more effectively than impairment focused approaches.[39]

Resistance training significantly improved grip strength and the motor capacity of the impaired hand compared with traditional therapeutic strategies (Bobath) aimed at reducing enhanced muscle tone (B).[40] Progressive resistive exercise studies have also been shown to improve gait, strength, activity, and mood.[41] There is some evidence that increased intensity of therapist input improves outcome but some patients cannot tolerate intense therapist input. The guidelines recommend that patients receive as much as they find tolerable and at least every working day (B). It is vital that patients have the opportunity to practise rehabilitation tasks.

The aim of rehabilitation is to regain patient independence and maximise ability in all activities of daily living. The need for special equipment such as a wheelchair or adapted cutlery should be assessed on an individual basis as review by an occupational therapist with specialist knowledge in neurological disability can significantly reduce disability and handicap (B).[42] The provision of hoists or adaptation of the home environment may prevent the patient going to institutional care.

Complications

One of the challenges of stroke care and rehabilitation is the management of complications. Mood disorders are common after stroke and can be difficult to diagnose in the presence of speech disturbance. Crying after minimal provocation may be related to emotionalism. It can be diagnosed by a few simple questions and may be treated effectively with fluoxetine (A).[43] A consensus statement from the guidelines recommends that patients should be screened for anxiety and depression within the first month after stroke and their mood kept under regular review (C). Patients diagnosed with a depressive disorder should be considered for antidepressive medication, even though the evidence for efficacy is very limited.[44]

Pain after stroke varies in type, origin, and modes of treatment. Some pain is related to stroke damage and is termed neuropathic or central pain. It has been shown to respond to tricyclic antidepressants (A).[45] More often pain is mechanical arising from reduced mobility or an exacerbation of pre-existing osteoarthritis. Shoulder pain is seen in up to 30% of patients after stroke and is not as previously thought related to subluxation of the shoulder. Treatment should begin with simple analgesia and proper handling techniques. Previous evidence for shoulder strapping, steroid injection, or cutaneous electrical stimulation has not been confirmed in recent trials.

Spasticity is a motor disorder characterised by a velocity dependent increase in tonic stretch reflexes. It may lead to secondary complications such as muscle and joint contractures. In practice the management of spasticity requires several coordinated interventions including physiotherapy, drug treatment, and patient education. Physiotherapy using isokinetic strength training can improve strength and gait velocity without increasing spasticity,[46] while drug therapy with either baclofen or tinzanadine as an adjunct to physiotherapy has been shown to reduce spasticity.[47] In patients with disabling or symptomatically distressing symptoms, botulinum toxin is safe and effective[48] and can be targeted to individual muscles. The guidelines indicate that spasticity should be treated if causing symptoms, though functional benefit is uncertain (B).

Venous thrombolism is common after stroke and studies using radiolabelled fibrinogen leg scanning suggest that deep vein thrombosis occurs in up to 50% of patients with hemiplegia. The guidelines recommend that aspirin (75–300 mg daily) should be used (A) (in non-haemorrhagic strokes) and that compression stockings should be applied to patients with weak or paralysed legs (A). The final recommendation on the length of stocking to be used awaits results from the ongoing CLOTs trial.

Secondary prevention

People who have a stroke have a 30% chance of experiencing a recurrent stroke in the next five years. They are also at increased risk of myocardial infarction and other vascular events. Control of vascular risk factors is of paramount importance and strong evidence has emerged in recent years to guide our secondary prevention strategies.

All patients should have their blood pressure checked and hypertension persisting for greater than one month should be treated (A). The treatment of hypertensive stroke survivors with blood pressure therapy decreases the recurrence of fatal and non-fatal stroke by 28% (95% CI 15 to 39).[49] The target blood pressure is that recommended by the British Hypertension Society of an optimal blood pressure of systolic <140 mm Hg and diastolic <85 mm Hg.[50]

A recent study on patients with a history of stroke or TIA looked at the benefit of treating patients with antihypertensive agents independent of baseline blood pressure. Patients treated with the angiotensin converting enzyme inhibitor, perindopril and a thiazide diuretic, indapamide, had a reduction in blood pressure of 12/5 mm Hg, and reduced stroke risk by 43%. There were similar reductions in the risk of stroke in hypertensive and non-hypertensive groups.[51] Further evidence of the efficacy of angiotensin converting enzyme inhibitors comes from the Heart Outcomes Prevention Evaluation (HOPE) study. Ramipril achieved a 32% relative risk reduction in primary and secondary stroke prevention in 9297 high risk patients. Baseline blood pressure was low at 139/79 mm Hg, while reduction in blood pressure seen was only 3.8 mm Hg systolic and 2.8 mm Hg diastolic.[52] The efficacy of angiotensin converting enzyme inhibitors may be explained by their antiinflammatory properties which lead to plaque stabilisation.[53]

Patients with a previous ischaemic stroke should be started on an antiplatelet agent, aspirin (75–325 mg) daily, clopidogrel 75 mg daily, or a combination of low dose aspirin (75 mg daily) and dipyridimole modified release 200 mg twice a day (A). Where patients are intolerant of aspirin, treatment with clopidogrel or dipyridamole modified release should be instituted. In patients with prior TIA or stroke, antiplatelet therapy produced a 25% reduction in non-fatal stroke.[54] There is no clear evidence for superiority of one antiplatelet agent over another or for combination antiplatelet therapy in cerebrovascular disease, but if a patient on one antiplatelet agent experiences a recurrent stroke then our practice is to add a second antiplatelet agent.

All patients with a history of stroke and atrial fibrillation should be considered for anticoagulation (A). Anticoagulant therapy decreases the odds of recurrent stroke in patients with atrial fibrillation by two thirds (OR 0.35; 95% CI 0.22 to 0.59). In those not suitable for anticoagulation, aspirin at a dose of 300 mg is a useful but less effective alternative.[55]

The evidence for treatment of raised cholesterol comes from secondary prevention studies in patients with ischaemic heart disease. In patients with average cholesterol levels, after myocardial infarction, treatment with pravastatin led to a 27% reduction in stroke or TIA (95% CI 4% to 44%).[56] The Royal College of Physicians' guidelines recommend treatment with a statin in any patient with a history of ischaemic heart disease and a cholesterol >5 mmol/l (A), however this may be reviewed in the light of the recently published Heart Protection Study. In this study over 20 000 high risk vascular patients aged 40–80 years (including a cohort of 1820 patients with a history of non-disabling stroke or TIA) were randomised to simvastatin 40 mg daily or placebo for five years, independent of baseline cholesterol levels. Allocation to simvastatin produced a highly significant 25% (SE%; 95% CI 15 to 34) proportional reduction in the incidence rate of first stroke. The benefits were seen across all age ranges and baseline cholesterol levels.[57] A report outlining the influence of the intervention on recurrent events is being prepared.

Carotid ultrasound or magnetic resonance angiography should be considered for any patient with a carotid area stroke, minor or no residual disability, and in whom carotid endarterectomy may be appropriate. The benefits of an endarterectomy are seen in patients with a carotid artery stenosis greater than 70% (A).[58] The operation should only be carried out by a specialist with a proved low complication rate (A).

Summary

There have been major advances in recent years in the management of stroke both acutely and during rehabilitation. Secondary prevention that is effectively implemented is likely to significantly reduce the risk of stroke recurrence below levels currently seen. The National Service Framework for Older People will require a revolution in the organisation of stroke care in England, both in the hospital and the community. If this is to be achieved it will require investment. Stroke is in the process of being recognised as a subspecialty in the UK. If this leads to every district having a well trained team of stroke physicians the prospects for stroke care in the 21st century are bright.

Questions

Answers can be found at the end of 'References'.
1. National stroke guidelines are published by?
2. What are the strengths of a stroke unit?
3. Most stroke patients can be managed in the community (true/false).
4. Who should be involved in making decisions concerning the patient?
(A) The doctor only.
(B) Anybody with an opinion.
(C) Patient, carers/family members, and health care staff.
5. Anticoagulation should be given immediately after cerebral infarction, especially if considered likely to be cardioembolic (true/false).
6. Patients with severe stroke get the most benefit from a stroke unit (true/false).
7. Crying after stroke following minimum provocation is called?
8. Thrombolysis will have a more dramatic effect on stroke mortality than any intervention introduced so far (true/false).

Box 19.1   Patient information websites

- Stroke Association: www.stroke.org.uk
- Young Stroke Patients: www.differentstrokes.co.uk
- Action for Dysphasic Adults (ADA): http://glaxocentre.merseyside.org/ada.ht

Box 19.2   Key references

- Stroke Unit Trialists' Collaboration. Organised inpatient (stroke unit) care for stroke (Cochrane review). The Cochrane Library, issue 1, 2002. Oxford: Update Software.
- Department of Health. *National service framework for older people*. London: Stationery Office, 2001.
- Wade D. Intercollegiate Working Party for Stroke. *National clinical guidelines for stroke*. London: Royal College of Physicians, 2000.
- Warlow CP, Dennis ME, Van Gign J, *et al. Stroke: a practical guide to management*. 2nd edn. London: Blackwell Sciences, 2001.
- Antithrombotic Trialists' Collaboration. Collaborative metaanalyses of randomised trials of antiplatelet therapy for prevention of death, myocardial infarction, and stroke in high risk patients. *BMJ* 2002; **324**: 71–86.

References

1 Wade D. Intercollegiate Working Party for Stroke. *National clinical guidelines for stroke*. London: Royal College of Physicians, 2000.
2 Rudd AG, Irwin P, Rutledge Z, *et al*. The national sentinel audit of stroke: a tool for raising standards of care. *J R Coll Physicians Lond* 1999; **33**: 460–4.
3 Clinical Standards Advisory Group. *Report on clinical effectiveness using stroke as an example*. London: Stationery Office, 1998.
4 Department of Health. *Saving lives: our healthier nation*. London: Stationery Office, 1999.
5 Department of Health. *National service framework for older people*. London: Stationery Office, 2001.
6 Scottish Intercollegiate Guidelines Network (SIGN). *Management of patients with stroke*. Edinburgh: Royal College of Physicians, 1998.
7 von Arbin M, Britton M, deFaire U, *et al*. Accuracy of bedside diagnosis in stroke. *Stroke* 1981; **12**: 288–93.
8 Stroke Unit Trialists' Collaboration. Organised inpatient (stroke unit) care for stroke (Cochrane review). *The Cochrane Library*, Issue 1, 2002. Oxford: Update Software.
9 Naylor M, Brooten D, Jones R, *et al*. Comprehensive discharge planning for the hospitalised elderly: a randomised clinical trial. *Ann Intern Med* 1994; **120**: 999–1006.
10 Jones A, Carr EK, Newham DJ, *et al*. Positioning of stroke patients. Evaluation of a teaching intervention with nurses. *Stroke* 1998; **29**: 1612–17.
11 Kalra L, Evans A, Perez I, *et al*. Alternative strategies for stroke care: a prospective randomised control trial. *Lancet* 2000; **365**: 894–9.
12 Indredavik B, Bakke F, Slordahl SA, *et al*. Stroke unit treatment. 10-year follow-up. *Stroke* 1999; **30**: 1524–7.
13 Early Supported Discharge Trialists'. Services for reducing duration of hospital care for acute stroke patients (Cochrane review). *The Cochrane Library*, issue 1, 2002. Oxford: Update Software.
14 Rudd AG, Wolfe CD, Tilling K, *et al*. Randomised controlled trial to evaluate early discharge scheme for patients with stroke. *BMJ* 1997; **315**: 1039–44.
15 Langhorne P, Dennis MS, Kalra L, *et al*. Services for helping acute stroke patients avoid hospital admission (Cochrane review). *The Cochrane Library*, issue 1, 2002. Oxford: Update Software.
16 Kelson M, Ford C, Rigge M. *Stroke rehabilitation: patient and carer views*. A report by the

College of Health for the Intercollegiate Working Party for Stroke. London: Royal College of Physicians, 1998.

17 Dennis M, O'Rourke S, Lewis S, *et al*. A quantitative study of the emotional outcome of people caring for stroke survivors. *Stroke* 1998; **29**: 1867–72.

18 Mant J, Carter J, Wade DT, *et al*. The impact of an information pack on patients with stroke and their carers: a randomised controlled trial. *Clinical Rehabilitation* 1998; **12**: 465–76.

19 Mant J, Carter J, Wade DT, *et al*. Family support for stroke: a randomised controlled trial. *Lancet* 2000; **356**: 808–13.

20 Dennis M, O'Rourke S, Slattery J, *et al*. Evaluation of a stroke family care worker: results of a randomised controlled trial. *BMJ* 1997; **314**: 1071–6.

21 Gubitz G, Counsell C, Sandercock P. Antiplatelet therapy for acute ischaemic stroke (Cochrane review). *The Cochrane Library*, issue 1, 2002. Oxford: Update Software.

22 Wardlaw JM, del Zoppo G, Yamaguchi T. Thrombolysis for acute ischaemic stroke (Cochrane review). *The Cochrane Library*, issue 1, 2002. Oxford: Update Software.

23 National Institute of Neurological Disorders and Stroke rt-PA Stroke Study Group. Tissue plasminogen activator for acute ischaemic stroke. *N Engl J Med* 1995; **333**: 1581–7.

24 Lenzer J. Alteplase for stroke: money and optimistic claims buttress the 'brain attack' campaign. *BMJ* 2002; **324**: 723–8.

25 Warlow C. Who pays the guideline writers? *BMJ* 2002; **324**: 728–30.

26 Gubitz G, Counsell C, Sandercock P, *et al*. Anticoagulants for acute ischaemic stroke (Cochrane review). *The Cochrane Library*, issue 1, 2002. Oxford: Update Software.

27 Stroke Prevention in Atrial Fibrillation Investigators. Adjusted-dose warfarin versus low-intensity, fixed-dose warfarin plus aspirin for high risk patients with atrial fibrillation: stroke prevention in atrial fibrillation 111 randomised clinical trial. *Lancet* 1996; **348**: 633–8.

28 Saxena R, Lewis S, Berge E, *et al.*, for the International Stroke Trial Collaborative Group: risk of early death and recurrent stroke and effect of heparin in 3169 patients with acute ischaemic stroke and atrial fibrillation in the International Stroke Trial. *Stroke* 2001; **32**: 2333–7.

29 Bousser MG. Cerebral venous thrombosis. Nothing, heparin or local thrombolysis? *Stroke* 1999; **30**: 481–3.

30 Wolfe CDA, Tilling K, Beech R, *et al*. Variations in case fatality and dependency from stroke in western and central Europe. *Stroke* 1999; **30**: 350–6.

31 Warlow CP, Dennis ME, Van Gign J, *et al*. *Stroke: a practical guide to management*. 2nd edn. London: Blackwell Sciences, 2001.

32 Stuck AE, Siu AL, Wieland GD, *et al*. Comprehensive geriatric assessment: a meta-analyses of controlled trials. *Lancet* 1993; **342**: 1032–6.

33 Odderson IR, Keaton JC, McKenna BS. Swallow management in patients on an acute stroke pathway: quality is cost effective. *Arch Phys Med Rehabil* 1995; **76**: 1130–3.

34 DePippo KL, Holas MA, Reding MJ, *et al*. Dysphagia therapy following stroke: a controlled trial. *Neurology* 1994; **44**: 1655–60.

35 Potter J, Langhorne P, Roberts M. Routine protein energy supplementation in adults: systematic review. *BMJ* 1999; **317**: 495–501.

36 Norton B, Homer-Ward M, Donnelly MT, *et al*. A randomised prospective comparison of percutaneous endoscopic gastrostomy and nasogastric tube feeding after acute dysphagic stroke. *BMJ* 1996; **312**: 13–16.

37 Robey R. The efficacy of treatment for aphasic persons: a meta-analysis. *Brain and Language* 1994; **47**: 582–608.

38 Poeck K, Humer W, Wilmess K. Outcome of intensive language treatment in aphasia. *Aphasiology* 1989; **54**: 471–9.

39 Wu C, Trombly CA, Lin K, *et al*. A kinematic study of contextual effects on reaching performance in persons with and without stroke: influences of object availability. *Arch Phys Med Rehabil* 2000; **81**: 95–101.

40 Butefisch C, Hummelsheim H, Denzier P, *et al.* Repetitive training of isolated movements improves the outcome of motor rehabilitation of the centrally paretic hand. *J Neurol Sci* 1995; **130**: 59–68.

41 Teixera-Salmela LF, Olney SJ, Nadeaus S, *et al.* Muscle strengthening and physical conditioning to reduce impairment and disability in chronic stroke survivors. *Arch Phys Med Rehabil* 1999; **80**: 1211–18.

42 Walker MF, Gladmam JF, Lincoln NB Occupational therapy for stroke patients not admitted to hospital: a randomised controlled trial. *Lancet* 1999; **354**: 278–80.

43 Brown KW, Sloan RL, Pentland B. Fluoxetine as a treatment for post stroke emotionalism. *Acta Psychiatrica Scandinavia* 1998; **98**: 455–8.

44 Anderson G, Vestergaard K, Lauritsen L. Effective treatment of post-stroke depression with the selective serotonin re-uptake inhibitor citalopram. *Stroke* 1994; **25**: 1099–104.

45 Leijon G, Boivie J. Central post-stroke pain: a controlled trial of amitryptline and carbamazepine. *Pain* 1989; **36**: 27–36.

46 Sharp SA, Brouwer B. Isokinetic strength training of the hemiparetic knee: effects on function and spasticity. *Arch Phys Med Rehabil* 1997; **78**: 1231–5.

47 Medici M, Pebet M, Ciblios D. A double-blind, long-term study of tizanidine in spasticity due to cerebrovascular lesions. *Curr Med Res Opin* 1989; **11**: 398–407.

48 Burbaud P, Wiart L, Dubos JL, *et al.* A randomised, double-blind, placebo-controlled trial of botulinum toxin in the treatment of spastic foot in hemiparetic patients. *J Neurol Neurosurg Psychiatry* 1996; **61**: 265–9.

49 Gueyffier F, Boissel F, Boutite B. Effect of antihypertensive treatment inpatients having already suffered from stroke. Gathering the evidence. The INDANA Project collaboration. *Stroke* 1997; **28**: 2557–62.

50 Ramsay L, Williams B, Johnston G, *et al.* Guidelines for the management of hypertension: report of the third working party of the British Hypertension Society. *J Hum Hypertens* 1999; **13**: 569–92.

51 PROGRESS Collaborative Group Randomised trial of a perindopril-based blood-pressure lowering regime among 6105 individuals with previous stroke or transient ischaemic attack. *Lancet* 2001; **358**: 1033–41.

52 Heart Outcomes Prevention Evaluation Study Investigators (HOPE). Effects of ramipril on cardiovascular and microvascular outcomes in people with diabetes mellitus: results of the HOPE and MICRO-HOPE substudy. *Lancet* 2000; **342**: 145–53.

53 Pepine CJ. Improved endothelial function with angiotensin-converting enzyme inhibitors. *Am J Cardiol* 1997; **79**: 29–32.

54 Antithrombotic Trialists' Collaboration. Collaborative meta-analyses of randomised trials of antiplatelet therapy for prevention of death, myocardial infarction, and stroke in high risk patients. *BMJ* 2002; **324**: 71–86.

55 Koudstall PJ. Anticoagulants versus antiplatelet therapy for preventing stroke in patients with non-rheumatic atrial fibrillation and a history of stroke or transient ischaemic attacks. *The Cochrane Library*, issue 1, 2002. Oxford: Update Software.

56 Plehn JF, Davis BR, Sacks FM, *et al.* Reduction of stroke incidence after myocardial infarction with pravastatin: the Cholesterol and Recurrent Events (CARE) study. The Care Investigators. *Circulation* 1999; **99**: 185–8.

57 Anoymous. MRC/BHF Heart Protection Study of cholesterol lowering with simvastatin in 20 536 high-risk individuals: a randomised placebo controlled trial. *Lancet* 2002; **360**: 7–22.

58 Cina CS, Clase CM, Haynes RB. Carotid endarterectomy for symptomatic carotid stenosis (Cochrane review). *The Cochrane Library*, issue 3, 1999. Oxford: Update Software.

Answers

1 The Royal College of Physicians, London.
2 Multidisciplinary teamwork with expertise in stroke care and rehabilitation.
3 False. Patients should only be managed at home if acute assessment guidelines can be adhered to and that services provided are part of an organised stroke service.
4 C.
5 False. One should not start anticoagulation until 10–14 days after the cerebral infarct.
6 True.
7 Emotionalism.
8 False. Stroke unit care is more powerful than any pharmacological agent.

Chapter Twenty

Management of neurogenic dysphagia

AMO Bakheit

Dysphagia is common in patients with neurological disorders. It may result from lesions in the central or peripheral nervous system as well as from diseases of muscle and disorders of the neuromuscular junction. Drugs that are commonly used in the management of neurological conditions may also precipitate or aggravate swallowing difficulties in some patients. Neurogenic dysphagia often results in serious complications, including pulmonary aspiration, dehydration, and malnutrition. These complications are usually preventable if the dysphagia is recognised early and managed appropriately.

Physiological mechanisms of neurogenic dysphagia

The act of swallowing may be viewed as three discrete but interrelated physiological stages: the oral, pharyngeal, and oesophageal phases. The oral phase is initiated voluntarily and serves to prepare the food bolus and deliver it to the pharynx. An adequately prepared and sufficiently large and cohesive food bolus triggers the swallow reflex by stimulating the sensory receptive field in the soft palate, dorsum of the tongue, epiglottis, and posterior pharyngeal wall. Simultaneously the larynx closes and the velum retracts upwards to prevent the entry of food and fluid into the nasal cavity. Coordination of respiration and swallowing is necessary to prevent the penetration of food into the airways. This is achieved by transient cessation of breathing, a process known as deglutition apnoea. The pharyngeal phase is followed by a prolonged expiration to avert mist aspiration, that is inhalation of air held in the pharynx (which is usually saturated with fluid and food particles). The swallow reflex triggers the oesophageal peristaltic movements and causes relaxation of the circopharyngeal sphincter. This, combined with the effects of gravity, facilitates the transmission of food down into the stomach.

Several factors contribute to the swallowing difficulties encountered in patients with neurogenic dysphagia. These include weakness of the oral musculature and tongue movements, failure to form a cohesive food bolus, reduced sensitivity of the pharyngeal receptors, and buccolingual apraxia. Although the abnormalities of swallowing associated with neurological disease predominantly affect the oropharyngeal phase, occasionally neurogenic dysphagia may result from disorders of innervation of the oesophagus.

Causes of neurogenic dysphagia

Normal swallowing depends on the anatomical and functional integrity of numerous neural structures and extensive pathways in the central and peripheral

301

nervous system. Lesions of the cerebral cortex, basal ganglia, brain stem, cerebellum, and lower cranial nerves may result in dysphagia. Degeneration of the myenteric ganglion cells in the oesophagus, muscle diseases and disorders of neuromuscular transmission, for example myasthenia gravis and Eaton-Lambers syndrome, are other less common causes.

Cerebral cortex

The commonest condition associated with dysphagia resulting from cortical lesions is stroke. Acute stroke is complicated by dysphagia in about 25–42% of all cases.[1] Dysphagia in these patients is usually associated with hemiplegia due to lesions of the brain stem or the involvement of one or both hemispheres. However, on rare occasions, dysphagia may be the sole manifestation of a cerebrovascular event. Dysphagia in the absence of other neurological symptoms and signs has been reported in patients with lacunar infarcts in the periventricular white matter[2] and after[3] discrete vascular brain stem lesions.

Dysphagia in stroke is usually transient. Recovery of the swallowing ability occurs in almost 90% of cases within two weeks. However, the symptoms persist in about 8% of patients for six months or more.[4] The occurrence of dysphagia in acute stroke does not appear to depend on the size or the site of the lesion. Interestingly, when it persists for a month or more after the stroke onset it is usually associated with right parietal lobe involvement.

Basal ganglia

Dysphagia is usually a late feature in Parkinson's disease but is sometimes reported by patients in the early stages and may even be the presenting symptom in some cases. More than 80% of patients with Parkinson's disease have dysphagia but, as a rule, this is mild and has little or no effect on the patient's nutritional status. However, in about 10% of dysphagic parkinsonian patients the symptoms are severe and this generally correlates with the severity and duration of the disease. Tremor and speech disturbances have been found to be the main predictors of dysphagia in these patients.[5]

The swallowing difficulties most frequently associated with Parkinson's disease relate to the oral phase (difficulties with lip closure and tongue movements) and the pharyngeal stage (complaints of food sticking in the throat). On videofluoroscopy these abnormalities are seen as abnormal bolus formation, multiple tongue elevations, delayed swallow reflex, and prolongation of the pharyngeal transit time with repetitive swallows to clear the throat. Drooling, which is commonly seen in patients with parkinsonism, is not due to excessive salivation but is an indication of bradykinesia of the oropharyngeal musculature. Other parkinsonian syndromes, for example Shy-Drager syndrome, multisystem atrophy, etc. result in similar, but usually more severe, symptoms. Dysphagia is also common in spasmodic torticollis. In one study it was observed on videofluoroscopy in more than 50% of a randomly selected patients' sample.[6] Interestingly, only two thirds of the study patients were symptomatic and the occurrence of dysphagia did not correlate with the patient's age or disease duration.

Cerebellum and brain stem

Cerebellar disease and brain stem lesions resulting in bulbar and pseudobulbar palsy mainly affect the oral phase of swallowing. Poor coordination of the activity of the orofacial musculature may lead to inadequate lip seal, difficulties with the timing of the voluntary initiation of the swallow reflex, preparation of a cohesive food bolus, and delivery of the bolus to the pharynx.

Peripheral nerves and muscles

Isolated peripheral nerve lesions and degeneration of autonomic ganglion cells in the lower two thirds of the oesophagus (which results in achalasia) are rare causes of dysphagia. Achalasia is characterised by stasis of food and dilatation of the oesophagus due to reduced peristalsis and incomplete relaxation of the lower oesophageal sphincter. In addition to dysphagia, patients typically present with halitosis. The diagnosis is confirmed with endoscopy and studies of oesophageal motility. Abnormalities of neuromuscular transmission, for example in myasthenia gravis, frequently cause difficulties with swallowing. In addition to dysphagia, patients with disorders of the neuromuscular junction often have dysphonia and dysarthria. Obvious weakness of oral and facial muscles may or may not be present. The diagnosis of the underlying disorder can usually be confirmed with single fibre electromyography.

Drugs and dysphagia

Many drugs may precipitate or aggravate swallowing difficulties. This effect is usually dose dependent and is often reversible with discontinuation of the drug. Sometimes reduction of the drug dose is sufficient. The mechanisms implicated in drug-induced dysphagia are diverse. These include depression of the level of consciousness (sedatives and hypnotics), interference with the oropharyngeal phase of swallowing, a direct effect on brain stem neurones or blocking of acetylcholine release at the neuromuscular junction. Some drugs mediate their effect on swallowing by more than one mechanism.

Neuroleptic drugs delay the initiation of the swallow reflex, sometimes in the absence of obvious extrapyramidal features. On the other hand, dopaminergic agents may cause orofacial dyskinesia which affects the preparation of the food bolus and its delivery to the pharynx. Dysphagia due to poor preparation of the food bolus may also result from xerostomia caused by anticholinergic drugs. The benzodiazepines can adversely affect swallowing in at least two ways. Dysphagia in patients taking these drugs is usually associated with depressed level of consciousness but has also been reported in alert subjects.[7] The latter effect could be explained by a direct inhibition of brain stem neurones that regulate swallowing. This is in keeping with observations from animal experiments.[8]

The most widely used drug that causes dysphagia due to inhibition of neural transmission at the neuromuscular junction is botulinum toxin type A. It is the drug of first choice for the treatment of spasmodic torticollis and may cause dysphagia in 10–28% of these patients. This adverse effect is usually mild and transient, lasting 10–14 days. Clinical observations suggest that the incidence of dysphagia is increased when a large dose of the drug is injected (for example 750 units or more of botulinum toxin type A), especially if the dose is divided between multiple sites in the muscle.

Clinical manifestations of dysphagia and pulmonary aspiration

Patients with mild or moderately severe neurogenic dysphagia may not be aware of their swallowing difficulties. However, on direct questioning most of these patients would admit that they have been avoiding certain foods which they found difficult to chew or swallow. Weight loss may be the first presentation in some cases. Drooling occurs in dysphagic patients when they are sitting up and aspiration is common in the recumbent position, especially during sleep. Occasionally interrupted sleep may be the only indication of swallowing difficulties. Pain on swallowing (odynophagia) is not a symptom of neurogenic dysphagia and suggests the diagnosis of oesophagitis, usually secondary to candida infections. Nasal regurgitation of fluids occurs when palatal weakness is present.

Assessment

Assessment of swallowing function starts with a careful examination of the oral cavity. The presence of dysphagia and its severity can then be confirmed at the bedside by observing the patient during 'trial swallows'. Swallowing behaviour can be observed while the subject is taking food and fluids of different consistencies under 'normal' everyday conditions. Coughing, splattering, and choking while eating are obvious signs. Change in the pattern of breathing or change in voice quality may also occur. Some patients attempt to compensate for their swallowing difficulties by taking small, frequent drinks during the meal in order to 'wash down' the food bolus. Inspection of the oral cavity usually reveals pooling of secretions or food residue in the mouth.

In recent years a simple bedside measurement of the swallowing speed has been suggested as a diagnostic test for neurogenic dysphagia.[9] The test, which has been shown to be specific and sensitive, consists of measuring the speed with which the patient drinks 150 ml of cold tap water while sitting up. A swallowing speed of less than 10 ml/s suggests the presence of dysphagia. This test has obvious advantages over other methods of assessment such as videofluoroscopy and nasendoscopy, especially when regular and frequent monitoring of the patient's condition is necessary.

Videofluoroscopy is considered the gold standard for the evaluation of dysphagia. It permits the observation of the oral preparatory phase, the reflex initiation of swallowing, and the pharyngeal transit of the food bolus. However, it is not suitable for repeated assessments because of the undesirability of frequent exposure to radiation and the cost of the procedure. An alternative method is fibreoptic nasendoscopy. This procedure consists of introducing an endoscope through the nose into the nasopharynx and placing the tip just above the soft palate. The patient is then given food and drink coloured with a dye and before and after swallowing pharyngeal pooling is observed. Nasal endoscopy is a reliable method for assessing dysphagia and the risk of pulmonary aspiration but special expertise is necessary to carry out the procedure and to interpret its results.

Another useful method of bedside diagnosis of dysphagia and pulmonary aspiration is pulse oximetry. The use of this method is based on the premise that aspiration of food or fluid in the airways causes reflex bronchoconstriction that leads to ventilation-perfusion mismatch. The resulting oxygen desaturation of arterial blood can be readily measured with pulse oximetry. In a recent study pulse oximetry predicted aspiration or the lack of it in 81.5% of dysphagic stroke patients.[10] This method is non-invasive, quick, and repeatable but its results must be interpreted with caution in smokers (high carboxyhaemoglobin concentrations may give false negative results) and in those with chronic lung disease.

Oesophageal manometry enables measurements of the intraoesophageal pressure gradient and is useful in the evaluation of dysfunction of the circopharyngeus muscle and abnormalities of oesophageal motility.

Differential diagnosis

A careful medical history and physical examination (supplemented by special investigations in some cases) are necessary to establish the cause of the swallowing difficulty and to exclude coincidental dysphagia due to obstructive lesions. In contrast to dysphagia due to oesophageal strictures or tumours, patients with neurogenic dysphagia find fluids more difficult to swallow than solids. This is probably because a solid (and more cohesive) food bolus is more likely to result in adequate pharyngeal stimulation and trigger a swallow reflex.

Dysphagia resulting from discrete brain stem lesions or confluent periventricular infarction may affect predominantly the volitional initiation of swallowing and spare reflexive deglutition. In these circumstances the patient's symptoms are often ascribed to globus hystericus. However, in the latter condition a 'lump in the throat' is a characteristic complaint and the symptoms are usually associated with emotional distress. Patients with globus hystericus have a normal bolus transit time and seldom complain of difficulties with eating or drinking.

Complications of dysphagia

A serious complication of dysphagia is pulmonary aspiration. Severe swallowing difficulties, even for relatively short periods, may also lead to dehydration, reduced calorie intake, and malnutrition.

Pulmonary aspiration is defined as penetration of food or fluid into the airways below the true vocal cords. It may result in severe morbidity and sometimes mortality. About a third of patients with dysphagia aspirate food or fluid into their airways and in 40% of them aspiration is silent, that is does not trigger coughing or cause symptoms or signs of distress. Paradoxically, aspirating patients frequently do not complain of swallowing difficulties and there are no reliable clinical signs of this complication. Interestingly, a weak cough, which is generally associated with the ability to protect the airways, is more likely to be present in aspirating rather than non-aspirating dysphagic patients.[11] Similarly, a diminished or absent gag reflex does not differentiate aspirating from non-aspirating patients. The detection of silent aspiration therefore depends largely on a high index of clinical suspicion and may be confirmed by non-invasive bedside investigations such as pulse oximetry.[10]

Management

The aim of management is to prevent pulmonary aspiration, to maintain adequate food and fluid intake, and to correct nutritional deficiencies when present. Oral feeding has important social and psychological significance to patients and their families and should be continued whenever possible. In some patients oral intake is often not adequate even in the absence of significant swallowing difficulties. This may be due to excessive fatigue or cognitive impairment. In these patients oral food intake may be supplemented with gastrostomy tube feeding. It is preferable that such supplements are given at night. Withholding morning gastrostomy feeds usually stimulates the patient's appetite. An interdisciplinary team approach is essential for the optimal management of patients with neurogenic dysphagia. The core team should consist of a speech and language therapist, a dietitian, a nurse, and a physician.

Dysphagia in some patients may result from poor preparation of the food bolus because of ill-fitting dentures or due to disease of the oral cavity, such as mouth ulcers or candida infections. These causes should be routinely looked for and treated. Care should be taken to avoid feeding when the patient is tired or distracted (for example while watching television). Talking while eating also increases the risk of aspiration and patients (and their carers) should be made aware of this. It is sometimes useful to plan the timing of meals so that they coincide with periods when the patient's functional abilities are maximal, for example, during the 'on periods' in parkinsonian patients with 'on/off' motor fluctuations. Frequent suction of copious saliva may be necessary in some cases. In dysphagic patients who have a tracheostomy, occlusion of the stoma with a speaking valve during swallowing reduces the risk of pulmonary aspiration presumably by normalising the pressure in the upper airways. The effects of posture on swallowing are well recognised. For example, 'chin tuck' decreases the pharyngeal transit time of the food bolus, whereas 'chin up' has the opposite effect. Head tilt to one side to maximise the effect of gravity on the unaffected side of pharynx is also a useful strategy on some occasions.

It has been shown that patients with weak tongue movements and those with poor pharyngeal clearance of the food bolus benefit from the use of gravity and posture to facilitate safe swallowing. Lying down on one side (at 45 degrees from flat) may be associated with less risk of aspiration than feeding in the upright position.[12,13]

Review of patient's medication

Sedative and other drugs that reduce the patient's level of arousal should be discontinued whenever possible. In patients with Parkinson's disease drug-induced dyskinesia may cause or aggravate dysphagia and the successful management of this complication usually improves swallowing. Sometimes it is sufficient to avoid feeding during periods of peak dose dyskinesia. Drooling in parkinsonian patients is primarily due to swallowing difficulties rather than the excessive production of saliva. Anticholinergic drugs should be avoided in these cases as they aggravate dysphagia by increasing the viscosity of oral secretions. Viscid secretions interfere with bolus preparation and predispose to the formation of a mucous plug. Prescribing of benzodiazepines to dysphagic patients is not desirable and it is sensible that anticonvulsants are taken as a single dose at bedtime if possible.

Dietary modification

Maintenance of hydration and nutrition can be achieved safely in most patients with neurogenic dysphagia with dietary modification. Simple, but effective, measures include avoidance of dry and sticky food and eating food with uniform consistency. The use of starch-based fluid thickeners, for example 'Thick and Easy' and Vitaquick, is also an important management strategy. Tube feeding is required in only a minority of patients.

Patients with neurogenic dysphagia experience more difficulties with fluids than with solid food. This is probably due to the difficulty in controlling a thin bolus and/or a delay or absence of triggering the swallow reflex. The rationale for the use of fluid thickeners is that by increasing the viscosity of ingested fluids the resistance to flow of the bolus is increased. In addition, the duration of cricopharyngeal opening and the oropharyngeal transit time are increased. However, the optimal viscosity of fluids that ensures safe swallowing in patients with neurogenic dysphagia has not been established. In practice the required fluid thickness is judged subjectively and recorded using descriptive terms such as syrup or yoghurt consistency. This has the disadvantage that fluids with low viscosity may be served and result in pulmonary aspiration. On the other hand, fluids that are too thick are usually unpalatable and are often rejected by patients. The use of a viscometer for the preparation of the prescribed fluid thickness has been shown to improve the dietary management in these cases.[14]

Tube feeding

The direct delivery of nutrients into the stomach (or rarely into the jejunum) via a feeding tube is frequently used as the sole method of nutritional support of severely dysphagic patients who are at risk of pulmonary aspiration if fed orally. Tube feeding should be considered if the subject aspirates approximately 10% or more of the food bolus (M Collins, personal communication) or shows evidence of slow transit of the food bolus, that is more than 10 seconds, on videofluoroscopy.[15] However, in some cases, for example when easy fatiguability makes swallowing unsafe, tube feeding can be used to supplement the daily oral intake. The patients will then be able to take their favourite foods orally and the rest of the calorie requirements will be given through the tube.

The use of a gastrostomy tube is preferred to naso-oesophageal intubation, especially when dysphagia is expected to be present for more than a few days. Nasogastric tube feeding is usually poorly tolerated and may make the patient irritable or even agitated. Extubation by patients is common and the volume of feeds delivered in this way is usually not adequate. In one study patients who were fed using a nasogastric tube received 55% of their feeds, whereas those fed with a gastrostomy tube had 93% of their prescribed daily intake.[16] When nasogastric tube feeding is prescribed the use of fine bore tubes, for example

Ryle's tube, is preferred to large bore ones. However, fine bore tubes are more likely to dislodge, kink, or block. They also deliver feeds at a relatively slow rate.

Some patients with neurological disease develop gastrointestinal ileus and in these patients enteral nutrition could be established with the intrajejunal administration of low residue solutions. Duodenal intubation is often facilitated by an intravenous injection of 20 mg of metoclopramide a few minutes before the procedure. (Metoclopramide increases stomach peristalsis and relaxes the pyloric sphincter.)

Prolonged nasogastric tube feeding is not desirable. It often results in numerous complications including nasopharyngitis, oesophagitis, oesophageal strictures, epistaxis, pneumothorax, and nasopharyngeal oedema with associated otitis media. Furthermore, nasogastric tube feeding does not fully protect against aspiration and the association between nasogastric tube feeding and this complication is well documented. Ciocon *et al.* have found that 43% of dysphagic patients aspirated in the first two weeks after nasogastric tube feeding was started.[17] Elevation of the head of the bed during and for 1–2 hours after bolus nasogastric tube gastric and intrajejunal feeding reduces the risk of aspiration in these patients.

Feeding via a gastrostomy tube should be considered when dysphagia is likely to be progressive or to persist for long periods. For example, most clinicians would consider gastrostomy tube feeding in stroke patients if there are no signs of recovery of swallowing after the first week. However, there are no conclusive data to support this at present, but the results of a large ongoing multicentre study are eagerly awaited.[18] In patients with motor neurone disease the option of percutaneous endoscopic gastrostomy (PEG) tube feeding should be offered early after the onset of dysphagia to supplement the oral intake and help maintain the muscle mass. Insertion of the feeding tube through a PEG, rather than a surgical gastrostomy, is a relatively simple, safe, and cost-effective technique. PEG tube feeding is effective and is usually acceptable to patients and their carers. Transient, self-limiting abdominal pain and diarrhoea may occur in the early postoperative period. Long-term complications include tube obstruction and wound infection.

In some patients who are fed via a PEG tube pulmonary aspiration may occur and routine intrajejunal feeding has been suggested for these cases. However, technically it is easier to insert a gastric rather than an intrajejunal feeding tube. An additional advantage is that bolus gastric tube feeding is more physiological, particularly with respect to insulin secretion. Furthermore, because the feeds can be given intermittently it allows greater patient freedom (intrajejunal feeding should be given continuously rather than intermittently). Direct intrajejunal delivery of nutrients should probably be reserved for patients with gastro-oesophageal reflux, hiatus hernia, or recurrent aspiration on gastrostomy feeding.

Entral feeding can be started a few hours after the insertion of the PEG tube. The volume of feed is usually restricted in the first 24 hours to one litre and is given at a rate of 50 ml/hour. The volume of feed and the rate of its administration are then gradually increased over the following 3–4 days until the patient's daily nutritional requirements are met. Some clinicians prescribe 'starter feeding regimens' in the first postoperative week. These are feeds diluted with sterile water. The concentration and osmolality are gradually increased over several days to full strength feeds. Starter regimens with clear water or diluted enteral solutions are thought to improve tolerance to feeds and reduce diarrhoea, but this has not been confirmed. In fact, a randomised controlled study demonstrated the poor relationship between osmolality of the feeds and the occurrence of diarrhoea in these patients.[19] Furthermore, patients who were randomised to the starter regimen group received 20% less nutrients in the first seven days than the control subjects. Diarrhoea in patients on enteral feeding is usually due to treatment with antibiotics for coincidental infections, bacterial contamination of the feed and bolus feeding (the use of enteral feeding pumps to control the rate of feeding may prevent diarrhoea, nausea, and vomiting).

Swallowing therapy

A range of remedial therapies and training in the use of compensatory strategies may be helpful in the treatment of neurogenic dysphagia. These include exercises to strengthen the orofacial musculature, manoeuvres to improve poor laryngeal elevation and laryngeal closure during swallowing, and techniques to stimulate the swallow reflex. These methods are usually used before starting direct swallowing practice.

Exercises to enhance the function of the orofacial muscles are used to improve lip seal, mastication, and tongue movements. A simple technique known as 'the supraglottic swallow' may improve the elevation and closure of the larynx during swallowing. During this manoeuvre the subject holds his/her breath and swallows and they release the air by coughing. Patients with delayed or absent swallow reflex often benefit from thermal stimulation of the oropharyngeal receptors. The procedure has been claimed to improve triggering of the swallowing action and to reduce the bolus transit time. It involves the repeated application of a small laryngeal mirror dipped in ice to the anterior faucial arch. Sensitisation may be repeated between swallows. Direct swallowing therapy can be started with small amounts of food (of the right consistency) under the supervision of a speech and language therapist when the risk of pulmonary aspiration is deemed to be low.

Surgical treatment of neurogenic dysphagia

Cricopharyngeal myotomy has been shown to be an effective method of treatment of dysphagia in a number of neurological disorders including stroke, muscular dystrophy, and a significant proportion of patients with motor neurone disease. However, the careful selection of patients for this procedure is essential and two conditions must be satisfied. First, failure of relaxation of the pharyngeal sphincter must be demonstrated on videofluoroscopy. Secondly, the oral phase of swallowing, that is lip seal, voluntary initiation of swallowing, and the propulsive action of the tongue must also be preserved. Poor tongue movements (demonstrated on videofluoroscopy by the inability to propel or retrieve the food bolus) is a contraindication to cricopharyngeal myotomy. Patients with absent pharyngeal peristalsis or delayed triggering of the swallow reflex by 10 seconds or more are also unlikely to benefit from this treatment. Surgery for cricopharyngeal dysfunction after stroke and traumatic brain injury should be considered after the first three months of the disease onset.

Relaxation of the cricopharyngeus can also be achieved with 'chemical cricopharyngeal myotomy' using botulinum toxin type A injections.[20] The location of the cricopharyngeal muscle is determined with direct oesophagoscopy and electromyography (using a hooked wire electrode) and the toxin is injected transcutaneously into the dorsomedial part and into the ventrolateral part of the muscle on both sides. A total dose of botulinum toxin type A of 80–120 units is usually sufficient and the mean beneficial effect of treatment is five months. The procedure usually requires a light general anaesthetic.

Summary

Dysphagia is a common impairment in patients with neurological disease and may be caused by lesions at any level of the neuroaxis. Frequently the swallowing difficulties are aggravated by sedatives and other drugs. The management as well as the clinical outcome of dysphagia depend on the underlying pathology. In stroke, for example, most patients recover in the first month and only a small minority will require long-term nutrition and hydration through a PEG feeding tube.

References

1 Kidd D, Lawson J, Nesbitt R, *et al*. Aspiration in acute stroke: a clinical study with videofluoroscopy. *Q J Med* 1993; **86**: 825–9.

2 Celifarco A, Gerard G, Faegenburg D, *et al*. Dysphagia as the sole manifestation of bilateral strokes. *Am J Gastroenterol* 1990; **85**: 610–13.

3 Buchholz DW. Clinically probable brain stem stroke presenting as dysphagia and nonvisualised by MRI. *Dysphagia* 1993; **8**: 235–8.

4 Smithard DG, O'Neill PA, Martin DF, *et al*. The natural history of dysphagia following stroke. *Dysphagia* 1997; **12**: 188–93.

5 Coates C, Bakheit AMO. Dysphagia in Parkinson's disease. *Eur Neurol* 1997; **38**: 49–52.

6 Riski JE, Horner J, Nashold BS. Swallowing function in patients with spasmodic torticollis. *Neurology* 1990,**40**: 1443–5.

7 Wyllie E, Wyllie R, Cruse RP, *et al*. The mechanism of nitrazepam-induced drooling and aspiration. *N Engl J Med* 1986,**14**: 35–8.

8 Hockman CH, Bieger D. Inhibitory effect of diazepam on reflexly-induced deglutition. *Proceedings of the Canadian Federation of Biological Sciences* 1979; **2**: 85.

9 Nathadwarawala KM, Nicklin J, Wiles CM. A timed test of swallowing capacity for neurological patients. *J Neurol Neurosurg Psychiatry* 1992; **55**: 822–5.

10 Collins MJ, Bakheit AMO. Does pulse oximetry reliably detect aspiration in dysphagic stroke patients? *Stroke* 1997; **28**: 1773–5.

11 Horner J, Massey W. Silent aspiration following stroke. *Neurology* 1988; **38**: 317–19.

12 Ekberg O. Posture of the head and pharyngeal swallowing. *Acta Radiol* 1986; **27**: 691–6.

13 Drake W, O'Donoghue S, Bartram C, *et al*. Eating in side lying facilitates rehabilitation in neurogenic dysphagia. *Brain Inj* 1997; **11**: 137–42.

14 Goulding R, Bakheit AMO. Evaluation of the benefits of monitoring fluid thickness in the dietary management of dysphagic stroke patients. *Clin Rehabil* 2000; **14**: 119–24.

15 Park RHR, Allison MC, Lang J, *et al*. Randomised comparison of percutaneous endoscopic gastrostomy and nasogastric tube feeding in patients with persisting neurological dysphagia. *BMJ* 1993; **304**: 1406–9.

16 Wilson PS, Johnson AP, Bruce-Lockhart FJ. Videofluoroscopy in motor neurone disease prior to cricopharyngeal myotomy. *Ann R Coll Surg Engl* 1990; **72**: 375–7.

17 Ciocon JO, Silverstone FA, Graver LM, *et al*. Tube feeding in elderly patients. Indications, benefits and complications. *Arch Intern Med* 1988; **148**: 429–33.

18 The FOOD trial (Feed Or Ordinary Diet) – a multicentre trial to evaluate various feeding policies in patients admitted to hospital with a recent stroke. National Research Register 2001, issue 2.

19 Keohane PP, Attrill H, Love M, *et al.* Relation between osmolality of diet and gastrointestinal side effects in entral nutrition. *BMJ* 1984; **288**: 678–80.

20 Schneider I, Thumfart WF, Potoschnig C, *et al.* Treatment of dysfunction of the cricopharyngeal muscle with botulinum A toxin: introduction of a new non-invasive method. *Ann Otol Rhinol Laryngol* 1994; **103**: 31–5.

Chapter Twenty-one

Pathophysiological and clinical aspects of breathing after stroke

RS Howard, AG Rudd, CD Wolfe and AJ Williams

Stroke may disrupt breathing either by:

1 causing a disturbance of central rhythm generation
2 interrupting the descending respiratory pathways leading to a reduced respiratory drive or
3 causing bulbar weakness leading to aspiration.

Pathophysiology of respiratory control in stroke

Neural control of respiration in man depends on a central drive to the respiratory muscles which is modulated by chemical and mechanical inputs.[1] While many of the factors controlling established respiratory rhythm in mammals are understood, the neural mechanisms of rhythm generation remain obscure.[2–4] It has proved difficult, in man, to attribute precise respiratory function to localised anatomical substrates because lesions are rarely localised and coexisting pulmonary, cardiovascular, or autonomic influences may complicate the clinical picture. Furthermore accurate diagnosis of respiratory insufficiency has led to earlier therapeutic intervention with controlled ventilation. Also there is probably considerable redundancy and plasticity of the neural substrate of respiratory control, thus congenital, long-standing, or slowly progressive and destructive mass lesions can have little or no functional consequence while acute discrete lesions in a similar distribution may lead to profound respiratory impairment. Finally much of the literature is flawed because the extensive experimental animal work has been applied to man without any evidence for anatomico-physiological correlates. However, in individual case studies abnormalities of respiration may be associated with small, discrete lesions of the central nervous system, defined by imaging or postmortem, particularly due to stroke. Such reports have complemented experimental animal work and have greatly increased our understanding of the mechanisms that control breathing in man.

Central respiratory drive is mediated by three pathways, which are largely anatomically and functionally independent above the segmental level,[1] although it is increasingly clear that these systems must interact with one another to some extent.[5,6]

Metabolic (automatic) respiration

Metabolic (automatic) respiration is the homoeostatic pathway by which ventilation may be mediated to maintain acid-base status and oxygenation to the metabolic requirements. Automatic control is mediated by localised areas in the dorsolateral tegmentum of the pons and medulla in the region of the nucleus tractus solitarius and nucleus retroambigualis (for review *see* Howard and Hirsch)[7]. As a consequence of lesions in this area automatic respiratory control is disrupted; the patient is voluntarily able to maintain his respiratory pattern and breathes normally while awake and alert but during sleep there is a sudden or progressive decline in tidal volume and respiratory rate culminating in central apnoea.

Abnormal patterns of rate and rhythm are also often a reflection of impaired automatic ventilatory control.[8] *Primary central neurogenic hyperventilation* is a rare condition characterised by rapid, regular hyperventilation which persists in the face of alkalosis, raised oxygen tension, low carbon dioxide tension, and in the absence of any pulmonary or airway disorder.[9,10] However, *hyperventilation* in the poststroke patient is common but is due to intrinsic pulmonary involvement.[11–13] In *apneustic* breathing there are sustained inspiratory cramps with a prolonged pause at full inspiration or alternating brief end inspiratory and expiratory pauses. The pattern has been associated with bilateral tegmental infarcts in the pons. *Ataxic respiration* is characterised by a completely irregular respiratory cycle of variable frequency and tidal volume alternating with periods of apnoea. It is particularly associated with medullary impairment either due to brainstem stroke or compression due to rapidly expanding lesions and may be an important sign of impending respiratory arrest. *Hiccups* consist of brief bursts of intense inspiratory activity involving the diaphragm and inspiratory intercostal muscles with reciprocal inhibition of the expiratory intercostals.[14,15] Glottic closure occurs almost immediately after the onset of diaphragmatic contraction thus minimising the ventilatory effect. Intractable hiccups may be the result of structural or functional disturbances of the medulla or its afferent or efferent connections with the respiratory muscles. This may be associated with structural lesions of the medulla including infarction in the territory of the posterior inferior cerebellar artery. The development of hiccups in this context may anticipate the development of irregularities of the respiratory rhythm culminating in respiratory arrest.

Behavioural (voluntary) respiration

Behavioural (voluntary) respiration operates during wakefulness and allows voluntary modulation of respiration in response, for example, to speaking, singing, breath holding, and straining. Volitional control is active during consciousness but quiescent during sleep, although it may be involved in the chaotic respiratory patterns seen during rapid eye movement sleep. Voluntary control may be impaired by bilateral lesions affecting the descending corticospinal or corticobulbar tracts,[5] and is particularly seen in association with destructive vascular lesions of the basal pons or of the medullary pyramids and adjacent ventromedial portion which may result in the 'locked in' syndrome.[16] Selective interruption of the voluntary pathways in man leads to a strikingly regular and unvarying respiratory pattern during wakefulness as well as sleep, with loss of the ability to take a deep breath, hold the breath, cough voluntarily, or initiate any kind of volitional respiratory movement. The tidal volume remains responsive to carbon dioxide and a reflex cough is preserved.[17] Diffuse cortical vascular disease may lead to selective abnormalities of voluntary breathing such that there is an inability to take a deep breath or to hold the breath to command. These *respiratory apraxias* may be associated with inability to initiate voluntary swallowing or with other behavioural apraxias.[1,18] *Cheyne-Stokes respiration* is characterised by a smooth waxing and waning of breath volume and frequency separated by periods of apnoea;[19,20] the hyperpnoeic phase is longer than the apnoea and the entire cycle typically lasts one minute or more. The respiratory oscillations are associated with phasic changes in cerebral blood flow, cerebrospinal fluid pressure, arterial and alveolar oxygen and carbon dioxide, level of alertness and pupillary size; periodic heart block and ventricular arrhythmias are also common. It has been suggested that Cheyne-Stokes respiration may occur in up to 50% of patients after unilateral supratentorial stroke[21,22] and, despite the observations of Plum and Posner, it may also be common after infratentorial stroke. Studies in these patients show the frequency variations of respiratory amplitude modulation is low suggesting that Cheyne-Stokes respiration represents a relatively uniform response to central nervous system injury regardless of infarct size or location. During Cheyne-Stokes respiration there are concomitant periodic drops in arterial oxygen saturation compromising the vulnerable hypoperfused peri-infarct tissue of the ischaemic penumbra.

Limbic (emotional) respiration

Limbic (emotional) respiration accounts for the preservation of respiratory modulation to emotional stimuli including laughing, coughing, and anxiety despite loss of voluntary control. This implies that descending limbic influences on automatic respiration are anatomically and functionally independent of the voluntary respiratory system. Munschauer *et al.* described a patient with locked in syndrome due to infarction of the basal pons. This led to loss of voluntary control but carbon dioxide responses remained normal.[23] This patient showed preserved respiratory modulation to emotional stimuli including coughing and anxiety and in another patient laughing.[17] Such an independent descending pathway, mediating limbic control of respiration, lies either in the pontine tegmentum or lateral basis pontis. Such limbic pathways are also suggested by the effect of limbic cortex stimulation and epileptic seizures.

Patterns of respiratory impairment due to stroke

Cortex

Hemispheric ischaemic strokes influence respiratory function to a modest degree. Reductions of both chest wall and diaphragm excursion contralateral to the stroke have been reported.[24,25] The latter association correlates well with the localisation of the diaphragm cortical representation found by transcranial magnetic stimulation and positron emission tomography scanning.[26–31] At present there is no clear evidence of cerebral dominance for diaphragm function.

Patients with bilateral hemispheric cerebrovascular disease show an increased respiratory responsiveness to carbon dioxide and are liable to develop Cheyne-

Stokes respiration suggesting disinhibition of lower respiratory centres. Such a response may persist months to years after the stroke. Diffuse cortical vascular disease may also lead to a selective inability of voluntary breathing (respiratory apraxia).[18] Intermittent upper airway obstruction and apnoea due to periodic fluctuations in the position of the vocal cords is associated with cortical supranuclear palsy due to bilateral lesions of the operculum.[32]

Brainstem

The effects of brainstem dysfunction on respiration depend on the pathology, localisation, and speed of onset of the lesion. In patients with bulbar lesions, particularly vascular, the combination of impaired swallow, abnormalities of the respiratory rhythm, reduced vital capacity, and reduced or absent triggering of cough reflex all increase the risk of aspiration pneumonia.[33] Nocturnal upper airway occlusion may also contribute to respiratory impairment. Unilateral or bilateral lateral tegmental infarcts in the pons (at or below the level of the trigeminal nucleus) may lead to apneustic breathing and impairment of carbon dioxide responsiveness,[34] while similar lesions in the medulla (for example, lateral medullary syndrome) may result in acute failure of the automatic respiration.[35,36] Infarction of the basal pons (locked in syndrome) or of the pyramids and the adjacent ventromedial portion of the medulla may lead to complete loss of the voluntary system with a highly regular breathing pattern but a complete inability to initiate any spontaneous respiratory movements.[36]

Acute vascular lesions in the lower brainstem compromise respiratory control, particularly during sleep, leading to irregularities of rate and rhythm of breathing which lead to Cheyne-Stokes respiration, hypopnoea, and obstructive apnoea.[37,38] It is likely that size and bilaterality of the lesions determine the type and severity of abnormalities of the respiratory pattern. In a series of 15 patients with vascular lesions of the lower brainstem, patients with unilateral lesions in the rostrolateral medulla showed a reduced ventilatory sensitivity to inhaled carbon dioxide. In these patients there was a minimal effect on breathing while awake, at rest or during exertion, however there was a high incidence of fragmented sleep and obstructive sleep apnoea associated with hypoxaemia. The authors concluded that patients with unilateral rostrolateral medullary lesions require monitoring during sleep to diagnose sleep apnoea.[37]

Isolated central sleep apnoea due to brainstem vascular disease is usually associated with bilateral lesions caudal to the V cranial nerve in the pons down to the ventral lateral, tegmental pons, medulla, and cervical spinal cord. Occasional reports have described central apnoea with unilateral lesions involving nucleus ambiguus but sparing nucleus tractus solitarius; however the relevance of these is difficult to assess with limited respiratory, imaging, and neuropathological information.[38]

Cervical cord

Infarction of the spinal cord at high cervical levels may selectively affect respiratory control.[39,40] Lesions of the anterior pathways, particularly descending reticulospinal, lead to loss of automatic control and sudden nocturnal death from apnoea while involvement of the dorsolateral corticospinal tracts may lead to automatic respiration of the type described earlier. Infarction of the spinal cord at high cervical levels is usually due to occlusion of the anterior spinal artery and may be due to fibrocartilaginous embolism.[41] Patients may present with neck or shoulder pain but then develop a rapidly evolving tetraplegia and respiratory insufficiency culminating in respiratory arrest. Complete anterior spinal artery occlusion causing infarction that extends up to C1 has a poor outlook, while incomplete occlusion at C3/4 may show significant recovery of respiratory and limb function.[42]

Respiration is commonly affected after stroke and the pattern of breathing may reflect the aetiology, localisation, and severity of the underlying cerebrovascular disease. However, the extent to which abnormal patterns of breathing after stroke may be of prognostic significance and the optimum management of post-stroke ventilatory sufficiency remain uncertain.

References

1 Plum E. Neurological integration of behavioural and metabolic control of breathing. In: Parker R, ed. *Breathing: Hering-Breuer centenary symposium*. Churchill: London, 1970: 314–26.

2 Monteau R, Hilaire G. Spinal respiratory neurons. *Progress Neurobiol* 1991; **37**: 83–144.

3 Richter DW, Mironov SL, Busselburg D, *et al*. Respiratory rhythm generation: plasticity of a neuronal network. *Neuroscientist* 2000; **6**: 181–98.

4 Bianchi AL, Denavit-Saubié M, Champagnat J. Central control of breathing in mammals: neuronal circuitry, membrane properties and neurotransmitters. *Physiol Rev* 1995; **75**: 1–45.

5 Murphy K, Mier A, Adams L, *et al*. Putative cerebral cortical involvement in the ventilatory response to inhaled CO_2 in conscious man. *J Physiol* 1990; **420**: 1–18.

6 Orem J, Netick A. Behavioral control of breathing in the cat. *Brain Res* 1986; **366**: 238–53.

7 Howard RS, Hirsch NP. The neural control of respiratory and cardiovascular function. In: Crockard A, Hayward R, Hoff JT, eds. *Neurosurgery – the scientific basis of clinical practice*. Oxford: Blackwell Scientific Publications, 2000: 289–309.

8 Plum F, Posner JB. Posthyperventilation apnoea. In: Plum F, Posner JB, eds. *Diagnosis of stupor and coma*. 3rd edn. Philadelphia: FA Davis, 1983: 33.

9 Rodriguez M, Beale PL, Marsh HM, *et al*. Central neurogenic hyperventilation in an awake patient with brain-stem astrocytoma. *Ann Neurol* 1982; **11**: 625–8.

10 Pauzner R, Mouallem M, Sadeh M, *et al*. High incidence of primary cerebral lymphoma in tumour-induced central neurogenic hyperventilation. *Arch Neurol* 1989; **46**: 510–12.

11 Mazzara JT, Ayres SM, Grace WJ. Extreme hypocapnia in the critically ill patient. *Am J Med* 1974; **56**: 450–6.

12 North JB, Jennett S. Abnormal breathing patterns associated with acute brain damage. *Arch Neurol* 1974; **31**: 338–44.

13 Leigh RJ, Shaw DA. Rapid, regular respiration in unconscious patients. *Arch Neurol* 1976; **33**: 356–61.

14 Newsom Davis J. An experimental study of hiccup. *Brain* 1970; **93**: 851–72.

15 Howard RS. The causes and treatment of intractable hiccups. *BMJ* 1992; **305**: 1237–8.

16 Patterson JR, Grabois M. Locked in syndrome: a review of 139 cases. *Stroke* 1986; **17**: 758–65.

17 Heywood P, Murphy K, Corfield DR, *et al*. Control of breathing in man; insights from the 'locked-in' syndrome. *Respir Physiol* 1996; **106**: 13–20.

18 Hebertson WM, Talbert OR, Cohen ME. Respiratory apraxia and anosogosia. *Trans Am Neurol Assoc* 1959; **84**: 176–9.

19 Tobin MJ, Snyder JV. Cheyne-Stokes respiration revisited. Controversies and implications. *Crit Care Med* 1984; **12**: 882–7.

20 Naughton MT. Pathophysiology and treatment of Cheyne-Stokes respiration. *Thorax* 1998; **53**: 514–18.

21 Lee MC, Klassen AC, Resch JA. Respiratory pattern disturbances in ischaemic cerebrovascular disease. *Stroke* 1974; **5**: 612–16.

22 Nachtmann A, Siebler M, Rose G. Cheyne-Stokes respiration in ischaemic stroke. *Neurology* 1995; **45**: 820–1.

23 Munschauer FE, Mador MJ, Ahuja A, *et al*. Selective paralysis of voluntary but not limbically influenced automatic respiration. *Arch Neurol* 1991; **48**: 1190–2.

24 Houston JG, Morris AD, Grosset DG, *et al*. Ultrasonic evaluation of movement of the diaphragm after acute cerebral infarction. *J Neurol Neurosurg Psychiatry* 1995; **58**: 738–41.

25 Cohen E, Mier A, Heywood P, *et al*. Diaphragmatic movement in hemiplegic patients measured by ultrasonography. *Thorax* 1994; **49**: 890–5.

26 Gandevia SC, Rothwell JC. Activation of the human diaphragm from the motor cortex. *J Physiol* 1987; **384**: 109–18.

27 Macefield G, Gandevia SC. The cortical drive to human respiratory muscles in the awake state assessed by premotor cerebral potentials. *J Physiol* 1991; **439**: 545–58.

28 Colebach JG, Adams L, Murphy K, *et al*. Regional cerebral blood flow during volitional breathing in man. *J Physiol* 1991; **443**: 91–103.

29 Maskill D, Murphy K, Mier A, *et al*. Motor cortical representation of the diaphragm in man. *J Physiol* 1991; **443**: 105–21.

30 Ramsay SC, Adams L, Murphy K, *et al*. Regional cerebral blood flow during volitional expiration in man: a comparison with volitional inspiration. *J Physiol* 1993; **461**: 85–93.

31 Similowski T, Straus C, Attali V, *et al*. Assessment of the motor pathway to the diaphragm using cortical and cervical magnetic stimulation in the decision making process of phrenic pacing. *Chest* 1996; **110**: 1551–7.

32 Besson G, Bogousslavsky J, Regle F, *et al*. Acute pseudobulbar or suprabulbar palsy. *Arch Neurol* 1991; **48**: 501–7.

33 Howard RS, Williams AJ. Chronic respiratory failure of neurogenic origin. In: Miller DH, Raps EC, eds. *Neurological intensive care*. Oxford: Butterworth-Heinemann, 1999: 249–79.

34 Stewart J, Howard RS, Rudd AG, *et al*. Apneustic breathing provoked by limbic influences. *Postgrad Med J* 1996; **72**: 559–61.

35 Levin BE, Margolis G. Acute failure of automatic respiration secondary to a unilateral brainstem infarct. *Ann Neurol* 1977; **1**: 583–6.

36 Bogousslavsky J, Khurana R, Deruaz JP, *et al*. Respiratory failure and unilateral caudal brainstem infarction. *Ann Neurol* 1990; **28**: 668–73.

37 Devereaux MW, Keane JR, Davis RL. Automatic respiratory failure associated with infarction of the medulla. *Arch Neurol* 1973; **29**: 46–52.

38 Askenasy JJM, Goldhammer I. Sleep apnoea as a feature of bulbar stroke. *Stroke* 1988; **19**: 637.

39 Nathan PW. The descending respiratory pathway in man. *J Neurol Neurosurg Psychiatry* 1963; **26**: 487–99.

40 Cheshire WP, Santos CC, Massey EW, *et al*. Spinal cord infarction: etiology and outcome. *Neurology* 1996; **47**: 321–30.

41 Srigley JR, Lambert CD, Bilbao JM, *et al*. Spinal cord infarction secondary to intervertebral disc embolism. *Ann Neurol* 1981; **9**: 296–300.

42 Howard RS, Thorpe J, Barker R, *et al*. Respiratory insufficiency due to high anterior cervical cord infarction. *J Neurol Neurosurg Psychiatry* 1998; **64**: 358–62.

Chapter Twenty-two

Thrombolysis in acute ischaemic stroke

AC Pereira, PJ Martin and EA Warburton

The primary deficit in acute ischaemic stroke is one of impaired blood flow. Part of the cerebral circulation is occluded either by *in situ* thrombosis, or embolism from the heart or a more proximal artery (for example, the ipsilateral internal carotid artery). Angiographic studies of the cerebral circulation in acute stroke demonstrate occluding thrombus in up to 80% of patients.[1] The aim of thrombolytic therapy therefore is to lyse an occluding thrombus or embolus and reduce the volume of cerebral tissue irreversibly damaged. Such an approach is of course successfully employed in the treatment of acute myocardial infarction.[2] However, a major complication of thrombolysis in stroke is cerebral haemorrhage which could offset any beneficial effects. Here we review the available evidence for thrombolysis in acute stroke and suggest imaging methods that could be used to aid future selection of patients who are most likely to benefit from such treatment.

Experimental rationale for thrombolysis in stroke

Data from animal stroke models confirm that cerebral blood flow can be restored to near normal levels after administration of recombinant tissue plasminogen activator (rtPA)[3] and that thrombolysis results in smaller infarcts and improved neurological function.[4–6] Comparison of streptokinase with rtPA suggested that, although their effectiveness in producing thrombolysis was comparable, strepto-kinase was less clot-specific and animals treated with it had increased frequency and severity of cerebral haemorrhage.[7] Animals treated with rtPA had the same frequency of cerebral haemorrhages as those treated with saline but the propor-tion of large haematomas was increased.[6]

In humans, thrombolytic therapy was first tried over 40 years ago but was largely abandoned due to excess mortality from major haemorrhagic complica-tions.[8] When computed tomography became widely available interest in the use of thrombolysis returned, leading to several larger randomised controlled trials. A dose escalation study using rtPA reported that the proportion of patients in whom recanalisation was demonstrated was independent of the dose of rtPA used.[1] The overall recanalisation rate immediately after rtPA infusion for extracranial in-ternal carotid artery occlusions was 8% and for major coronary artery occlusions was 26–38%. Patients who had a cerebral haemorrhage received rtPA signific-antly later than those who had no haemorrhage (6.1(1.5) compared with 5.3(1.7) hours, p=0.006). This suggested that six hours might be the latest time after the onset of stroke where it was safe to use rtPA. Animal experiments also showed that increasing the duration of ischaemia up to three hours yielded progressively larger infarcts but, beyond three hours, final infarct size was independent of the duration of ischaemia. This suggested that three hours was the time window for intervention before cells became irreversibly damaged.[9] As the primary pathology in ischaemic stroke is severe reduction of blood flow, it seemed logical to try to reverse this as soon as possible. Therefore, a further dose escalation study of urgent thrombolysis within 90 minutes from onset of stroke using rtPA was started.[10] A dose-related effect on intracranial haemorrhage was noted: no patient treated with 0.95 mg/kg rtPA suffered an intracranial haemorrhage but 3/26 patients treated with higher doses did, suggesting that doses up to 0.9 mg/kg may be safely administered to acute stroke patients. Further studies suggested that the time window for treatment could be safely extended to three hours.[11] In summary this evidence suggested that rtPA was an appropriate thrombolytic agent when administered at a dose of 0.9 mg/kg to patients within three hours of the onset of acute stroke. It is of interest that the only trial that has shown a benefit of thrombolysis is also the only trial to have adhered to these criteria.[12]

Recent randomised controlled trials

In stroke patients seven major randomised trials of urgent thrombolytic therapy have been published. Three used streptokinase as the thrombolytic agent: the Australian Streptokinase Trial (ASK),[13] the Multicentre Acute Stroke Trial-Italy (MAST-I),[14] and the Multicentre Acute Stroke Trial-Europe (MAST-E).[15] Four used rtPA as the thrombolytic agent: the National Institute of Neurological Disorders and Stroke (NINDS)[12] trial, the first and second European Co-operative Acute Stroke Studies (ECASS 1[16] and ECASS 2)[17], and the Alteplase Thrombolysis for Acute Noninterventional Therapy in Ischaemic Stroke (ATLANTIS) Study.[18] The most important data in studies such as these are the safety of the treatment (indicated by the early death or haemorrhage rate) and the efficacy (death or dependency at the end of trial follow-up). Table 22.1 shows these figures for each trial.

Streptokinase trials

The three streptokinase trials were all stopped early because of concerns over safety. The ASK trial randomised patients to either streptokinase or placebo administered within four hours from symptom onset; 340 patients were enrolled in the trial. However, there was a significant increase in mortality in patients given streptokinase compared with placebo, particularly after three hours (43.4% v 22.1%, $p<0.001$).[19] Interestingly, there was no such increase in hazard in patients treated within three hours, but these patients represented only 21% of all the patients in the trial.[13] Similarly in MAST-E, there was a significant increase in haemorrhage and early death in the streptokinase-treated group. This result was confounded by the concomitant use of heparin (which now is known to independently increase the risk of haemorrhage)[20] in about 60% of the patients in each group. MAST-I was slightly different in that it had a 2 × 2 factorial design with patients randomised to streptokinase or placebo and/or aspirin or placebo. Therefore, half of the patients receiving streptokinase also received aspirin, as did half of the patients receiving placebo. Again, there was an increase in haemorrhage and early deaths with no significant improvement in the outcome of the survivors. Those patients who received aspirin as well as streptokinase did particularly badly (case fatalities of streptokinase plus aspirin, streptokinase and neither drug were 34%, 19%, and 13% respectively). These data strongly suggest that streptokinase is unacceptably hazardous in acute stroke and has no apparent long-term efficacy.

Table 22.1 Randomised controlled trials and meta-analysis of thrombolysis in acute stroke showing rates of early death up to 30 days, dependency (usually defined as a Rankin score greater than 2 (inclusive) or death at up to 6 months and rates of symptomatic intracranial haemorrhage)

Trial	No	Drug/time	Thrombolytic (%)	Control (%)
ASK[13]	340	SK		
Early death (7 days)*		<4 hours	17.8	10.9
Death/dependency (3 months)			42.3	44.6
Haemorrhage*			12.6	2.4
MAST-E[15]	310	SK		
Early death (10 days)*		<6 hours	34.0	18.2
Death/dependency (6 months)			79.5	81.8
Haemorrhage*			21.2	2.6
MAST-I[14]	622	SK		
Early death (10 days)*		<6 hours	26.5	11.7
Death/dependency (6 months)			62.6	64.7
Haemorrhage*			8.0	1.3
ECASS 1[16]	620	rtPA		
Early death (30 days)*		<6 hours	17.9	12.7
Death/dependency (3 months)			63.3	71.7
Haemorrhage*			19.8	6.5
NINDS[12]	624	rtPA		
Early death (30 days)		<3 hours	12.8	15.7
Death/dependency (3 months)*			57.4	73.4
Haemorrhage*			6.4	0.6
Meta-analysis[22]				
Early death*	3435	SK/rtPA	20.9	11.8
Death/dependency*			61.5	68
Haemorrhage*			9.6	2.6
ECASS 2[17]	800	rtPA		
Early death (7 days)		<6 hours	6.1	4.9
Death/dependency (3 months)			59.7	63.4
Haemorrhage*			8.8	3.4
ATLANTIS[18]	613	rtPA		
Early death (30 days)		3–5 hours	7.6	4.2
Death/dependency (3 months)			58.3	59.5
Haemorrhage*			6.7	1.3

The asterisks (*) signify that the difference between the two groups reached statistical significance. No is the number of subjects in each study; SK is streptokinase and rtPA is recombinant tissue plasminogen activator.

Recombinant tissue plasminogen activator (rtPA) trials

The data were much more promising from the rtPA trials, the most important of which was the NINDS study. Altogether 624 patients were randomised to receive either 0.9 mg/kg rtPA or placebo within three hours of the onset of their symptoms. The overall result showed that patients treated with thrombolysis were at least 30% more likely to have minimal or no disability at three months and this benefit was sustained to one year.[21] Furthermore, although there was a significant increase in the frequency of symptomatic intracerebral haemorrhage, this did not produce an increase in the early death rate. The frequency of asymptomatic haemorrhage was similar in both groups (4% treated with rtPA and 3% in controls). The frequency of serious extracranial haemorrhage was about 1%.

The European trial comparable to the NINDS study was ECASS 1. This randomised 620 patients to receive either 1.1 mg/kg of rtPA or placebo within six hours of the onset of stroke. A target population of patients was defined with moderate to severe stroke with only minor signs of ischaemia on the randomisation computed tomogram. The intention to treat analysis demonstrated a significant increase in early mortality and haemorrhage and a non-significant improvement in final outcome. However, retrospective analysis of the randomisation data highlighted 109 patients who had a protocol violation, usually more extensive changes on randomisation computed tomography than desired. These patients' data were removed *post hoc* and analysis of the target population was repeated. This suggested that, had only members of the target population been randomised, there would have not been an increase in early mortality and their final outcome would have significantly improved. This was particularly true for those patients in the target group randomised within three hours.[22] However, this *post hoc* procedure clearly was biased: 21% of rtPA treated patients were removed (of whom 30% died) compared with 14% of controls (of whom 19% died). In ECASS 2, therefore, centres underwent training to standardise the interpretation of early computed tomograms. Furthermore, the lower dose of rtPA (as used in the NINDS study) was administered. ECASS 2 demonstrated a significant increase in symptomatic intracerebral haemorrhage but without a significant increase in early mortality; there was no significant improvement in final outcome. This result was disappointing. However, the strict inclusion criteria may have yielded a population of stroke patients with less severe strokes. Compared with the control groups of the NINDS study and ECASS 1, of whom 73.4% and 71.7% respectively had poor final outcomes, the figure in ECASS 2 was 63.4%.

The ATLANTIS study provided data on thrombolysis from three to five hours after the onset of stroke. Some caution is needed when interpreting the results as two changes in trial protocol were made during recruitment of patients. The initial study in 1991 was a comparison of rtPA (0.9 mg/kg) against placebo for acute stroke patients within six hours of the onset of symptoms. However, in 1993, safety concerns regarding patients randomised after five hours resulted in the trial being halted. Recruitment later restarted (as ATLANTIS B) using a new zero to five hours time window. In 1996, after publication of the NINDS trial, the time window was further modified to three to five hours. Data from these 'target group' patients have been published recently.[18] The results do not show any benefit for the thrombolysis over placebo for patients randomised between three and five hours after stroke.

Overall, therefore, the trials suggest that streptokinase is more hazardous to the cerebral circulation than rtPA. None of the streptokinase trials reached completion. The major differences between the NINDS study and ECASS 1 were the dose of rtPA used and the time interval from stroke onset and treatment. When the issue of dose was addressed in ECASS 2, a positive treatment benefit was still not confirmed but there was no increase in early mortality. These data suggest that rtPA given within six hours of stroke onset may be safe but may not be effective after three hours. A meta-analysis of the data from all the thrombolysis trials except ECASS 2 (3435 patients) confirmed the early hazard from thrombolysis (mainly from streptokinase) but suggested there may be a significant overall benefit of 6.5%.[22] A more recent overview from the Cochrane database which added data from patients in ECASS 2 and ATLANTIS confirmed the findings of the first meta-analysis.[23] In 4236 patients, thrombolysis increased the risk of symptomatic intracranial bleeding from 2.5% to 9.4% but against this was the benefit that a significantly smaller proportion of patients (55.2% compared with 59.7%) were dead or dependent at three to six months. This means that for every 1000 patients treated, 65 extra patients would be independent by three to six months. This means that for every 1000 patients treated, 44 extra patients would be independent by three to six months. Both these meta-analyses may be criticised for combining the results from both, streptokinase and rtPA, trials.

On the basis of the NINDS trial, the US Food and Drug Administration licensed rtPA for treatment of acute stroke patients within three hours of onset of their symptoms. Although a recent series from centres in the USA suggested that favourable clinical outcomes and low rates of symptomatic intracerebral haemorrhage could be achieved using rtPA,[24] the other negative trials have tempered enthusiasm for the use of thrombolysis in routine practice in Europe and means that a further trial will be necessary before this treatment is widely accepted as beneficial.[25] Furthermore, a recent survey of 3948 stroke patients admitted to 29 hospitals in Cleveland, Ohio, showed that 10.4% were admitted within three hours and 1.8% were given rtPA. Half of these patients deviated from the national treatment guidelines.[26] The incidence of symptomatic intracerebral haemorrhage was 15.7%, much higher than in comparable trials, thus highlighting the need to know the risks and benefits of thrombolysis in a more general and representative clinical setting.

Problems in the design and interpretation of human trials

Part of the problem in judging the utility of thrombolysis is that often the underlying pathology is not taken into consideration. Clearly an important principle of rational treatment is to ensure that the patient has the target problem: there seems little point treating patients with thrombolysis if the occlusion has already dissipated.[27] Other considerations such as whether thrombolysis was successful in individual patients (that is, broke down the occluding clot) and identification of patients at most risk of haemorrhage have been poorly addressed.

Ischaemic stroke is a heterogeneous clinical condition. Patients presenting with lacunar syndromes or large vessel occlusion syndromes have different prognoses[28] and these need to be considered when interpreting the results of treatment trials. In the NINDS trial, 16% of patients given rtPA had lacunar infarcts while 38% had large vessel occlusions compared with 10% and 43% respectively in the control group. Therefore, it is possible that some of the apparent benefit attributed to thrombolysis may reflect the different mix of pathology in the two groups. Future stroke trials should take these pathological subtypes of stroke into account during randomisation.

There is no routine practice to ensure that thrombolysis has successfully produced recanalisation. Reperfusion is less likely to be achieved with proximal internal artery occlusions rather than more distal middle cerebral artery occlusion.[1] Reperfusion rates after intravenous thrombolysis are reported to be 30% immediately after infusion,[1,29] 53% 12–24 hours later,[29] and 65% within three days.[30] Reperfusion is associated with smaller infarcts and better clinical outcome.[29,30] Intra-arterial thrombolysis produces a higher rate of recanalisation (58%) immediately after the infusion but has not been shown to improve clinical outcome.[31] Therefore, in future, it may be important to include a measure of perfusion to ascertain whether recanalisation has occurred and to aid decisions regarding further thrombolysis.

The major adverse effect of thrombolysis is intracranial haemorrhage. Haemorrhage is a common sequelae of stroke and the spontaneous haemorrhage rate in stroke patients is high. In ECASS 2, the frequency of all haemorrhage was similar in the rtPA and control groups (48.4% v 40.2% respectively), but, in the rtPA group, there was a significant increase in parenchymal haemorrhage (11.8% v 3.1%) and large haematomas (8.1% v 0.8%). The larger parenchymal haemorrhages were more likely to cause neurological worsening.[32] Therefore, rtPA seems to increase the severity of haemorrhage rather than the incidence of haemorrhage. Haemorrhage is more likely to occur late after the onset of stroke when cell necrosis causes blood vessels to break down.[33] In the NINDS trial, haemorrhage was more likely in patients with a more severe neurological deficit at randomisation, a mass effect, or cerebral oedema on randomisation computed tomography.[34] There does seem to be evidence to suggest that if an infarct is visible on the initial computed tomography that the infarction process is advanced and that the risk of haemorrhage is higher than for patients with normal or mildly abnormal computed tomograms.[35] However, even patients with extensive abnormalities on the initial scan or more severe clinical deficits can benefit from thrombolysis.[36–38] Therefore, more sophisticated methods of assessing the underlying pathology of cerebral ischaemia are required.

Imaging in acute stroke

Most trials have used unenhanced computed tomography as the necessary imaging investigation before randomisation. In the early phase of stroke, computed tomography is very good at demonstrating haemorrhage but up to 50% of computed tomograms may be normal and not show the area of infarction.[39–41] Furthermore, computed tomography provides no information about perfusion or about cellular function. Therefore, it has major disadvantages in the early stage of stroke. Single photon emission tomography (SPECT) or xenon computed tomography can address some of these deficiencies and provide a measure of perfusion.[42,43] A more informative technique is positron emission tomography (PET), which provides measures of perfusion and cellular metabolism.[44] In fact, PET has demonstrated that substantial ischaemic regions survive for up to a month after the onset of stroke in humans, suggesting that there was hope of cell recovery for quite a prolonged period of time.[45,46] This has very important treatment implications as it suggests that some patients may still benefit from therapy at extended time periods.[46] As it is unlikely that many stroke patients will undergo a PET scan, a more widely available and useful investigation is the use of magnetic resonance imaging. Magnetic resonance angiography can show the occluded artery.[47] Diffusion weighted imaging (DWI) demonstrates the region of infarction within minutes of the onset of stroke,[48] while perfusion imaging can demonstrate a region of low cerebral blood flow.[49,50] Magnetic resonance spectroscopy (^{1}H MRS) demonstrates biochemical changes occurring in the region of infarction[51] and may be used to identify surviving neuronal tissue in a region of ischaemia that may be salvageable using thrombolysis (*see* Figure 22.1).[52]

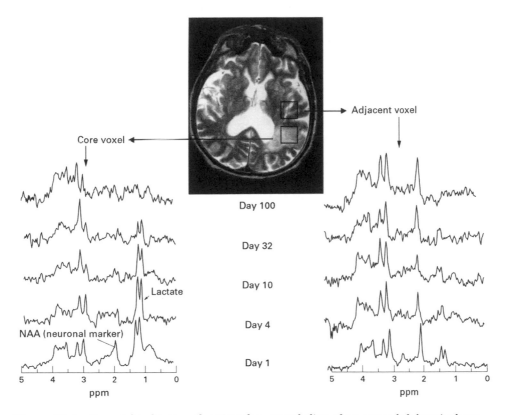

Figure 22.1 T_2-weighted image showing the central slice of an acute left hemisphere middle cerebral artery infarct. Two voxels are identified: a 'core' voxel and an 'adjacent' voxel. Each voxel was studied on five occasions at the times shown. The ^{1}H MR spectra from each voxel are shown and the metabolites, *N*-acetyl aspartate (NAA, a neuronal marker) and lactate (a marker of ischaemia) are labelled. The area under each metabolite peak in the spectrum is proportional to the metabolite concentration. The figure demonstrates that in the core voxel, lactate is present for several weeks and neuronal loss continues until virtually no NAA is detectable. In the voxel adjacent to the visible infarct, even though there is no abnormal T_2-weighted signal, lactate is present implying ischaemia of this adjacent tissue. This technique may in future play a part in identifying viable neuronal tissue or ischaemic tissue that may benefit from thrombolysis.

The size of the defect visible on DWI correlates with the size of the infarct pathologically[53] and the volume of the infarct measured early using DWI,[54] T_2-weighted images,[55] perfusion imaging,[56] or combination with ^{1}H MRS[57] correlates with clinical outcome. Infarcts where the perfusion deficit is larger than the DWI lesion are likely to increase in size, suggesting that regions having decreased perfusion without DWI changes may be most suitable for thrombolysis.[58,59] These new techniques may improve the acute assessment of stroke patients and allow individual patients to be assessed and given thrombolysis at more prolonged time intervals after the onset of stroke.[46,60]

Summary

In conclusion, thrombolysis with rtPA given within six hours of the onset of stroke in carefully selected patients is a safe therapy. However, efficacy has only been demonstrated within three hours after stroke onset. At present, only 6%[61]–12%[62] of all stroke patients are likely to be eligible for thrombolysis. Improved methods for investigating acute stroke, particularly magnetic resonance techniques, may improve the appropriate targeting of this treatment to those patients most likely to benefit. What is certain is that any increasing use of thrombolysis will have major effects on stroke services. The emphasis will have to be on early assessment and referral, if only to reach an imaging facility for a treatment decision to be made.

References

1 del Zoppo GJ, Poeck K, Pessin MS, *et al.* Recombinant tissue plasminogen activator in acute thrombotic and embolic stroke. *Ann Neurol* 1992; **32**: 78–86.
2 ISIS-2 Collaborative Group. Randomised trial of intravenous streptokinase, oral aspirin, both or neither among 17187 of acute myocardial infarction. *Lancet* 1988; **ii**: 349–60.
3 Papadopoulos SM, Chandler WF, Salamat MS, *et al.* Recombinant human tissue-type plasminogen activator therapy in acute thromboembolic stroke. *J Neurosurg* 1987; **67**: 394–8.
4 del Zoppo GJ, Copeland BR, Waltz TA, *et al.* The beneficial effect of intracarotid urokinase on acute stroke in the baboon model. *Stroke* 1986; **17**: 638–43.
5 Zivin JA, Lyden PD, DeGirolami U, *et al.* Tissue plasminogen activator. Reduction in neurologic damage after experimental embolic stroke. *Arch Neurol* 1988; **45**: 387–91.
6 Lyden PD, Zivin JA, Clark WM, *et al.* Tissue plasminogen activator-mediated thrombolysis of cerebral emboli and its effect on haemorrhagic infarction in rabbits. *Neurology* 1989; **39**: 703–8.
7 Lyden PD, Madden KP, Clark WM, *et al.* Incidence of cerebral haemorrhage after antifibrinolytic treatment for embolic stroke in rabbits. *Stroke* 1990; **21**: 1589–93.
8 Sussman BJ, Fitch TSP. Thrombolysis with fibrinolysin in cerebral arterial occlusion. *JAMA* 1958; **167**: 1705–9.
9 Memezawa H, Smith M-L, Siesjo BK. Penumbral tissues salvaged by reperfusion following middle cerebral artery occlusion in rats. *Stroke* 1992; **23**: 552–9.
10 Brott TG, Haley ECJ, Levy DE, *et al.* Urgent therapy for stroke. Part I. Pilot study of tissue plasminogen activator administered within 90 minutes. *Stroke* 1992; **23**: 632–40.
11 Haley ECJ, Levy DE, Brott TG, *et al.* Urgent therapy for stroke. Part II. Pilot study of tissue plasminogen activator administered 91–180 minutes from onset. *Stroke* 1992; **23**: 641–5.

12 National Institute of Neurological Disorders and Stroke rt-PA Stroke Study Group. Tissue plasminogen activator for acute ischemic stroke. *N Engl J Med* 1995; **333**: 1581–7.

13 Donnan GA, Davis SM, Chambers BR, *et al.* and for the Australian Streptokinase (ASK) Trial Study Group. Streptokinase for acute ischaemic stroke with relationship to time of administration. *JAMA* 1996; **276**: 966.

14 Multi-centre Acute Stroke Trial – Italy (MAST-I) Group. Randomised controlled trial of streptokinase, aspirin and combination of both in treatment of acute ischaemic stroke. *Lancet* 1995; **346**: 1509–14.

15 Multicenter Acute Stroke Trial – Europe Study Group. Thrombolytic therapy with streptokinase in acute ischemic stroke. *N Engl J Med* 1996; **335**: 145–50.

16 Hacke W, Kaste M, Fieschi C, *et al.*, and for the ECASS Study Group. Intravenous thrombolysis with recombinant tissue plasminogen activator for acute hemispheric stroke. *JAMA* 1995; **274**: 1017–25.

17 Hacke W, Kaste M, Fieschi C W, *et al.* Randomised doubleblind placebo controlled trial of thrombolytic therapy with intravenous alteplase in acute ischaemic stroke (ECASS II). *Lancet* 1998; **352**: 1245–51.

18 Clark WM, Wissman S, Albers GW, *et al.* and for the ATLANTIS Study Investigators. Recombinant tissue-type plasminogen activator (alteplase) for ischaemic stroke 3 to 5 hours after symptom onset. *JAMA* 1999; **282**: 2019–26.

19 Donnan GA, Davis SM, Chambers BR, *et al.* Trials of streptokinase in severe acute ischaemic stroke. *Lancet* 1995; **345**: 578–9.

20 International Stroke Trial Collaborative Group. The International Stroke Trial (IST): a randomised trial of aspirin, subcutaneous heparin, both, or neither among 19 435 patients with acute ischaemic stroke. *Lancet* 1997; **349**: 1569–81.

21 Kwiatkowski TG, Libman RB, Frankel M, *et al.* Effects of tissue plasminogen activator for acute ischaemic stroke. *N Engl J Med* 1999; **340**: 1781–7.

22 Wardlaw JM, Warlow CP, Counsell C. Systematic review of evidence on thrombolytic therapy for acute ischaemic stroke. *Lancet* 1997; **350**: 607–14.

23 Wardlaw, JM Yamaguchi T, del Zoppo GJ. Thrombolytic therapy versus control in acute ischaemic stroke. *Cochrane database of systematic reviews*. Stroke Module, 1997.

24 Albers GW, Bates VE, Clark WM, *et al.* Intravenous tissue-type plasminogen activator for treatment of acute stroke. The standard treatment with alteplase to reverse stroke (STARS) study. *JAMA* 2000; **283**: 1145–50.

25 Lindley RI, Waddell F, Livingstone M, *et al.* Can simple questions assess outcome after stroke? *Cerebrovasc Dis* 1994; **4**: 314–24.

26 Katzan IL, Furlan AJ, Lloyd LE, *et al.* Use of tissue-type plasminigen activator for acute ischaemic stroke. *JAMA* 2000; **283**: 1151–8.

27 Caplan LR, Mohr JP, Kistler JP, *et al.* Should thrombolytic therapy be the first-line treatment for acute ischemic stroke? Thrombolysis – not a panacea for ischemic stroke. *N Engl J Med* 1997; **337**: 1309–10 (*see* discussion 1313).

28 Bamford JM, Sandercock PAG, Dennis MS, *et al.* Classification and natural history of clinically identifiable subtypes of cerebral infarction. *Lancet* 1997; **337**: 1521–6.

29 von Kummer R, Hacke W. Safety and efficacy of intravenous tissue plasminogen activator and heparin in acute middle cerebral artery stroke. *Stroke* 1992; **23**: 646–52.

30 Ringelstein EB, Biniek R, Weiller C, *et al.* Type and extent of hemispheric brain infarctions and clinical outcome in early and delayed middle cerebral artery recanalization. *Neurology* 1992; **42**: 289–98.

31 del Zoppo G, Higashida RT, Furlan AJ, *et al.* and the PROACT Investigators. PROACT: a phase II randomised trial of recombinant pro-urokinase by direct arterial delivery in acute middle cerebral artery stroke. *Stroke* 1998; **29**: 11.

32 Fiorelli M, Bastianello S, von Kummer R, *et al.* Hemorrhagic transformation within 36 hours of a cerebral infarct. Relationships with early clinical deterioration and 3 month

outcome in the European Cooperative Acute Stroke Study (ECASS I) cohort. *Stroke* 1999; **30**: 2280–4.

33 del Zoppo GJ, von Kummer R, Hamann GF. Ischaemic damage of brain microvessels: inherent risks for thrombolytic treatment in stroke [editorial]. *J Neurol Neurosurg Psychiatry* 1998; **65**: 1–9.

34 Anonymous. Intracerebral hemorrhage after intravenous t-PA therapy for ischemic stroke. The NINDS t-PA Stroke Study Group. *Stroke* 1997; **28**: 2109–18.

35 Wardlaw JM, Lewis SC, Dennis MS, *et al*. Is visible infarction on computed tomography associated with an adverse prognosis in acute ischaemic stroke? *Stroke* 1998; **29**: 1315–19.

36 Trouillas P, Nighoghossian N, Getenet JC, *et al*. Open trial of intravenous tissue plasminogen activator in acute carotid territory stroke. Correlations of outcome with clinical and radiological data. *Stroke* 1996; **27**: 882–90.

37 Trouillas P, Nighoghossian N, Derex L, *et al*. Thrombolysis with intravenous rtPA in a series of 100 cases of acute carotid territory stroke: determination of etiological, topographic, and radiological outcome factors. *Stroke* 1998; **29**: 2529–40.

38 Anonymous. Generalized efficacy of t-PA for acute stroke. Subgroup analysis of the NINDS t-PA Stroke Trial. *Stroke* 1997; **28**: 2119–25.

39 Bryan RN, Levy LM, Whitlow WD, *et al*. Diagnosis of acute cerebral infarction: comparison of CT and MR imaging. *AJNR* 1991; **12**: 611–20.

40 Lindgren A, Norrving B, Rudling O, *et al*. Comparison of clinical and neuroradiological findings in first ever stroke: a population based study. *Stroke* 1994; **25**: 1371–7.

41 Mohr JP, Biller J, Hilal SK, *et al*. Magnetic resonance versus computed tomographic imaging in acute stroke. *Stroke* 1995; **26**: 807–12.

42 Lassen NA, Fieschi C, Lenzi G-L. Ischaemic penumbra and neuronal death: comments on the therapeutic window in acute stroke with particular reference to thrombolytic therapy. *Cerebrovasc Dis* 1991; **1**: 32–5.

43 Wolfson SK, Clark J, Greenberg JH, *et al*. Xenon-enhanced computed tomography compared with ^{14}C iodoantipyrine for normal and low cerebral blood flow states in baboons. *Stroke* 1990; **21**: 751–7.

44 Baron JC. Pathophysiology of acute cerebral ischaemia: PET studies in humans. *Cerebrovasc Dis* 1991; **1**: 22–31.

45 Marchal G, Beaudouin V, Rioux P, *et al*. Prolonged persistence of substantial volumes of potentially viable brain tissue after stroke: a correlative PET-CT study with voxel-based data analysis [*see* comments]. *Stroke* 1996; **27**: 599–606.

46 Baron JC, von Kummer R, del Zoppo GJ. Treatment of acute ischemic stroke. Challenging the concept of a rigid and universal time window [editorial]. *Stroke* 1995; **26**: 2219–21.

47 Prichard JW. Nuclear magnetic resonance methods in stroke. *Stroke* 1994; **24**(suppl I): I-70-I71.

48 Moseley ME, Butts K, Yenari MA, *et al*. Clinical aspects of DWI. *NMR in Biomedicine* 1995; **8**: 387–96.

49 Fisher M, Prichard JW, Warach S. New magnetic resonance techniques for acute ischemic stroke. *JAMA* 1995; **274**: 908–11.

50 Baird AE, Warach S. Magnetic resonance imaging of acute stroke. *J Cereb Blood Flow Metab* 1998; **18**: 583–609.

51 Howe FA, Maxwell RJ, Saunders DE, *et al*. Proton spectroscopy in vivo. *Mag Reson Q* 1993; **9**: 31–59.

52 Back T, Hoehn-Berlage M, Kohno K, *et al*. Diffusion nuclear magnetic resonance imaging in experimental stroke. Correlation with cerebral metabolites. *Stroke* 1994; **25**: 494–500.

53 Warach S, Dashe JF, Edelman RR. Clinical outcome in ischemic stroke predicted by early diffusion-weighted and perfusion magnetic resonance imaging: a preliminary analysis. *J Cereb Blood Flow Metab* 1996; **16**: 53–9.

54 van Everdingen KJ, van der Grond J, Kappelle LJ, *et al.* Diffusion-weighted magnetic resonance imaging in acute stroke. *Stroke* 1998; **29**: 1783–90.

55 Saunders DE, Clifton AG, Brown MM. Measurement of infarct size using MRI predicts prognosis in middle cerebral artery infarction. *Stroke* 1995; **26**: 2272–6.

56 Barber PA, Darby DG, Desmond PM, *et al.* Prediction of stroke outcome with echoplanar perfusion- and diffusion-weighted MRI. *Neurology* 1998; **51**: 418–26.

57 Pereira AC, Saunders DE, Doyle VL, *et al.* Measurement of initial N-acetyl aspartate concentration using magnetic resonance spectroscopy and initial infarct volume using MRI predicts outcome in patients with middle cerebral artery territory infarction. *Stroke* 1999; **30**: 1577–82.

58 Busza AL, Allen KL, King MD, *et al.* Diffusion-weighted imaging studies of cerebral ischaemia in gerbils. *Stroke* 1992; **23**: 1602–12.

59 Baird AE, Benfield A, Schlaug G, *et al.* Enlargement of human cerebral ischaemic lesion volumes measured by diffusion weighted magnetic resonance imaging. *Ann Neurol* 1997; **41**: 581–9.

60 Albers GW. Expanding the window for thrombolytic therapy in acute stroke. The role of acute MRI for patient selection. *Stroke* 1999; **30**: 2230–7.

61 Chiu D, Krieger D, Villar-Cordova C, *et al.* Intravenous tissue plasminogen activator for acute ischemic stroke: feasibility, safety, and efficacy in the first year of clinical practice [*see* comments]. *Stroke* 1998; **29**: 18–22.

62 Grond M, Stenzel C, Schmulling S, *et al.* Early intravenous thrombolysis for acute ischemic stroke in a community based approach. *Stroke* 1998; **29**: 1544–9.

Index